Nursing the Infant, Child & Adolescent

INTERACTIONS AND CARE

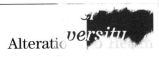
Anne Adams

RN BA MA DNE Cert Paed N FRCNA FCN(NSW)

Senior Lecturer, Faculty of Nursing
University of Technology, Sydney

Carmel McQuellin

RN Dip Teach (Nurs) BHS(Nurs) CertPaed Cardio-Thoracic Nurs
Cert Acute Care Nurs MRCNA MCN(NSW)

Co-ordinator, Graduate Certificate in Paediatric Nursing Course
Woden Valley Hospital, ACT

Sue Nagy

RN PhD FRCNA FCN(NSW)

Professor of Paediatric Nursing
University of Western Sydney
and Royal Alexandra Hospital for Children, Sydney

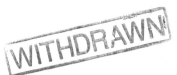
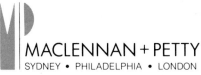
MACLENNAN + PETTY
SYDNEY • PHILADELPHIA • LONDON

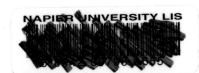

First published 1996

MacLennan & Petty Pty Limited
809–821 Botany Road, Rosebery, Sydney NSW 2018 Australia

National Library of Australia
Cataloguing-in-Publication data:

Nursing the infant, child & adolescent: interactions and care.
Bibliography.
Includes index.

ISBN 0 86433 126 6.
ISBN 0 86433 105 3 (v. 1).
ISBN 0 86433 124 X (v. 2).

1. Teenagers — Medical care. 2. Pediatric nursing.
I. McQuellin, Carmel. II. Adams, Anne, 1940– . III. Nagy, Sue.
610.7362

Printed and bound in Australia

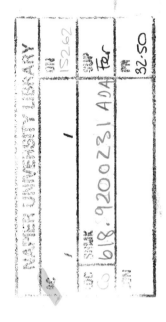

The authors, editors and publisher have done everything possible to make this book accurate up, to
date and in accord with accepted standards at the time of publication. They, however, are not
responsible for errors or omissions or for consequences arising from the use of the book. Information
in this book should be applied by the reader in accordance with professional standards of care
relevant to individual circumstances.

NOTE FROM THE PUBLISHER

In consideration of the range of readership and for ease of handling,
Nursing the Infant, Child & Adolescent is published in two volumes.

Volume 1 consists of PART ONE *Growth and Development: Body, Mind,
Relationships and Emotions* and PART TWO *Alterations to Health in Infancy,
Childhood and Adolescence* (ISBN 0–86433–105–3).

Volume 2 consists of PART THREE *Alterations to Health in Infancy,
Childhood and Adolescence: Special Problems* (ISBN 0–86433–124–X).

Page, table and figure numbers run continuously through the two volumes
and both contain the complete Contents, Appendices and Index.

Dedication

To

the many children and their families who have given our endeavours purpose and meaning

and

to paediatric nurses everywhere who through their commitment, sensitivity, optimism and capacity for joy continue to make differences in the lives of others

Editors and Contributors

Anne Adams RN BA MA DNE Cert
Paed N FRCNA FCN(NSW)
Senior lecturer, Faculty of Nursing
The University of Technology, Sydney

Gail Anderson RN CM BN Grad Dip
Child Health Nursing, Adolescent Mental
Health Certificate, MCN(NSW)
Clinical Nurse Consultant,
Adolescent Health
Westmead Hospital NSW

Jennifer Backhouse RN CM Grad
Dip Child Health Nursing
Children's ward
Hills Private Hospital, Sydney

Julie Bleasdale RN
formerly Clinical Nurse Specialist
Royal Alexandra Hospital for Children,
Sydney

Katrina Brereton RN MRN ND
Pain Management Nurse Consultant
Royal Children's Hospital, Melbourne

Lynne Brodie RN BA Cert Paed N MRN
Nursing Unit Manager
Royal Alexandra Hospital for Children,
Sydney

Kim Burke RN LLB
Barrister-at-Law, formerly Clinical
Nurse Consultant, Oncology
Royal Alexandra Hospital for Children,
Sydney

Sue Casanelia RN BN Grad Dip
Adv Nsg(Comm Hlth) Cert in Genetic
Counselling
Genetics Department
Royal Children's Hospital, Melbourne

Kuei Meei Chen RN
Clinical Nurse Specialist
Royal Children's Hospital, Melbourne

Patricia Comerford RN BN Cert
Paed N
formerly Nurse Unit Manager
Department of Paediatrics
John Hunter Hospital, Newcastle NSW

Marilyn Cruickshank RN
BA(Hons) Neuro Cert PICU Cert
FCN(NSW) FRCNA
Clinical Nurse Consultant
The Prince of Wales Children's
Hospital, Sydney

Victoria Cullins RN BN Cert NIC
Clinical Nurse Educator
Christchurch Women's Hospital,
New Zealand

Helen Dickinson RN
Clinical Nurse Specialist
Royal Children's Hospital, Melbourne

Laurence Dubourg RN Grad Dip
Neuro Cert
Neuro Unit Manager — Nursing
Royal Children's Hospital, Melbourne

Jill Farquhar RN BHS(Nurs) Renal
Certificate
Clinical Nurse Consultant
Renal Treatment Centre
Royal Alexandra Hospital for Children,
Sydney

Glenys Goodwin RN CM PICU Cert
Occ Health Management Cert IBCLC
formerly Clinical Nurse Consultant
Home Ventilation/Oxygen Support
Program
Royal Alexandra Hospital for Children,
Sydney

Maurice Hennessy RN RSCN B
AppSci Ad Nsg(Ed)
Nurse Educator
Royal Children's Hospital, Melbourne

Angela Jones RN BEd Grad Dip
Neurosciences CNRN
Case Manager — Neurosciences
The George Washington University
Medical Center, Washington DC

Tina Kendrick RN BN MN PICU
Cert FCN(NSW)
formerly Nurse Educator, Intensive Care
Royal Alexandra Hospital for Children,
Sydney

John Leach RN Grad Dip Nurs Mgt
Cert Paed N
formerly Nurse Unit Manager
Isolation ward/infectious diseases
Royal Alexandra Hospital for Children,
Sydney

Paul Longridge RN Dip N
Clinical Nurse Specialist
Royal Children's Hospital, Melbourne

Jane Lush RN
Registered Nurse
Royal Children's Hospital, Melbourne

Carmel McQuellin RN BHS(Nurs)
Dip Teach(Nurs) Cert Paed Cardio-thoracic
N Cert Acute Care N MRCNA MCN(NSW)
Co-ordinator, Graduate Certificate in
Paediatric Nursing Course
Woden Valley Hospital, Canberra ACT

Irene Mitchelhill RN, RMN,
BHS(Nurs), Cert Paed & Child & Family
Health
Clinical Nurse Consultant — Paediatric
Endocrinology
Prince of Wales Children's Hospital,
Sydney

Jill Molan RN BA Dip Ed(Nurs) Cert
Opth N
formerly Course Co-ordinator
NSW College of Nursing

Sue Nagy RN PhD FRCNA FCN(NSW)
Professor of Paediatric Nursing
University of Western Sydney
and Royal Alexandra Hospital
for Children, Sydney

Gill Patterson RN MN Cert Paed N
Nurse Unit Manager
Royal Alexandra Hospital for Children,
Sydney

Robyn Pedersen RN RM BA(Hons)
Certified Genetic Counsellor (HGSA)
Clinical Nurse Consultant (Genetics)
Prince of Wales Children's Hospital,
Sydney

Mary Perisanidis-Douros
RN Dip N
Clinical Nurse Specialist
Royal Children's Hospital, Melbourne

Helen Sharp RN BN Cert Paed N
Clinical Nurse Specialist
Royal Alexandra Hospital for Children,
Sydney

Kaye Spence RN CM BEd(N) Cert
NIC Cert Paed N MRCNA
Clinical Nurse Consultant, Neonatology
Royal Alexandra Hospital for Children,
Sydney

David Sutton RN BHS(Nurs)
Associate Charge Nurse
Royal Children's Hospital, Melbourne

Lean Muar Tan RN BN MN
Registered Nurse
Royal Alexandra Hospital for Children,
Sydney

Isobel Taylor RN Dip Teach(Nurs)
Orth Cert
Lecturer, Faculty of Nursing
University of Sydney

Sandy Wales RN Cert Paed N
Clinical Nurse Specialist (Asthma
Resource Nurse)
Prince of Wales Children's Hospital,
Sydney

Margaret Yates RN Dip Teach(Nurs)
formerly Paediatric Nurse Educator
John Hunter Hospital, Newcastle NSW

Contents

**PART ONE   Growth and Development: Body, Mind, Relationships
                    and Emotions**

Forewords

I

The care of the sick child has seen many changes since the inception of the first hospitals for the care of sick children in Australia between 1870 and 1880. The evolution and development of nursing knowledge that is distinctly paediatric nursing is readily seen within the collective writings of this book.

Paediatric nursing is a discipline which builds upon the knowledge of the normal child as a basis for care and caring. It is therefore a tribute to the writers that the foundation of the text is that of growth and development, body and mind, relationships and emotions.

Keeping children healthy is more than nursing practice within the hospital. The writers of this book have given us to understand a function of wellness through health management, which includes the avoidance of infectious diseases through adequate and timely immunisation programs. The concept of health promotion extends the role of the paediatric nurse beyond the early aspirations of a nurse to care for sick children to that of a nurse caring for a child in illness and in health.

Care of the paediatric patient today requires a nurse who is a skilled professional member of a health team, able to keep pace with technical and scientific changes. The challenge is to acquire not only the technical skills of caring but a highly developed power of accurate observation which together with the knowledge of growth and development makes the nurse who cares for the child a specialist within the broader category of nursing.

Paediatric nursing practice, in keeping pace with changes in
health service delivery, has recognised that while the majority
of paediatric nurses continue to practise within a hospital
there is an increasing need to support the child and family
within their home. Every nurse must become familiar with
teaching of patient, parents and the community at large to
keep the continuity of care.

The challenge to paediatric nursing today is not the limitation
of a nurse practising within a specialty, it is the opportunity
for a nurse who has a responsibility of providing care for the
infant, child and adolescent to influence the health of
successive generations.

A defined paediatric nursing text written and edited by
Australian nurses which, drawing on the knowledge of the
nurse in clinical paediatric practice, embraces this challenge,
is to be commended.

Jan Y. Minnis
Director of Nursing
Royal Alexandra Hospital for Children
Sydney

II

The paediatric nurse of the 1990s is a sophisticated clinician
working as part of the health care team. The changing
patterns of childhood disease and the focus of health
promotion and maintenance are altering the way that nurses
practise. The specialist paediatric nurse functions as clinical
expert, educator of other staff and the family, role model,
resource person and change agent. There has also been a
change in community expectations of care and an explosion
of knowledge and technology which contribute to a rapidly
changing and increasingly complex health environment. Owing
to the rapidity of change in the health sector, we need
paediatric nurses who are well informed, open to change,
capable of moving freely between practice settings and able
to meet the needs of diverse cultural populations.

The changes in the focus and delivery of nursing care are also reflected in a broader educational preparation for nurses. However, in a bid to cover the breadth of clinical practice, nursing practice is often represented in a fragmented fashion to students of nursing. This may impede the development of an holistic understanding of, and approach to, the child and family with multiple needs for care. The demand for nurses with advanced clinical knowledge and skills imposes an imperative for quality educational activities and resources to foster and support competency in the nursing work force.

An effort has been made over the last decade to return care and caring to their essential places in nursing practice and education. Benner[1], who has written widely on the subject of practice, believed in the transformation of nursing practice through the exploration of the meaning of nursing. She also believed that nursing is a practice-based discipline with a knowledge base which should derive from and be explored through practice.

The editors are to be congratulated on their efforts in bringing together the clinical expertise of nurses caring for children in the Australian context. **Nursing the Infant, Child & Adolescent** aims to present a view of paediatric nursing which is practice-based. It is designed to meet the needs of all general and specialist nurses in the paediatric area. The book is a significant development in the history of nursing in Australia and encourages each learner to look beyond the immediate appearances in a nursing situation to consider medical, social, personal and other relationships.

Sandra Willis
Principal Nurse Educator
Mackinnon School of Nursing
Royal Children's Hospital
Melbourne

1. Benner, P. *From Novice to Expert: Excellence and Power in Clinical Nursing Practice*, Menlo Park: Addison Wesley, 1984.

Preface

The thinking in producing a text about the nursing care of infants, children, adolescents and their families began with the idea that a text written by nurses who could draw on their expert knowledge and experience in the Australian context would be a valuable resource and make a contribution to the practice of nurses who care for infants, children and adolescents in a range of settings. The editors were convinced that such a text was timely and have been encouraged throughout its production by the many expressions of affirmation for this work. Since that first idea was formed, the text has taken on a momentum of its own, reminiscent of the processes of growth and development. In content, there has been a steady growth in the scope and number of contributions and the detail within each section.

The content of the text has been arranged in three main parts in order to achieve a logical sequence. The first part is concerned with healthy growth and development and the management of health needs from birth to adolescence. Those alterations to health which nurses can expect to encounter in their care of infants, children and adolescents and the nursing management of such alterations are the concern of the second section. The third section is concerned with special problems which require highly specialised nursing. The content of the text is designed to meet the range of needs and interests of readers.

We are conscious that while the contributions in the text cover many topics there are some we have not been able to include. There is, however, a commitment to nursing throughout the text. Knowledge is presented as the basis for care and nursing management is the focus within each topic.

It is our belief that the text will be a useful source of information and a contribution to good practice in paediatric nursing.

The editors have been helped in their task in bringing this text to fruition. We are deeply grateful for the support, encouragement and direction we have received from Jenny Curtis. Her patience and constancy have sustained us. Jeremy Fisher has been a friend to the project and his positive approach is appreciated. We have been impressed by the efforts and perseverance of the many contributors and applaud their determination through numerous drafts and requests. We record our thanks for their efforts and commitment.

Anne Adams

Carmel McQuellin

Sue Nagy

ALTERATIONS TO HEALTH IN INFANCY, CHILDHOOD AND ADOLESCENCE: SPECIAL PROBLEMS

In this age of specialisation, paediatric nursing accommodates a range of specialised areas of practice. Each of these areas of practice has a specific knowledge base and requires clinical expertise in the care required by infants, children and adolescents with special problems.

Part Three contains contributions from expert nurses who have explored highly specialised areas of practice across the spectrum. The first chapter in this section (Chapter 10) addresses the care of newborn infants with special needs. The care of infants, children and adolescents with an alteration to cardiovascular function (Chapter 11), requiring intensive care (Chapter 12) and with burns (Chapter 13) follow. Chapter 14 discusses the care of adolescents with special needs.

In each of the chapters in Part Three the authors have included detailed information about the health breakdown and practice issues which arise within their specialty and have emphasised the specific nursing approaches to care. Their writing reveals the knowledge and skills of expert clinicians and offers a rich and informative reference for each of the speciality areas.

Chapter 10

Care of the Newborn Infant with Special Needs

Kaye Spence

Neonatal nursing is practised in a variety of settings. The newborn with special needs can range from the smallest of premature infants to the term infant with a complex congenital abnormality. No matter what the problem, certain basic principles of care need to be applied in all infants. These basic principles of care centre around resuscitation, oxygenation, ventilation, thermoregulation, fluid therapy and nutrition.

This chapter will describe these basic principles and then apply them to some of the specific conditions found in neonatal nurseries.

Principles of Care

RESUSCITATION

Neonatal resuscitation involves a series of actions aimed at the initiation or restoration of normal respiratory rate and pattern, heart rate, colour, blood pressure and general activity level. Resuscitation may be required in the delivery room or in the nursery where the infant can suddenly show signs of respiratory failure.

Approximately 5% to 10% of infants require some form of assistance with ventilatory or circulatory adaptation at birth.[1] All nurses who work with the newborn need to have a basic understanding of fetal and neonatal pathophysiology and to master resuscitation techniques. At birth, the newborn must adapt to the transition from a fluid-filled to an air-filled lung, and the time during labour, delivery and immediately after birth carries a high risk of asphyxia. Skilful resuscitation of the asphyxiated newborn can prevent brain damage and minimise subsequent neonatal problems such as hypoxic brain injury.

Asphyxia has four main groups of causes.[2]

1. Fetal asphyxia from the interruption of umbilical blood flow, e.g., cord compression during labour or prolapsed cord.
2. Fetal asphyxia from failure of exchange across the placenta because of placental separation, e.g., abruption.
3. Fetal asphyxia from inadequate perfusion of the maternal side of the placenta, e.g., maternal hypertension.

4. Neonatal asphyxia from failure to inflate the lungs and complete the transition from a fetal to a neonatal circulation. Neonatal asphyxia may occur because of airway obstruction, excessive fluid in the lungs or a weak respiratory effort. It may also occur as a sequela to fetal asphyxia and is often a progressive process which is potentially reversible. In early, mild stages the asphyxia may reverse spontaneously if the cause is removed.

Survival before 24 weeks' gestation is almost impossible due to the structural immaturity of the alveoli and the capillaries. Gas exchange becomes possible between 24 and 28 weeks' gestation as the alveolar–capillary membrane matures. Sufficient surfactant phospholipid must be produced to prevent collapse of the alveoli at the end of expiration. Surfactant secretion does not begin until the 24th week of gestation. Circulatory maturity makes perfusion possible. At birth, the infant must rapidly effect the transition from the fetal to the neonatal circulation.[3] Many interruptions can occur to this transition, for example structural cardiac abnormalities and persistence of pulmonary hypertension with resultant right-to-left shunting of blood (see Chapter 11, Cardiac Abnormalities).

Resuscitation techniques for the newborn differ for full-term and preterm infants. The term infant is at risk for cerebral damage and the resuscitation is aimed at preventing this complication. The preterm infant with immature body systems requires expert management to avoid complications from the procedure.[1,4]

The principles of resuscitation are as follows:

1. Prevention. The nurse needs to be prepared by having the resuscitation equipment checked and ready for use, and knowing how to use it. The correct-sized masks and endotracheal tubes are identified for individual infants. Assessment includes fetal factors, intrapartum monitoring, gestation and pulmonary maturity. Recognition of the high-risk infant or pregnancy aids in this preparation.

2. Adequate resuscitation. Requires skilled nursing and medical personnel to resuscitate all newborn infants. Effective mask and bag resuscitation is achieved by having the infant in the correct position with the appropriate-sized mask. The stomach is vented with a wide-bore (8 fg) gastric tube. Adequate inflation of the lungs will ensure good chest movement and air entry, which can be detected on auscultation. Newborn resuscitation in the majority of cases is ventilatory in origin, therefore the establishment of good respiratory function avoids the need for more invasive techniques.

3. Avoid cold stress. The infant who is cold is extremely difficult to revive. Keep the infant dry and warm by nursing in an appropriately warm environment. Use of a 'resuscitaire' with an overhead radiant heater is ideal.

4. Ensure a patent airway by firstly suctioning the nose and then the oropharynx with a size 10 or 12 fg catheter and aspirating the gastric content. Avoid suction to the posterior oropharynx as this may induce apnoea and/or bradycardia. Position the infant in a left lateral decubitus position and check that there are no anatomical abnormalities which could be a potential obstruction, e.g., microganthia with a large tongue.

5. If the infant is not breathing, he will require artificial ventilation using a bag and mask. Artifical ventilation requires care to avoid injury. Poor technique may cause a pneumothorax from the delivery of excessively high inflating pressures. Inadequate pressures may result in underexpansion of the alveoli. If the rate is too slow it may be insufficient to produce oxygenation. Bag and mask ventilation should be commenced immediately if the infant is making no respiratory effort on his own and his

heart rate is below 100 beats per minute. A pressure gauge with the rebreathing bag is recommended so that the pressures can be documented. A pressure of 20 cmH$_2$O at a rate of 30 breaths per minute with an inspiratory phase of one second is recommended to start.

6. If the infant is cyanosed or hypoxaemic, 100% oxygen is administered. Extra precautions must be taken when administering 100% oxygen to the premature infant. These include incremental decreases in oxygen when the infant responds.

7. Successful hand bagging is determined by assessment of bilateral air entry, chest excursions with deflation of the bag and improvement of colour and heart rate. If, despite a good technique, the infant does not respond, intubation by a skilled practitioner is necessary.

8. If the heart rate remains below 100 beats per minute after intubation, and ventilation has been established, chest compressions should begin in order to improve cardiac output.

9. Closed chest cardiac massage is best performed by compressing the lower sternum 1 to 2 cm with the resuscitator's first and second fingers at a rate of 100 to 120 times per minute. This procedure should be alternated with positive pressure ventilation at a ratio of 3:1.[5]

In summary, the goals of resuscitation are:[5] to allow expansion of the lungs by clearing the upper airways; to increase the partial pressure of arterial oxygen (PaO$_2$) by providing adequate alveolar ventilation with supplementary oxygen if necessary; ensuring adequate cardiac output; and minimising oxygen consumption by reducing heat loss.

OXYGENATION

Oxygen is necessary for cell growth and metabolism. In sick infants, supplementary oxygen may be required for these functions to occur. The nurse needs to identify the necessity for oxygen, understand the benefits and hazards of its use, and be able to operate the equipment necessary for the controlled delivery of oxygen therapy.

Hypoxia is a reduction in the oxygen supply to the tissues to below physiological levels, despite adequate perfusion of the tissues. Tissue hypoxia can be caused by heart failure, anaemia, hypotension, abnormal affinity of the haemoglobin for oxygen or a fall in the PaO$_2$.

Hypoxaemia is a deficiency of oxygen in the circulating blood, resulting from lung disease or cyanotic heart disease. The most common reason is lung disease which results in intrapulmonary right-to-left shunting.

Oxygen therapy is required in the following groups of infants:

- Those with central cyanosis indicated by a blue appearance of the mucous membranes.
- Those requiring resuscitation for apnoea or those with bradycardia and cyanosis. Oxygen alone may not be sufficient and other resuscitative measures may be needed.
- Those with respiratory distress due to lung disease.
- Those with an inappropriate elevation of their pulmonary vascular resistance.
- Following cardiac surgery, where oxygen is used to induce pulmonary vasodilation or prevent pulmonary vasoconstriction.

Oxygen is not indicated in some conditions, namely: acrocyanosis (blue hands and feet) as this condition may be due to other causes such as cold stress or poor peripheral blood flow; prematurity without respiratory distress or cyanosis; congenital heart disease with a significant left-to-right shunt, when oxygen therapy may increase the shunt and precipitate increased heart failure.

Complications of oxygen therapy may occur when inadequate oxygen administration has resulted in organ damage; high PaO_2 levels have been implicated in the genesis of retinopathy of prematurity.

Principles of oxygen administration

1. All infants receiving supplementary oxygen should be monitored using a saturation monitor, transcutaneous oxygen monitor or by regular blood gas measurements. By using the trend facility, early detection of deterioration in the infant's condition can be made. The electrodes should be resited every 4 to 6 hours and the skin examined for pressure sores, burns or skin abrasions. Blood gases are measured using arterial collection in the acute stage.
2. The inspired gases should be a blend of oxygen and medical air to enable the oxygen concentrations to be adjusted. An oxygen analyser placed near the infants' face allows checking of the required concentration. The analyser needs to be calibrated to air and 100% oxygen each shift to ensure accuracy.
3. All gases should be administered through a humidifier and into a head box of appropriate size for the infant. The temperature measured in the head box should be within the infants' neutral thermal zone to avoid excessive cooling from dry, cool gases. Administration of oxygen directly into the incubator is not recommended as fluctuations occur when the portholes are opened. Some newer incubator models compensate for this fluctuation with an altered air flow.
4. Fluctuations in oxygenation can be prevented by ensuring that the infant remains in the correct concentration at all times. If the infant needs to be removed from the incubator for weighing or x-ray, ensure that an alternative means is available to provide the same concentration of oxygen.
5. A minimum flow of 8 L/minute is recommended when using a head box, to avoid the rebreathing of expired carbon dioxide.

All nurseries need to be adequately equipped with facilities and staff so that acute oxygen therapy can be provided in the case of an unexpected deterioration or emergency. The equipment includes: headbox, oxygen analyser, humidifier, oxygen and medical gas, transcutaneous oxygen or saturation monitor. Facilities should be nearby for the measurement of blood gas levels.[5]

FLUIDS AND NUTRITION

There is only a narrow margin of safety when calculating the fluid and electrolyte requirements of the newborn, as a number of factors influence the infant's ability to maintain fluid balance.

- The newborn infant has a high metabolic rate.
- The renal system is immature and the renal function does not develop at the same rate. For example, the glomerular filtration rate is low at birth and rises rapidly during the next 6 weeks.
- The excretion of urinary sodium increases slowly during the first 2 years. The urinary sodium losses are influenced by the sodium intake and gestational age. Very low

birthweight (<1500 g) infants tend to lose more sodium and therefore are likely to require supplements.

- The insensible water loss, which occurs through the skin and lungs, is influenced by environmental factors such as temperature, use of radiant warmers, phototherapy, activity, gestational age and weight. The factors that influence insensible water loss must be identified early and the maintenance needs of the individual infant should be adjusted to prevent problems with water and electrolyte imbalance.

The following points are important when administering fluids to the newborn infant:

- Intravenous fluids must be administered by an infusion pump capable of delivering 0.1 to 99.9 mL/hour. Care needs to be taken to ensure that the pump is set to deliver the correct amount each hour.
- Fluid intake is measured and recorded every hour.
- Urinary specific gravity and output are evaluated every 4 to 8 hours; desirable ranges are specific gravity 1005 to 1015 and urine output 2 to 4 mL/kg/hour.
- The infant is assessed for clinical signs of overhydration or dehydration. The infant needs to be weighed daily when receiving intravenous fluids as it is easy to overload the infant with fluid.
- The cannula must be patent, the strapping non-restrictive, the site visible and the limb restrained.
- A blood glucose level is measured with a reagent strip and recorded frequently over the first 48 hours. Caution must be taken in the interpretation of these results when the infants' haematocrit is greater than 0.60, as falsely low readings may be obtained. A laboratory blood glucose level may be required to verify a result of less than 2 mmol/L.

The fetus receives a constant supply of glucose across the placenta. At birth, this supply is stopped and the infant must regulate his own glucose concentration. Glycogen stores in the newborn infant are greater than adults, but the newborn infant uses glucose at twice the rate of adults. Within 2 to 3 hours after birth or sooner, the neonate uses his stores, which then remain low for several days, when they slowly increase to adult levels.

The use of glucose is influenced by several factors. In asphyxia, anaerobic glycolysis is an inefficient means of energy production. Other factors such as abnormal body temperature, increased activity, perinatal asphyxia, prematurity, maternal diabetes and delayed feeding may contribute to hypoglycaemia. Small-for-gestational-age (SGA) infants are a particularly high-risk group for hypoglycaemia because of their decreased glycogen and bodyfat stores.[6]

The attainment of growth and development is the goal of nutritional management. The sick or small infant may not be able to be fed by the enteral route and nutritional requirements are then given by the parenteral route, using total parenteral nutrition (TPN). The decision to delay enteral feeds is determined by several factors: an instability in the overall clinical condition of the infant; increasing gastric residuals, vomiting and abdominal distension; an increase in the infant's respiratory rate; and apnoea and bradycardia.

If TPN is used in the small infant it is often for a short period and used to complement the cautious introduction of enteral feeds. TPN may be administered via a peripheral vein, with restriction of glucose concentration to 10% or less. This avoids the complications of infiltration and burns from hypertonic solutions. Centrally placed catheters are preferred for the more hypertonic solutions as the fluid is diluted by the blood flow in the large vessel. The infant should be monitored for complications such as catheter-related sepsis and hyperglycaemia.[7]

TPN is also used for those newborn infants in whom gastrointestinal dysfunction is the result of congenital abnormalities (e.g., gastroschisis, long segment Hirshsprung's disease) or in cases of acquired abnormalities such as necrotising enterocolitis (NEC). There are a number of reasons why the newborn infant receiving TPN should be cared for in a Level III/IV neonatal unit. The infant needs close observation and monitoring for potential complications. The catheter must be properly maintained and a very small sample of blood must be taken for chemical analysis. Pharmacy and laboratory facilities must also be available for adequate preparation and monitoring of the use of the TPN.

Small preterm infants who are unable to suck may be fed enteral feeds once their general condition has stabilised. Enteral feeds are commenced in small volumes (30 mL/ kg every 2 to 3 hours) and slowly increased as the infant demonstrates tolerance of the volumes given. Feeds are given by orogastric tube and allowed to flow by gravity to avoid milk aspiration.

THERMOREGULATION

The newborn infant's body temperature is maintained by a delicate balance between the amount of heat produced and the amount of heat lost. If production exceeds loss, then the body temperature will rise. Conversely, if loss exceeds production, then the body temperature will fall.

The infant loses heat in 2 ways. First, heat is transferred from the interior of the body to the skin from the circulating blood. Second, heat is transferred from the body to the external environment by evaporation, conduction, convection and radiation. Understanding the mechanisms of heat loss is an important basis for nursing care.

The evaporation of moisture on the skin has a cooling effect. A wet newborn infant in a delivery room will decrease body temperature at a rate of 0.2°C of skin temperature per minute. Thus, over 10 minutes the infant's body temperature will drop by 2°C. This reflects a heat loss of 210 J/kg/minute. To avoid this loss, the infant must be dried immediately and kept in a warm environment. Evaporative loss can occur if the infant remains in a wet nappy, if the hands of attendants are wet or if cool swabbing solutions are used for antiseptic skin care.

Conductive heat loss occurs through direct contact with the immediate environment. Materials differ in the extent to which they conduct heat away from the body. Air is a poor conductor of heat, whereas water is an excellent conductor. An infant placed in a cool bath will loose heat very rapidly. Conductive heat loss is minimised when clothing and blankets provide insulation.

Convective heat loss occurs when a cool draught blows over the infant. An infant who is nursed under a radiant heat source is still subject to convective heat loss from air currents created by air conditioners and movement of personnel.

Radiant heat travels through air without appreciably changing the temperature of the air. An infant who is placed near a cold wall or surface will radiate heat to that surface. Thus an infant in an incubator set at 34°C can still radiate heat to a cooler window located behind the incubator. To minimise this loss, the environmental temperature in the nursery should be kept to within 7°C of the infant's incubator temperature.[8]

Heat production

All tissues are capable of metabolising or burning food materials for the production of heat within the body. This heat production derives from general metabolic changes when the body is cooled or warmed. The newborn infant has another mechanism for heat production which is known as brown fat metabolism. The brown fat tissue is located in the upper thorax, in the axilla and beneath the skin in the upper part of the back. It differs from normal yellow fat in that it has a primary function of generating heat under cold stress. When the infant is cooled, the brown fat deposits are stimulated by the autonomic nervous system to release the stored fat. As this heat is combusted it is transferred throughout the body by the bloodstream.[9]

Effects of cooling on the infant

Cooling has an adverse effect on oxygen consumption, caloric requirements, glucose utilisation, blood pH and surfactant production. When cooled, in an attempt to generate sufficient heat to maintain body temperature conditions, the newborn infant increases brown fat metabolism and also stimulates his general metabolism. Oxygen consumption is increased to supply fuel for metabolism. The aim, therefore, is to maintain the infant in a state requiring minimal oxygen consumption by keeping him normothermic in a neutral thermal environment.

Cooling also affects the rate of calorie use and the rate that glucose is metabolised. While the term infant has reasonably large glucose stores, the premature or small-for-gestational-age infant has very small stores which are easily depleted. Under cold stress, the premature infant may exhaust his stores within 2 to 6 hours and become hypoglycaemic. Under these conditions, the infant is at risk for sustaining brain damage.[8]

When the infant is cooled and the brown fat metabolism is stimulated, fatty acids are released into the bloodstream. In the presence of adequate oxygen, glucose is metabolised to carbon dioxide and water for excretion. If, however, adequate oxygen is not available, glucose is metabolised into lactic acid which is released into the bloodstream. The combination of both lactic acid and fatty acids can result in the infant becoming acidotic. If sufficiently severe, acidosis can interfere in the normal processes required for life and death can result.[8]

Controlling the environment

The optimal thermal environment is known as the neutral thermal environment (NTE). This zone is bounded by an upper and lower critical temperature. The upper critical temperature is the ambient temperature above which thermoregulatory evaporative heat loss is stimulated. The lower critical temperature is the ambient temperature below which the rate of metabolic heat production increases to maintain thermal balance.

Each infant has his own NTE and this is determined by the infant's postnatal age in hours and days, his bare weight, and the state of his health. The range given is that of thermoneutrality. The ambient air temperature is adjusted to keep the infant in the lower end of this range.[8] The NTE can only be measured when using a closed incubator and every effort should be made to avoid fluctuations in the environmental temperature by keeping the doors closed. Care must be coordinated to minimise opening the doors.

Some convective incubators, and most open care radiant warmers, can provide servo control. Servo control is a method of maintaining the infant's surface (skin) temperature at a constant predetermined level (mostly 36.2 to 36.8°C). The environmental (air) temperature in the incubator or the output from the radiant heaters are controlled by the predetermined skin temperature setting. By using servo control, the infant's temperature is kept within a desired range. There are, however, many precautions that need to be observed when using this mode of temperature control. Firstly, the control of the heating output relies on the surface probe adhered to the upper surface of the infant. The probe needs to be covered with a heat reflective disc. Secondly, any fluctuations in the infant's temperature are disguised, especially under open care systems when it is difficult to monitor heat output.[10] In closed convective incubators, fluctuations in the ambient air temperature can alert the nurse to an unstable temperature in the infant.

The Newborn Infant Requiring Short-term Assisted Ventilation

Some infants will require intubation and ventilation for a short period (less than 6 hours) while awaiting transfer to a tertiary centre. The nurse caring for the infant needs to have an understanding of the particular ventilator, the basic principles of ventilation and the care the infant will require. It is beyond the scope of this chapter to cover assisted ventilation in the intensive care nursery, however the same basic principles apply. For more information the reader is referred to the numerous excellent texts that cover assisted ventilation in more detail.[11]

As early recognition of changes in vital signs can avert major complications,[12] an infant requiring assisted ventilation needs meticulous nursing care. An infant should only be disconnected from the ventilator for suctioning when an adaptor is not used and the time of disconnection should be minimal. All procedures, such as suctioning and turns, require 2 nurses, one of whom should have some experience in managing a ventilated infant.

Nasotracheal tubes are preferred in the intensive care nursery and on transport as they are easier to secure in order to avoid movement and extubation. However, orotracheal tubes are easier to insert and will suffice in the short term. Occasionally, an orotracheal tube may be used for the very low birthweight infant. All the equipment for intubation should be checked and ready for use. Following intubation, the tube should be securely strapped to the infant's face and the ventilator tubing secured to the bed. Chest auscultation for bilateral air entry, supported by a chest x-ray, is used to ensure that the tube has been correctly placed. The position of the endotracheal tube at the nares or mouth should be noted and recorded on the infant's chart.

ASSESSMENT OF ADEQUATE VENTILATION

The following points may indicate that the infant's ventilatory requirements are being met:

- Symmetrical and synchronous chest movement.
- Equal air entry on chest auscultation.
- Heart rate within normal range, 120 to 160 bpm.
- Colour pink with good perfusion.

- Transcutaneous oxygen within the range 60 to 90 mmHg.
- Arterial blood gas measurement within acceptable range — PaO_2 50 to 80 mmHg, $PaCO_2$ 35 to 45 mmHg, pH 7.35 to 7.45.

The infant's condition should be monitored continuously. The following observations should be recorded hourly:

- Skin colour, chest movement and air entry.
- Heart rate. Any instability, such as a drop in the heart rate on handling or during suctioning should be notified.
- Respirations should synchronise with the ventilator. The chest should move equally on both sides.
- Transcutaneous oxygen levels and trends. Look for changes during procedures or after alteration in ventilation.
- Endotracheal tube:

  a) Taping must be secure. If the strapping is loose and lifts from the face, inform the medical officer immediately so that he or she can restrap the tube. If this is not attended to, accidental extubation may occur.

  b) Position. The tube position at the nose or mouth and vocal cords is recorded in centimetres on the chart. Check this reading frequently. Record, in centimetres, the length of the tube from the nostril or mouth to the external tip of the tube.

  c) Kinking. Position ventilator tubing to avoid kinking or twisting, and secure to the mattress. The tube should be angled down to avoid pressure on the nostril.

  d) Mobility. If the tube can move in and out through the nostril more than 1 cm, then the tube needs to be restrapped.

- Ventilator observations — Always check against the instructions on the ventilator order chart:

  a) Flow. Combined oxygen and air flow is normally between 8 and 12 L/minute.

  b) Oxygen concentration (F_iO_2). This is set with the blender in the ventilator and checked with an oxygen analyser. The analyser is calibrated each shift in air (0.21) and 100% (1.0) oxygen. The alarm limits are set 3% above and 3% below the required percentage.

  c) Pressures. Peak airway or inspiratory pressure (PIP) and positive end expired pressure (PEEP) should correlate with the ventilator orders. The mean airway pressure (MAP) is a derived pressure and is recorded from the ventilator. If any change in pressure is noticed, the circuit must be checked for leaks and the accumulation of water in the tubing. The alarms are set appropriate to the ordered pressures, usually 3 cmH_2O below the peak inspiratory pressure.

  d) Inspiratory time. This should read between 0.6 seconds and 1.0 second for standard ventilation. Check the inspiratory/expiratory ratio to ensure that the ratio has not been reversed.

  e) Rate. The rate should coincide with the order chart.

  f) Humidity. The humidifier should be refilled with sterile water when the water level falls below the recommended level. Excessive water in the ventilator tubing will alter the pressures being delivered to the infant. Check the tubing for condensation and empty any water. All ventilator tubing should be placed below the level of the infant to avoid water accumulation at the elbow connection and accidental drainage into the patient's endotracheal tube.

g) Manifold (inspired gas) temperature. The sensor in the circuit needs to be placed away from any direct heat source such as incubator air flow. The temperature is read on the humidifier and should be maintained at 0.5 to 1.0°C below body temperature, usually 36°C.

Nursing care

The need for endotracheal tube suction is assessed every 4 hours and carried out when there are audible rales on chest auscultation or there is suspicion of a blocked endotracheal tube. Assess the infant's response and quantity of secretions in order to determine the frequency of suction. Record the amount, consistency and colour of secretions. A technique which is swift and thorough is essential to avoid compromising the infant during the procedure.

If the infant's condition permits, reposition the infant every 4 hours, alternately from supine to either side supported with a rolled towel.

A rebreathing bag and pressure manometer must be connected to oxygen and airflow or a blender and positioned in the infant's incubator at all times. The desired oxygen concentration is dialled on the blender or obtained by mixing the oxygen and air flow.

A size 8 fg gastric tube is passed orally and left on free drainage and aspirated every 4 hours to relieve gastric distension. Ensure the tube is correctly positioned in the stomach. The position may be confirmed by viewing the x-ray.

Complications

Complications may arise from the tube or the ventilator, and may also be a result of suctioning or other causes.

* Tube — blocked, kinked or displaced into a main stem bronchus, the oesophagus or the pharynx.[12]
* Ventilator — mechanical failure, inadequate humidification, disconnection in the circuit, flow meter turned off.[13]
* Suctioning — mucosal damage, hypoxaemia, arrhythmia, hypotension, lung collapse, infection or poor technique.[12,14]
* Other complications — gastric distension, pneumothorax, pneumomediastinum, pulmonary interstitial emphysema, atelectasis, pneumonia, septicaemia, hypotension, post extubation stridor and subglottic stenosis.[15]

Ventilator Emergencies

In an emergency, action should proceed in the following order:
* Summon help.
* Check the ventilator is working; if not, disconnect the ventilator.
* Connect the bag with or without the mask and hand ventilate. Ensure the chest is moving.
* If the endotracheal tube appears blocked, use suction to clear it, or remove it.
* Check ventilator circuit for leaks.
* If in doubt, seek advice and assistance.

X-ray Interpretation

When caring for a ventilated infant, the chest x-ray can be a useful aid in determining the correct position of the endotracheal tube and gastric tube, the state of the lung fields and in detecting complications such as a pneumothorax.

The x-ray is interpreted for the following:

- Both sides of the chest (lungs) are of similar radiolucency.
- The endotracheal tube is straight and positioned in the trachea, below the clavicles and above the carina.
- The gastric tube tip lies within the gastric bubble.
- Dark areas within the chest may indicate a pneumothorax and light areas collapse or consolidation.

Extubation Procedure

Extubation should proceed at the convenience of the staff looking after the infant. Unplanned extubation should not occur, is considered an accident and is therefore to be avoided. Extubation should only be considered if the infant is making good respiratory effort and able to sustain adequate gas exchange and acid-base balance. Premature extubation can result in a deterioration in the infant's condition and expose the infant to the risk of trauma from reintubation.

When preparing to extubate an infant, all equipment must be checked and ready for use. This includes: headbox with humidifier, flow meters and/or blender, oxygen analyser, suction catheters 10 to 12 fg for oropharyngeal suction and resuscitation equipment for reintubation if necessary.

Place the infant in the prone position and empty the stomach by aspirating the gastric tube. Position the tcPO$_2$ electrode or SaO$_2$ probe and ensure the monitor is working. Suction the endotracheal tube before removal. Suction the pharynx as the tube is removed, and suction the nose. Ensure oxygen is being delivered at the correct concentration into the headbox. Minimal handling allows the infant sufficient time to recover.

Following extubation, the infant needs to be closely monitored for signs of increasing respiratory effort or episodes of apnoea. A chest x-ray may be required following extubation if there is doubt that the lung fields are clear. Consider withholding enteral feeds if the respiratory rate is greater than 40 breaths per minute or for at least 4 hours following extubation.

The Low Birthweight Infant

DEFINITIONS

A preterm infant is one who is born before 37 completed weeks of gestation.
A low birthweight infant weighs less than 2500 g.

A very low birthweight infant weighs less than 1500 g.
An extremely low birthweight infant weighs less than 1000 g.
A small-for-gestational-age infant is when the weight is below the 10th percentile.
A large-for-gestational-age infant is when the weight is above the 90th percentile.

Infants born preterm or with a low birthweight are at risk for particular problems and diseases. The more immature the infant, the higher the risk for certain conditions. The following conditions form some of the more common problems specific to the preterm infant.

HYALINE MEMBRANE DISEASE

Hyaline membrane disease (HMD) is a condition of lung immaturity due to a deficiency of surfactant, which results in stiff, non-compliant lungs which are difficult to inflate. The condition presents with respiratory distress and poor oxygenation that may require assisted ventilation for a period of time. The infant recovers from HMD once surfactant is produced, at approximately 72 hours after delivery. The aim of the treatment is to have the infant survive and avoid the complications of treatment, namely air leak, chronic lung disease, intraventricular haemorrhage and necrotising enterocolitis.[3,7] Surfactant replacement therapy is used for premature infants with the disease and is commenced within 24 hours of birth.

SEPSIS

Sepsis should be considered in any high-risk infant and following premature or prolonged rupture of membranes and maternal fever. Prematurity, an immature immune system and complicated medical or surgical problems contribute to the infant's increased susceptibility to infection. Clinical signs include respiratory distress, abnormal temperature, poor feeding, apnoea, jittery movements, and a general unwellness. Common organisms include Group B beta haemolytic streptococci, *Staphylococcus aureus*, *Escherichia coli*, *Klebsiella pneumoniae* and *Pseudomonas aeruginosa*. Infection control practices are necessary for the prevention of nosocomial infections. These practices include handwashing, removal of environment hazards, skin and umbilical cord care and aseptic procedures.[16]

ANAEMIA

Anaemia present at birth or in the immediate neonatal period can be caused by blood loss, a haemolytic process or decreased red cell production. For the majority of newborns, the normal haematocrit range is 48% to 60%, and the normal haemoglobin range is 160 to 200 g/L for the term infant and 140 to 150 g/L for the preterm infant.[17] A newborn infant with suspected anaemia should be examined for pallor, hypotension and tachycardia and observed for the signs of shock. An acute blood loss of 20% of the blood volume, which may not be reflected in the haemoglobin immediately after birth, is sufficient to produce shock. The premature infant is at risk of blood loss from repeated sampling for laboratory investigations. An infant with anaemia may be lethargic or have episodes of apnoea and bradycardia.

INTRAVENTRICULAR HAEMORRHAGE

Small preterm infants have fragile cerebral blood vessels, which can dilate and rupture as a result of hypoxic episodes. This is known to occur in 40% of infants of less than 28 weeks' gestation and 17.3% of infants with gestation between 28 and 31 weeks.[18] If the haemorrhage is small, the baby is usually asymptomatic. A common complication of a severe intraventricular haemorrhage is hydrocephalus. Regular weekly measurements of head circumference should be taken and plotted on a graph to aid early detection. Nursing observations should include checking the fontanelles for fullness, and the sutures for abnormal separation. The intraventricular haemorrhage (IVH) can be diagnosed by head ultrasound. Many factors contribute to an IVH, including some nursing procedures, therefore nursing routines should be aimed at avoiding sudden alterations in oxygenation, which may result in alterations to the cerebral blood flow.

CHRONIC LUNG DISEASE

Chronic lung disease is characterised by prolonged oxygen requirements, beyond 28 days of life, with abnormal chest x-ray findings. It occurs secondary to a period of mechanical ventilation.[15] The fluid balance in these infants is monitored closely to avoid fluid overload. An adequate nutritional status is important to help with the added work of breathing.[19] As these infants require prolonged periods of hospitalisation, the attending nurse must facilitate the infant's psychological development through planned and appropriate interventions.[20] Long-term management includes the administration of oxygen therapy by nasal cannulae and the possibility of a home oxygen program.

PERSISTENT DUCTUS ARTERIOSUS

The ductus arteriosus normally constricts within 72 hours of birth in response to the rise in the pressures on the left side of the heart. If the infant is premature or the oxygen tension does not rise after birth, the ductus may remain patent. Persistent ductus arteriosis (PDA) is common in the very low birthweight infant with an incidence of 28.9% among newborns of less than 28 weeks' gestation.[18] The presence of a PDA allows blood to shunt from the aorta to the pulmonary artery (left-to-right shunt). When pulmonary resistance falls, the result is an increase in pulmonary blood flow, resulting in signs of pulmonary congestion. The infant's symptoms are dependent on the size of the ductus and the difference between pulmonary and systemic resistance. The administration of increased fluid volumes can contribute to symptoms in the premature infant.[21] Clinical signs include: bounding peripheral pulses; a characteristic harsh murmur; and an increase in the work of breathing. The infant becomes tachypnoeic with increased respiratory effort with chest retractions and nasal flaring. Other signs of congestive heart failure include tachycardia, hepatomegaly and an enlarged heart on chest x-ray.[22]

RETINOPATHY OF PREMATURITY

Premature infants receiving oxygen therapy are at risk of developing retinopathy of prematurity (ROP). The immature retina has sections that remain unvascularised at 8 months of gestation. Fluctuations in oxygen levels and exposure to high PaO_2 in the presence of vascular immaturity can damage the developing capillary bed. Oxygen acts on the immature retina by causing arterial vasoconstriction and resultant hypoxic retinal oedema, the vessels proliferate as a reaction to the hypoxia and haemorrhages can occur. The result is the formation of a fibrovascular tissue and eventual retraction of this tissue. The international classification of the stages of progress of ROP places emphasis on the size and the site of the lesion.[15,23]

Infants at risk of developing ROP need to be monitored during oxygen administration. The PaO_2 needs to be kept within 60 to 80 mmHg and periods of hyperoxygenation avoided. All premature infants receiving supplemental oxygen should be monitored using a $tcPO_2$ monitor. SaO_2 monitors do not inform the caregiver if the infant has high partial pressure levels as the saturation curve flattens out at 95%.

NECROTISING ENTEROCOLITIS

Necrotising enterocolitis (NEC) is a multifactoral disease. It is an ischaemic disease of the gut, which can extend from the stomach to the rectum. Numerous clinical factors are associated in the development of the disease, but the exact relationship is not known and approximately 80% of infants with NEC are premature. The main contributing factor appears to be mucosal injury associated with intestinal hypoperfusion secondary to perinatal asphyxia, shock, umbilical catheters, polycythaemia and hyperosmolar feeds in the sick infant. Early signs of the disease include: increased volume of gastric aspirates; vomiting; abdominal distension; stools positive to haematest (blood) and clinitest (glucose); lethargy; hypothermia; and apnoea. Late signs include: abdominal tenderness and erythema; the passage of blood per rectum; septic appearance; and shock.[24] Nursing care should aim at prevention. This may be achieved by minimal handling, maintaining the $tcPO_2$ within the therapeutic range, monitoring blood pressure (report if systolic less than 40 mmHg) and feeding cautiously. Feeds may be delayed for 5 days in the at-risk infant. They should be stopped in the following circumstances: when bile is aspirated; in the presence of abdominal distension; and when there is an acute collapse irrespective of the cause.

APNOEA OF PREMATURITY

Periodic breathing is common in preterm infants. In some infants, the pauses between breaths are prolonged, that is, for longer than 20 seconds. These apnoeic episodes lead to hypoxaemia and bradycardia. Metabolic disturbances, particularly hypoglycaemia, and conditions such as anaemia, infection, asphyxia, and drug depression contribute to apnoea. Management includes adequate monitoring of ventilatory movement and heart rate and correction of any aggravating factors. Cutaneous stimulation is often sufficient to terminate the apnoea. Ambient oxygen, however, may be cautiously increased. If the apnoeic episodes are frequent, (4 or more a day) then xanthanes may be prescribed or the infant may require assisted ventilation or continuous positive airway pressure (CPAP).[25]

JAUNDICE

Hyperbilirubinaemia is an elevated level of bilirubin in the blood. *In utero*, a baby's unconjugated bilirubin is removed by the placenta and at birth the total bilirubin is usually below 50 μmol/L. After birth, conjugation must occur in the baby's own liver. In every baby there is a rise of serum bilirubin in the first few days of life, after which the level should fall. Jaundice, common in the preterm infant, is usually harmless and does not require investigation. The contributing factors for physiological jaundice are that the red blood cells have a shortened life span, therefore twice as much bilirubin is produced. Also, the preterm infant has a greater red cell mass, a deficiency of gluconyrol transferase, and a lower plasma bilirubin binding capacity. The bowel of the preterm infant is sterile, therefore unconjugated bilirubin is absorbed and re-enters the circulation. Treatment is maintaining hydration. The infant should be nursed under phototherapy lights and the bilirubin levels should be monitored. An exchange transfusion may be indicated for the removal of excessive unconjugated bilirubin. Indications will vary according to the presence of perinatal asphyxia, respiratory distress, metabolic acidosis, hypothermia, low serum protein level, sepsis, birthweight less than 1500 g or any other condition that may interfere with the binding of bilirubin to albumin.

Nursing Care of the Low Birthweight Infant

ENVIRONMENT

The primary nurse's role is to provide an optimal environment that will promote normal physical growth and psychological development.

The appropriate incubator/cot will enable the infant to be nursed in his neutral thermal environment to conserve energy and to minimise insensible fluid losses. Therefore, it is recommended that infants weighing less than 2500 g be nursed in a forced convection, double-walled incubator. For infants weighing less than 1000 g, the ambient humidity is increased by adding water to the environment. This is achieved by placing warmed sterile water in the incubator reservoir. Radiant warmers on open-care systems are considered more convenient by some staff, but they do not provide an optimal environment for the low birthweight infant. Other warming aids such as bubble wrap and heat shields may be considered on an individual basis.

Caregivers play an important role in providing an appropriate environment. The lights in the nursery need to be regulated to avoid daylight constantly shining in the infant's eyes. By covering part of the crib with a cloth, the individual infant's environment can be modified and at the same time a level of lighting suitable for the rest of the nursery is maintained. The noise in the nursery may be sufficiently loud and continuous to have a detrimental effect on the infant. Noxious noise may create a stress response in a sick infant, leading to changes in blood pressure and oxygen desaturation. Studies[10] have shown that the main source of noise is human voices, telephones and alarms.

Inflicted pain may be avoided by altering the procedure or giving the infant analgesia. Morphine infusions are being used more often in the intensive care nursery, but some health professionals still resist prescribing or administering narcotic infusions.[26] The difficulty in obtaining an objective assessment of the newborn's pain remains a dilemma for the attending nurse. Knowledge of the capabilities of the newborn brain is limited and there is a need for more research in this area.[27]

The premature infant is often hospitalised for many weeks or months. During this time the nurse needs to consider his psychological and emotional needs together with the appropriate interventions to facilitate development. This is particularly important for the chronically ill infant. Primary nursing may be the best way of meeting these goals as the primary nurse is more able to provide continuing care based on familarity with the particular infant. Planned intervention programs based on both short and long-term care are required to meet the individual needs of the infant.[10]

POSITIONING

The small infant requires optimal positioning for positive effects on various body systems and for his developmental needs.

Various aids and interventions can help prevent contractures and promote appropriate body alignment.[28]

- The position needs to be changed regularly. These changes can be incorporated with other routines to avoid overhandling.
- Hand-to-mouth behaviour where the infant can place his hand in his mouth and suck needs to be promoted. Try to ensure that at least one limb is not restricted and that other devices such as oxygen head boxes are not obstructing this process.
- Use rolled towels or bean bags to provide a nesting shape to support the spine and the limbs. When placing the infant prone, use hip rolls to promote flexion of the hips. The aim is to create a position of flexion to reduce the tendency to extension.
- Encourage the parents to cuddle and hold their infant as this encourages a normal flexed position.

SKIN CARE

There are several developmental factors that influence skin care for the low birthweight infant. Firstly, the skin of the immature infant has an underdeveloped stratum corneum which diminishes its barrier function. There is an increased risk for the absorption of toxins. Care should therefore be taken in applying swabbing solutions and soap products to the fragile skin. Secondly, there is a tendency to oedema due to decreased fibrin and elastin fibres. Oedema makes the skin very fragile and likely to tear when adhesive tapes and friction are applied. Thirdly, the acid mantle that develops in the term infant is not present in the skin of the premature infant. The acid mantle is thought to have a bactericidal effect and the premature infant is susceptibile to infection. Greater emphasis on handwashing is required. Fourthly, the nutritional stores are decreased. The premature infant lacks fat. As zinc stores are laid down in the 3rd trimester, an essential fatty acid deficiency can present in the form of skin disruptions.[10,29]

Nursing routines need to be modified to protect the skin of these infants. Routine practices of bathing or washing with soap should be omitted for the first week and then slowly introduced. As solvents used for tape removal will be absorbed, olive oil is a useful substitute. Tears and abrasions in the skin from the use of tapes can be avoided by using a pectin-based barrier under all tapes.[30] These are available from a variety of suppliers and can be cut to any size. Many manufacturers of monitoring leads are suppling adhesive with non-abrasive properties. Particular care needs to be taken when using transcutaneous electrodes. The heating of the electrode can burn a poorly perfused skin and lead to skin breakdown.

OUTCOME AND FOLLOW-UP

Survival trends over the past decade have increased. More than 50% of infants with birthweights over 750 g and 90% of infants with birthweights over 1000 g are now surviving. The emphasis of management is shifting from survival to a concern for some of the complications of survival. Most NICUs have a follow-up program to monitor the outcome of intensive care, particularly developmental and neurological outcomes. Risk factors for poor developmental outcome include birthweight, being transported from place of delivery to a neonatal unit, low gestational age, prolonged time receiving mechanical ventilation, and a history of asphyxia, intraventricular haemorrhage and sepsis.[31] Studies have shown that 50% of surviving infants weighing less than 1000 g at birth will have normal cognitive and motor development at 2 years of age. In the 1000 g to 1500 g group, 75% can expect to be normal at 2 years, and for infants weighing more than 1500 g, 90% could expect to be normal.[32]

The neurological follow-up of these infants includes assessment of auditory and visual responses together with monitoring for cerebral palsy. Prematurity remains an important risk factor for the development of cerebral palsy. The incidence of cerebral palsy in infants weighing less than 1500 g at birth is 15%.[32]

Often the low birthweight infant has had an extended period in hospital and this in turn can have an effect on the behaviour of the infant and the needs of the parents. Many intervention programs have been devised[20] to reduce the effects of extended hospitalisation; these programs can be instituted within the neonatal nursery. They include environmental modification to light and noise, interactive play periods, appropriate stimuli and regular routines for feeds, baths and sleeping. Parents can be encouraged to provide care for their infants. Support programs can be established to help parents adapt to the care of their convalescing infant.

In New South Wales, survival rates for infants weighing 400 g to 999 g depend on their place of birth and gestational age. In 1992, survival rates for infants born at less than 28 weeks' gestation were 72.4% when transferred in utero, compared with 59.56% when transferred *hospital ex utero*. The 1-year survival increased dramatically as birthweight increased, with infants weighing more than 700 g and less than 1000 g having a 61.8% to 82.8% chance of survival. In infants weighing 1000 g to 1200 g and those weighing 2500 g to 2990 g, the 1-year survival rates were 90% and 95% respectively.[18]

The commonest morbidity for infants of less than 28 weeks' gestation were lung diseases requiring surfactant (57.1%), patent ductus arteriosis (28.9%), infection (45.2%), Grade 3 retinopathy of prematurity (15.4%) and Grade 1 intraventricular haemorrhage (13.2%).[18]

The Newborn Infant with Specific Conditions

MECONIUM ASPIRATION

Meconium aspiration is a complication of intrapartum asphyxia and occurs mostly in term infants and those small for gestational age. To avoid respiratory distress, the meconium needs to be aspirated from the pharynx as soon as the head is delivered. The trachea must be aspirated with the cords in direct view. The infant presents with tachynopea, an overinflated chest with coarse opacities on chest x-ray. Treatment consists of liberal use of oxygen to avoid the complication of increased pulmonary vascular resistance. In severe cases, ventilation may be indicated. Pneumothoraces are a complication of overinflation and may require draining with an intercostal catheter.[1,25]

INFANTS OF DRUG-DEPENDENT MOTHERS
(The neonatal abstinence syndrome)

Most drugs, including those of addiction, readily cross the placenta. The fetus of the drug-addicted mother becomes similarly dependent. The pattern of infant withdrawal depends on a number of factors. Withdrawal may take up to several weeks, as babies generally take longer to metabolise the drug. The nurse needs to be aware of the antenatal drug history so that the problem can be anticipated and then the signs of withdrawal can be recognised. A baby who is showing clinical signs of agitation should always be suspected of suffering drug withdrawal. Various scoring charts are available which aid in the assessment of central nervous system and metabolic, vasomotor, respiratory and gastrointestinal disturbances. Morphine or phenobarbitone will settle the infant. The dose is gradually reduced over a period of weeks.[33]

INFANT OF DIABETIC MOTHERS

While the infant of a diabetic mother (IDDM) may be premature, or large for gestational age, most are appropriate for gestational age following control of the maternal diabetes. On admission to the nursery, an assessment needs to be undertaken in order to identify the potential problems likely to develop. These problems include hypoglycaemia, hypocalcaemia, hyperbilirubinaemia and polycythaemia. Respiratory distress, as seen with prematurity, may also be present. The infants may be asymptomatic with normal blood glucose levels (2.5 to 5.2 mmol/L) or symptomatic with low blood glucose levels (<2 mmol/L). In either case, careful and frequent monitoring of glucose levels using reagent strips should to be undertaken for the first 48 hours or until stable. Early feeding or intravenous glucose is required.[34]

THE SMALL-FOR-GESTATIONAL-AGE INFANT

These infants fall below the 10th percentile of weight for gestational age. The assessment includes identifying the possible cause, particularly placental insufficiency, chromosomal abnormalities, malformations and congenital infections. Evaluation for hypoglycaemia, hypocalcaemia, polycythaemia, meconium aspiration, hypoxia, and the effects of asphyxia should be undertaken as a matter of routine. These infants are at risk for poor postnatal growth and developmental handicaps. As glucose stores are inadequate, they require feeding as soon as possible after birth and frequent estimates of blood glucose levels using reagent strips.[6]

POST-ASPHYXIA

Asphyxia that has not been corrected can result in damage to the major organs of the body. The complications are often life-threatening and include cerebral palsy. The fetus and newborn respond to asphyxia and poor tissue perfusion by switching to anaerobic glycolysis.[15] Metabolic acidosis develops from the accumulation of acids after glucose stores are exhausted. The situation is exacerbated by respiratory acidosis which follows retention of carbon dioxide during asphyxia.

The effect of asphyxia on the infant is varied and can include respiratory failure, persistent pulmonary hypertension, meconium aspiration syndrome, renal failure, bleeding disorders such as disseminated intravascular coagulation (DIC), necrotising enterocolitis and congestive cardiac failure from damage to the myocardium.

Most infants who experience severe asphyxia for 10 minutes or longer are at risk of cerebral damage with long-term consequences. Amiel-Tison and Ellison[35] have categorised neurological damage in the neonatal period into 3 stages, which are identified by the infant's behaviour. In Stage 1 the infant is irritable with abnormal tone, poor head control and exaggerated stretch reflexes. Infants who suffer no further neurological damage usually develop normally. In Stage 2 there is depression of the central nervous system and lethargy. The infant is hypotonic, has a poor suck and difficulty in swallowing. There may be seizures and the prognosis is fair. In Stage 3 the infant is deeply comatose, hypotonic with weak or absent stretch reflexes, a poor respiratory effort, seizures and the prognosis is poor.

The Newborn Infant with a Congenital Abnormality

Conditions presenting in the neonatal period can be grouped according to the need for immediate intervention. Group 1 are those infants with a life-threatening condition for whom a surgical operation is necessary within the 1st day of life. Group 2 are those infants with an obvious abnormality but for whom a surgical operation may be deferred for days or months. Group 3 are infants who have an obvious abnormality but management may consist of interventions after due consideration. In most cases, the infant needs to be transferred to a regional surgical unit for assessment and intervention.

CONGENITAL DIAPHRAGMATIC HERNIA

This abnormality occurs when the pleural and abdominal cavities fail to separate; the abdominal contents herniate into the thoracic cavity. This causes compression of the lungs. Congenital diaphragmatic hernia occurs in approximately 1 in 2000 to 3000 live births with a sex ratio at 1:1. Left-sided defects are 5 times more common than right.[36]

Most infants with congenital diaphragmatic hernia present with respiratory distress within the first 24 hours of birth. The abdomen may appear scaphoid and a chest x-ray confirms the diagnosis. A wide-bore (8 fg) gastric tube needs to be passed orally to decompress the stomach. These infants present as a neonatal emergency and require rapid transfer to a surgical unit for stabilisation before surgery.

The mortality rate following operative repair remains high (20% to 40%) and is influenced by the degree of lung hypoplasia.[37] Infants who present with symptoms of respiratory failure within the first 4 hours of birth generally have a poor prognosis.[38,39]

These infants should be intubated for resuscitation. Resuscitation by face mask is avoided because of the risk of inflating the stomach. If the stomach is overinflated and is positioned in the thoracic cavity, further respiratory distress can result. Care centres on the provision of warmth and oxygenation.

Survival depends on the degree of lung hypoplasia present. Infants with small lungs mostly develop pulmonary hypertension that is often fatal.

TRACHEO-OESOPHAGEAL FISTULA AND OESOPHAGEAL ATRESIA

There are many types of malformation which have their origin in the first 6 weeks of embryological development. Tracheo-oesophageal abnormalities occur in approximately 1 in 3000 live births and tend to present in clusters associated with other defects. The Vater syndrome of associated defects includes vertebral, anal, cardiac, renal and limb abnormalities.[40]

The infant presents with respiratory distress and increased saliva. Abdominal distension and cyanosis during feeding may also be present. Oesophageal atresia is suspected when a 8 fg gastric tube cannot be passed more than 10 cm. The diagnosis is confirmed on x-ray when air outlines the oesophageal pouch.

Surgery can be undertaken in several stages, depending on the type of defect and the extent of the atresia. Survival with operation is 96%. The goal of care is to avoid the potential complications of infection and aspiration. Immediate management consists of using frequent suction to keep the pouch clear of secretions. The infant is pacified to prevent crying, which can aggravate reflux of stomach secretions via the distal fistula. The administration of intravenous fluids is necessary to ensure the infant remains adequately hydrated.[36,41] The infant is nursed with his head elevated to 45° and positioned either prone or supported on the right side.

ANTERIOR ABDOMINAL WALL DEFECTS

These defects form in the first 10 weeks of gestation when the yolk sac fails to return to the abdominal cavity or when there is a defect in the abdominal wall. The 2 defects are often confused with each other and need to be differentiated at birth.

Exomphalos

This is a congenital herniation of the structures surrounding the attachment of the umbilical cord. The defect may vary in size from 2 cm to around 20 cm when the defect is comprised of most of the abdominal wall and most of the abdominal contents. The defect is covered with a membranous sac which hardens and becomes necrosed within a day, at which time there is danger of rupture and evisceration. Nearly 40% of infants have associated malformations, the majority of which are congenital cardiac disease or malrotation of the midgut.[42] Exomphalos is also associated with Beckwith-Wiedemann syndrome, where hypoglycaemia can be a problem.

Initial management consists of wrapping the defect in plastic kitchen wrap to avoid evaporative heat loss and fluid loss. Insulation can be provided by placing dry wool over the plastic wrap. The infant should be positioned on his side with the left side uppermost, to avoid hypotension secondary to inferior vena caval compression and reduced venous return and cardiac output. This is more likely to occur when the defect is large. The stomach should be vented with a wide-bore (8 fg) gastric tube.

Gastroschisis

Gastroschisis is a protrusion of the abdominal viscera, usually the entire midgut loop, through a defect in the anterior abdominal wall at the level of the umbilicus. The defect is small, 1 to 2 cm in diameter and located to the right of the umbilicus. It is often separated by a thin bridge of skin. The protruding loops of intestine become thickened, oedematous and shortened because of the effects of venous congestion and contact with the amniotic fluid. The chronic oedema of the bowel interferes with gut function. Most infants with gastroschisis do not present with other abnormalities.[42]

Initial management is to gently untwist (wearing sterile gloves) any loops of bowel causing ischaemia and to cover the defect with plastic kitchen wrap. This ensures that the defect is supported and protected and at the same time fluid loss and evaporative heat loss are reduced. The stomach should be vented using a wide-bore gastric tube and an intravenous infusion commenced. Immediate transfer for corrective surgery is necessary.

Outcome for these infants is influenced by the condition of the bowel, complications such as atresia, and malabsorption due to the shortened thickened bowel.

EXTROPHY OF THE URINARY BLADDER

This is a rare abnormality caused by the failure of fusion of the lateral mesodermal elements of the lower anterior abdominal wall. There is a midline gap between the rectus and pubic bone. The dorsal urethral wall, the anterior aspect of the bladder and the bladder neck fail to develop and produce an epispadias in the male and extroversion of the exposed vesical mucosa.

Initial management consists of protecting the defect, keeping the infant dry and reducing heat loss. Surgery is indicated early in the neonatal period to reduce the risk of infection from the exposed viscera.

INTESTINAL OBSTRUCTION

Intestinal obstruction and associated alterations in the gastrointestinal system occur for a number of reasons. Most are due to embryological factors and result in some form of obstruction due to stenosis, atresia, plugs or reduced function. Detection of early signs and symptoms, diagnosis and early intervention are essential for a favourable long term outcome.

Signs and symptoms are as follows:

- Polyhydramnios may be present in upper bowel obstructions, such as duodenal or oesophageal atresia.
- Vomiting is suggestive of obstruction, but is not diagnostic. Bile-stained vomitus is suggestive of obstruction below the Ampulla of Vater. A high obstruction would be indicated by clear or milky vomitus.
- Abdominal distension is prominent in obstructions of the large bowel or the distal sections of the small bowel.
- The gas pattern in the intestine on an abdominal x-ray may also suggest the level of the obstruction.
- Delayed passage or failure to pass meconium.

Initial management consists of the passage of a wide-bore gastric tube to deflate the stomach and proximal bowel. An intravenous line should be inserted and any fluid and electrolyte deficiencies corrected. Restoration of an adequate circulating blood volume is achieved by colloid infusion. In some types of obstruction (e.g., volvulus) the infant may be in pain and shock. Supportive analgesia and ventilation may be necessary.

MYELOMENINGOCELE

This cystic swelling filled with cerebrospinal fluid overlying a spinal defect contains neural elements. The defect is commonly lumbosacral, sometimes cervical and rarely thoracic in position and may be open or closed. Initial management involves protection of the defect from infection. It is covered with sterile non-adherent gauze and care is taken to avoid any direct injury. The infant is positioned prone or supported on his side. Surgery may be required for some lesions to provide comfort for the infant. Hydrocephalus and paraplegia are complications of the condition and supportive counselling needs to be offered early after the diagnosis has been confirmed.

CONGENITAL HEART DISEASE

The incidence of congenital heart disease is approximately 1 in 100, with transposition of the great arteries and hypoplastic left heart syndrome being the most common abnormalities to present in the first week of life. As congenital heart disease often presents initially with respiratory signs, any infant presenting with respiratory distress should be assessed in order to exclude heart disease. Cyanosis, respiratory distress, congestive cardiac failure, abnormal cardiac rhythm and cardiac murmurs are the common signs and symptoms of severe congenital heart disease in the newborn. Optimal management of infants with congenital heart disease requires expertise. The infant needs to be closely monitored and observed for hypoxia, hypoglycaemia, acidosis and cardiac failure.[22,43] (See Chapter 6 for more detailed information on cardiac defects).

UPPER AIRWAY OBSTRUCTIONS

Choanal atresia

This is a membranous or bony atresia of the openings of the posterior nasal cavity into the pharynx. Unilateral atresia is more common than bilateral, which causes extreme respiratory obstruction with stridor and periods of cyanosis. The defect should be suspected when the symptoms are relieved by the insertion of an oral airway. The diagnosis is confirmed by failure to pass a nasal catheter. A unilateral defect may have no symptoms. Initial management aims at creating an oral airway and keeping it well secured.

Robin sequence

Robin sequence is the combination of cleft palate with micrognathia (small jaw) and glossoptosis. The micrognathia causes the tongue to be displaced backwards so there is a high risk of obstruction. This risk is present for several months until growth of the mandible and other structures ensure a clear airway. The essence of management is to ensure a clear airway, which can be achieved by nursing the infant prone. More often the infant requires an artificial airway. This may be a pharyngeal tube, an endotracheal tube or a tracheotomy.

The Newborn Infant Requiring Transport

ORGANISATION

Regionalisation has been implemented in Australia so that the available resources for neonatal intensive care services can be provided. In Australia, intensive care nurseries are located in supraregional obstetric hospitals (Level 6)[44] and at children's hospitals where infants may undergo surgery. Therefore, infants born in other hospitals and who require intensive or special care will require transfer to a hospital with a nursery with the appropriate level of care.

To facilitate the organisation of the service and to enable resources to be allocated appropriately, all nurseries providing care for the newborn have been graded into levels of care.[45]

Level 1 provides for the healthy newborn with rooming-in facilities with the emphasis on parenting skills and education.

Level 2 provides staff and services to look after an infant of 32 weeks' gestation or more who requires oxygen and cardiorespiratory monitoring, parenteral fluid therapy, tube feeds, phototherapy and long-term convalescence in an incubator.

In several states, the Level 2 nurseries have been divided into low and high dependency units.[46] The high-dependency (2a) units provide staff and facilities for short-term (<6 hours) ventilator care before transfer to a Level 3 unit. Some country centres have also been given this grading because of their geographic isolation.

Level 3 provides for all aspects of neonatal care including intensive care for the critically ill baby and medium/long-term ventilation and total parenteral nutrition.

Level 4 is as Level 3 but also provides neonatal surgery and related care.

The successful organisation of nurseries at these levels relies on the hospital having appropriately trained nursing and medical staff and ancillary support services such as radiology and pathology, providing care over 24 hours. Facilities and equipment must be sufficient for the nursery to function at the determined level.

PRINCIPLES OF STABILISATION

The basic principles of transport aim to provide an environment which is close to optimal, meeting the basic needs of an infant for warmth, oxygenation and hydration. Sick infants may be transferred safely provided the following 5 basic rules are met:[5]

- Perinatal transport advice is available on a 24-hour basis, and requires direct access to a transport consultant.
- Response to requests for transport are expeditious.
- Resuscitation and stabilisation are effective.
- Full intensive care support and monitoring equipment are available in a mobile form.
- An appropriate and skilled team manages the infant during transfer from the referring hospital to the referral hospital.

The stabilisation process is initiated with the referral call to the Newborn Emergency Transport Service (NETS).

HOW TO CALL NETS

In some states of Australia, a Newborn Emergency Transport Service is available. Telephone hotline services allow the staff in referring centres to seek assistance and guidance for the initial management of a sick or small newborn infant while awaiting the transport team. The delay between the time of the call and the arrival of the team is kept to a minimum. This time will vary according to the geographic location of the referring hospital. Staff can utilise this time to prepare the infant and family for the team's arrival.

WAITING FOR THE TRANSPORT TEAM TO ARRIVE

Space

Most transport trolleys are the size of an adult stretcher, therefore adequate room around the infant's incubator will be required. The system will require electrical, oxygen, air and suction outlets for the stabilisation process. It will also be helpful to have an empty procedure trolley with a supply of syringes, needles and swabs available for the team's use. X-ray technician and laboratory staff should be alerted in case it becomes necessary for them to operate equipment or perform tests when the team arrives.

Environment

In most cases it is more convenient to have the infant nursed on an open-care system which allows easy access for stabilisation. When nursing the infant under the heater, care must be taken to avoid overheating the infant. A skin probe placed securely on the infant's abdomen to monitor his temperature is essential. If a servo control facility is available, the probe should be set to 36.5°C. Care must be taken to avoid evaporative heat loss in small infants. For infants less than 2000 g, a convective crib set to the infant's neutral thermal environment may be more suitable. When the team arrives, the infant can be transferred to an open-care system. It is desirable to have a nurse allocated to care for the infant on a one-to-one basis so that subtle changes in the infant's condition can be detected and appropriate interventions implemented. A policy of minimal handling needs to be instituted to ensure that the sick infant does not become exhausted.

The infant

The basic principles of care as discussed earlier (**Chapter 1**) need to be met and maintained. Sick infants can have unpredictable oxygen requirements and present with respiratory distress for a variety of causes. The infant's oxygenation is monitored with a transcutaneous oxygen monitor placed on the upper right quadrant of the thorax. The ambient oxygen needs to be adjusted to maintain the $tcPO_2$ between 60 and 90 mmHg. The readings may be affected by decreased perfusion, an improperly adhered probe or a clinical condition such as cyanotic heart disease. An arterial blood sample should be taken to determine the infant's acid-base status.

The nurse needs to make frequent assessment of the infant's respiratory status and look for signs of deterioration that may indicate the necessity for intubation and ventilation. These signs include a respiratory rate of 60 per minute or greater, chest recession, grunting, nasal flaring and decreased peripheral perfusion as indicated by a sluggish capillary refill time (>3 seconds). The infant's colour is observed in response to handling, as changes may be an early indicator of increasing respiratory distress.

Fluids

The infant needs to be kept nil-by-mouth and the stomach vented with a size 8 fg gastric tube passed orally, with the correct position determined. An intravenous infusion of a dextrose/saline solution is administered through the umbilical or a peripheral vein. The catheter needs to be secured firmly. The site and the infusion rate are monitored. Blood glucose levels are measured regularly as a sick infant may become hypoglycaemic very quickly. Enteral feeds should be avoided as they can be poorly tolerated in a sick infant and the risk of pulmonary aspiration is a concern.

Abnormalities

Any obvious abnormalities need to be dealt with to avoid complications. A thorough physical assessment should enable the nurse to determine which abnormalities need immediate intervention. The position in which the infant is nursed will be determined by the abnormality. As a general guide, infants with abdominal distension and/or masses are at risk of respiratory embarrassment and should be nursed with their body and head elevated to 30° and in the right lateral position.

Documentation

All charts, x-rays, investigation results and a consent form should be available for the transport team. It is important that information such as the obstetric, labour and infant histories be included, together with any other details that may aid the diagnosis and/or management.

Parents

The parents will be anxious about the necessity for their infant to be transferred. Arrange for them to be available when the team arrives so that they can meet the staff and ask any further questions. An instant photograph of the infant gives the parents something tangible of their infant despite the separation.

Practical information such as the location of the referral hospital, transport routes and parking, accommodation details and visiting policies can help allay some concerns for the parents and their families. The mother should be advised about lactation and the routine if expressing. This is a shared responsibility with the referral centre.

WHEN THE TRANSPORT TEAM ARRIVES

Staff should be available to assist the transport team with the stabilisation process. The team will not be familiar with the nursery/ward and the available facilities. Staff in the referring hospitals have a valuable learning opportunity. Questions can be answered by the specialists in the transport team.

AFTER THE TRANSPORT TEAM DEPARTS

Staff should take the opportunity to evaluate the management of the infant in order to determine if some aspect of care should be revised. Maintain contact with the referral hospital for progress of the infant. Often problems develop that may have been overlooked initially and feedback to the staff can alert them to similar problems that may occur in the future. Reassure the family if they are unable to travel with the infant.

The optimal time for referral is before birth, so that the mother can be transferred to a perinatal centre, the baby delivered and both cared for in the same hospital.

The Newborn Infant Requiring Intensive Care

VENTILATION

Over the past 20 years or so, innovations and advances in neonatal assisted ventilation have been aimed at improving survival and preventing short-term complications, such as pulmonary interstitial emphysema and pneumothorax, and the long-term problem of bronchopulmonary dysplasia. These advances include a better understanding of conventional mechanical ventilation and the development of newer modes, such as high-frequency jet ventilation, high-frequency oscillation, extracorporeal membrane oxygenation,[47,48] and nitric oxide.[49,50]

Whichever mode of ventilation is chosen, the infant requires meticulous care and support. The objectives of ventilation are to:

* Maintain adequate gas exchange and normal arterial acid-base values.
* Reduce oxygen consumption by keeping energy use to a minimum.
* Permit recovery from a treatable condition without causing damage to the lungs.
* Keep the risk of pulmonary barotrauma to a minimum.

In general, during ventilation of infants with severe hyaline membrane disease, the PaO_2 is maintained at 60 to 80 mmHg by alterations to the inspired oxygen concentration and peak inspiratory pressure. The positive end expired pressure (PEEP) is usually maintained at 4 to 5 cmH_2O with the inspiratory time (IT) at less than 1.0 second and the inspiratory:expiratory ratio at 1:1 or 1:2. The $PaCO_2$ is maintained at 35 to 45 mmHg.[40]

Hyperventilation, that is, induced hypocapnoea ($PaCO_2$ 20 to 30 mmHg), is used in the treatment of persistent pulmonary hypertension. It is achieved by increasing the peak inspiratory pressure and/or the rate, with concomitant reductions in the PEEP and inspiratory time, in order to avoid pulmonary overdistension and a reduction in systemic venous return, pulmonary blood flow and cardiac output.[13]

Most infants requiring ventilation have a peripheral artery cannula inserted and attached to a pressure transducer for measurement of arterial blood pressure and blood sampling. The attending nurse measures the arterial blood gases every 2 to 4 hours, more frequently in a labile infant, and within 15 minutes of alterations in ventilation. To help with the monitoring of blood gases, transcutaneous oxygen and carbon dioxide monitoring are used. Because frequent blood sampling can result in anaemia, a check needs to be kept on the volume removed and the infant's haemoglobin level.

A persistent ductus arteriosus (PDA) is often present in infants weighing less than 1200 g. Together with an increasing left-to-right shunt, this may produce a need for ventilation beyond 24 hours. A widening arterial pulse pressure and bounding peripheral pulses are signs of a significant persistent ductus arteriosis.

Infants who require assisted ventilation may receive a morphine sulphate infusion of 10 to 20 mg/kg/hour. This is often increased in infants with labile pulmonary hypertension. The morphine sedates the infant and reduces asynchronous breathing. Muscle relaxation can also be used to control ventilation and reduce ventilation/perfusion (V/Q) inequality by abolishing asynchronous breathing or increasing chest wall compliance. These effects are suspected when adequate gas exchange is not achieved despite an inspired oxygen of 100% and peak inspiratory pressure greater than 30 to 35 cmH$_2$O or if the infant seems to be at risk of developing a pneumothorax or there is persistent pulmonary hypertension.

Hypothermia is known to increase oxygen consumption and to increase pulmonary vascular resistance.[40] The infant's abdominal skin temperature is maintained within a range of 36.2 to 36.8°C. Infants weighing more than 2500 g are nursed under servo controlled radiant warmers while lighter weight infants are nursed in forced convection double-wall incubators.

One of the nurse's most important tasks in caring for the ventilated infant is to maintain patency of the endotracheal tube and to ensure the tape on the ETT is dry and secure. The nurse assesses the frequency of and need for ETT suction by chest auscultation and observation of the trends on the transcutaneous oxygen and carbon dioxide monitors. It may be necessary to increase the inspired oxygen before the procedure to avoid hypoxaemia. Suction adaptors that do not require disconnection from the ventilator can be used. It is recommended that 2 nurses perform the procedure. Each catheter passage is limited to 10 seconds.[12,14,51] Physiotherapy is not used routinely for the acutely ill infant, but is important for the recovering or chronically ventilated infant.

Water balance is important in the ventilated very low birthweight infant as overhydration may lead to complications such as bronchopulmonary dysplasia and symptomatic persistent ductus arteriosus.[20] An infant is considered to be normally hydrated if the serum sodium ranges from 130 to 150 mmol/L, the urine output is 2 to 4 mL/kg/hour, the urine specific gravity is 1005 to 1015 and the weight falls by 1.0% to 1.5% of the birthweight over the first 5 to 7 days. Urine output can be measured by nursing the infant on disposable pads and weighing the pads every 1 to 2 hours. The specific gravity is recorded every 4 hours. All intake, including drug infusions and arterial flushes, is measured. As volume of fluid for nutrition is often limited, the necessary calories are supplied by total parenteral nutrition (TPN), using central or peripheral catheters. Ventilated infants are usually weighed daily. This procedure requires 2 nurses, and the infant needs to be fully monitored throughout the procedure. In the chronically ventilated infant, nutrition can be provided by the enteral route with cautious introduction of feeds of expressed breast milk or a premature infant formula.

Vasoactive drugs are sometimes used as an adjunct to conventional ventilation in infants with pulmonary hypertension and low cardiac output. Indications include: hypoxaemia and the inability to achieve hypocapnoea with hyperventilation; hypoxaemia despite hypercapnoea and an adequate circulating blood volume with arterial hypotension and/or circulatory failure. Drugs used may include either one or a combination of dopamine, isoprenaline, tolazoline and dobatumine. The implications for the nursing care are related to the difficulty of maintaining vascular access when there is a need to avoid mixing drugs in a cannula because of known or suspected incompatibilities. Central venous multilumen catheters can help overcome this problem. These are mostly inserted into the umbilical vessels. Care needs to be taken in their management. They need to be securely taped and observed for leaking, catheter migration and infection. Infection is indicated by erythema at the insertion site or an unexplained instability in the infant's temperature. Nurses need to be aware of the numerous side effects associated with this form of treatment. It is particularly important to be aware of peripheral ischaemia.

Bronchopulmonary dysplasia is a concern with ventilation. However, through close monitoring of water balance, closure of the ductus arteriosis with indomethacin, monitoring blood gases and reducing ventilator pressures the severity of the problem may be reduced. Diuretics and the glucocorticoid steroid, dexamethasone, are used in the management of bronchopulmonary dysplasia.[40]

Very low birthweight infants have a high incidence of symptomatic persistent ductus arteriosus, which may prevent them from being weaned from the ventilator. The magnitude of the left-to-right shunt can vary with hypoxia from suctioning or fluid overload. Management may consist of closure with indomethacin or surgical ligation if the former is unsuccessful.

Pneumothoraces, with an incidence of 20%, are a concern and a serious complication of conventional ventilation. They increase the incidence of bronchopulmonary dysplasia and are associated with subependymal and intraventricular haemorrhages.[52] Skilled observation of the infant who is considered at risk of air leak, and the use of sedation and muscle relaxation, may help prevent the infant resisting ventilation by breathing against the ventilator cycles. Careful selection of ventilator parameters, particularly pressure and inspiratory time, may help prevent this serious complication.

An important aspect in the care of the ventilated infant is the involvement of parents. An open visiting policy for all members of the family and extended family can facilitate visits. Parents need to be encouraged to help in the basic care of their baby and an open information policy is recommended.

NEONATAL SURGERY

The newborn infant who requires surgery needs meticulous preoperative and postoperative management. The aim of care is to minimise the effects of transfer, anaesthesia and the operative procedure itself. Neonatal surgery is performed in hospitals with specialist paediatric services and a sufficient turnover of surgical patients is necessary to maintain skills. Because these infants may show subtle signs of organ dysfunction, it is essential that nurses with specialised assessment skills continuously monitor the physiological data and intervene when appropriate.

Infants are prepared for surgery within the environment of the neonatal unit. This enables them to be adequately prepared while their vital signs and fluid management continue to be monitored. Preparation includes washing the skin with a mild antiseptic preparation and ensuring that the infant remains normothermic. All newborns undergoing an operation or a general anaesthetic need to have an intravenous cannula *in situ* with a maintenance infusion of fluids attached to an infusion pump. Infants who are less than 34 weeks' gestation who require oxygen therapy and/or ventilation will require transcutaneous oxygen monitoring. A pulse oximeter is used for infants whose gestation is greater than 34 weeks or the infant who has a cardiac defect that needs monitoring of the oxygen saturation levels. This equipment ensures that the infant's oxygenation remains satisfactory throughout the surgery. Transferring the infant to the operating theatre in a closed incubator with an internal battery allows full monitoring en route. The aim is to avoid compromising the infant through hypothermia or hypoxia from an unstable transfer.

Postoperative management aims at maintaining thermoneutrality, monitoring respiratory effort and ensuring that the infant remains pain free. The newborn infant at risk of postoperative apnoea is often left intubated and ventilated for 24 to 48 hours. This practice avoids an unscheduled intubation and allows adequate analgesia, such as a morphine infusion, to be administered.

NEONATAL PAIN

Over the past few years, clinicians have become increasingly aware of the neonate in pain. Several factors have contributed to this change, namely an increase in the knowledge of the capabilities of the newborn brain, the advent of neonatal intensive care nurseries where many invasive procedures are carried out, and a growing concern regarding the effects of inappropriate environmental stimuli on the developing central nervous system.

Several myths about newborn pain remain. These include the beliefs that there is no direct correlation between tissue damage and pain, that the infants do not feel pain as adults do and thus do not need pain relief, and that medication for pain relief will cause addiction.

Nurses caring for infants in the intensive care nursery must take responsibility for the assessment and management of pain. Assessment of neonatal pain should include both behavioural and physiological components.

Some authors describe crying as the most useful index for assessing pain. However, it needs to be understood that sick newborns may not always be able to show pain by crying.[26] It is therefore useful to recognise other behavioural expressions of pain, such as facial expression, posture, body movements and palmar sweating in the mature infant. In assessing the infant for pain, the nurse needs to take into consideration other factors which may influence the infant's behaviour, such as abnormal movements caused by seizures or hypoglycaemia.

Useful physiological measures of pain are heart rate, blood pressure and transcutaneous oxygen levels. It is important to have continuous measurements of these indices in order to relate them to the various procedures/interventions.

At present there is a heightened interest in developing more objective and reliable methods for assessing pain in the newborn.[53] This is because there is no method suitable for sick or premature infants.

Discomfort in infancy is not only caused by internal factors, but can also be influenced by external factors. In the intensive care environment, noise from incubators, phones and voices together with bright lights and frequent handling for many invasive procedures constitute some of these factors. In recent years, there has been an increase in the attention paid to the modification of the infant's environment. Some hospitals have started to modify noise and light levels by using shades in the incubator, dimming lights, introducing quiet periods for the whole unit and encouraging people to speak softly. It may also be useful to introduce earplugs for the baby.

Nurses in the intensive care unit often experience emotional distress at having to inflict pain on their patients. Traditionally, nurses have been carers. However, with the expansion of the nursing role, nurses are acquiring more advanced technical skills, such as intravenous cannulation, and they also find themselves in the position of inflicting pain. At the same time, they provide comfort and try to soothe the infant. These 2 activities may evoke conflict. There is a need for peer support to help nurses cope with this situation of conflict and confusion.

THE FAMILY

The holistic care of the sick infant requires that his psychosocial needs are met as well as his physical needs.

The parents of an infant requiring admission to the newborn nursery are anxious for their infant and require support from the nursing staff.[54] These parents are often in a crisis situation and many hours of patience and explanation from the staff will be required. Most neonatal nurseries have an open visiting policy that gives parents the freedom to visit at their convenience and to bring in members of the extended family. Information on their infant is freely given with explanations of the disease process and encouragement in ways that the parents can contribute to the infant's care.

The importance of establishing and maintaining the initial bond between the parents and infant remains a priority for the nurse in the neonatal nursery. This may be fostered by encouraging the parents to touch their baby and to have regular cuddles. Even infants requiring ventilation may be taken out of the incubator for a cuddle once their condition is stable. The expression of milk by the mother is encouraged from the initial visit. Often these mothers require support and a gentle, caring attitude as they try to establish lactation and the infant cannot initially be put to the breast. Helpful hints on expressing can be given. The availability of a breast pump in the unit with information and direction about the correct method of use may help alleviate difficulties.

Many articles have been written on the need for siblings to visit in the neonatal nursery.[55,56] It is held that if the sibling sees and touches their new brother or sister they are helped in adjusting to his or her arrival. This is particularly important if the baby has been born prematurely and the 'promise' of a 9-month wait has been broken. Children are often more curious than frightened by intensive care and they can easily adapt to the routines of handwashing and gently stroking their new sibling through the incubator doors.

The provision of precious items such as small toys and family photographs is encouraged. The parents often place a lot of emphasis on providing a 'homely' environment for their baby. All such items can help in the establishment of family ties and need to be encouraged by the staff.

Many nurseries now have an early discharge program which aims at supporting the parents through instruction and guidance when taking their baby home when the weight may still be below 2 kg. These programs rely on a nurse or team of nurses to establish contact in the hospital and follow-up through home visits for the first few weeks after discharge. Infants requiring long-term oxygen therapy, stoma care, gastrostomy feeds, central catheters and complex dressings can be managed by these support nurses.

REFERENCES

1. Karotkin EH, Goldsmith JP. Resuscitation. *In:* Goldsmith JP and Karotkin EH, eds. *Assisted ventilation of the neonate.* 2nd ed. Philadelphia: Saunders, 1988: 70–85.
2. Phibbs RH. Delivery room management. *In:* Avery GB, Fletcher MA, Macdonald MG, ed. *Neonatology: pathophysiology and management of the newborn.* 4th ed. Philadelphia: Lippincott, 1994: 182–200.
3. Hagedorn M, Gardner S, Abman S. Respiratory diseases. *In:* Merestein GB, Gardner SL, eds. *Handbook of neonatal intensive care.* 3rd ed. St Louis: Mosby, 1993: 311–364.
4. Goldsmith JP. Advances in neonatal resuscitation and stabilisation. Paper presented at 5th Annual National Meeting, NANN, Atlanta, Georgia, 1989.
5. Department of Health, NSW. *Maternal and perinatal care in New South Wales.* 3rd ed. State Health Publication No. (HP) 88–013. Sydney: The Department, 1989: 64–78.
6. Digiacomo JE, Hagedorn MI, Hay WW. Glucose homeostasis. *In:* Merestein GB, Gardner SL, eds. *Handbook of neonatal intensive care.* 3rd ed. St Louis: Mosby, 1993: 169–183.

7. Sterk MB. Understanding parental nutrition: a basis for neonatal nursing care. *J Obstet Gynecal Neonatal Nurs* 1983; May/June (Suppl): 45s–50s.

8. Merestein GB, Gardner SL, Woods Blake W. Heat balance. *In:* Merestein GB, Gardner SL, eds. *Handbook of neonatal intensive care.* 3rd ed. St Louis: Mosby, 1993: 100–114.

9. Brueggemeyer A. Neonatal thermoregulation. *In:* Kenner C, Brueggemeyer A, Gunderson LP, eds. *Comprehensive neonatal nursing: a physiologic perspective.* Philadelphia: Lippincott, 1993: 247–262.

10. Peabody JL, Lewis K. Consequences of newborn intensive care. *In:* Gottfried AW, Gaiter JL, eds. *Infant stress under intensive care.* Baltimore: University Park Press, 1985: 204.

11. Goldsmith JP, Karotkin EH. *Assisted ventilation of the neonate.* Philadelphia: Saunders, 1988.

12. Turner BS. Maintaining the artifical airway: current concepts. *Pediatric Nursing* 1990; 16: 487–493.

13. Fox W, Spitzler AR, Shutack J. Positive pressure ventilation: pressure and time cycled ventilators. *In:* Goldsmith JP, Karotkin EH. *Assisted ventilation of the neonate.* Philadelphia: Saunders, 1988: 146–170.

14. Cassani VL. Hypoxaemia secondary to suctioning in the neonate. *Neonatal Network* 1984; June: 8–16.

15. Hodson WA, Troug WE. Principles of management of respiratory problems. *In:* Avery GB, Fletcher MA, Macdonald MG, eds. *Neonatology: pathophysiology and management of the newborn.* 4th ed. Philadelphia: Lippincott, 1994: 496–498.

16. Bruhn FW, Jones B, O'Donnell JP. Infection in the neonate. *In:* Merestein GB, Gardner SL, eds. *Handbook of neonatal intensive care* 3rd ed. St Louis: Mosby, 1993: 287–310.

17. Merenstein GB, Gardner SL. *Handbook of neonatal intensive care.* 3rd ed. St Louis: Mosby, 1993.

18. Department of Health, NSW. *Report of the NSW NICUS 1986–1987 infants.* State Health Publication No (EHSEB) 91–61. Sydney: The Department, 1991: 11.

19. Platzker AC. Chronic lung disease in infancy. *In:* Ballard RA, *Pediatric care of the ICN graduate.* Philadelphia: Saunders, 1988: 129–156.

20. Ails H, Lawhon G, Duffy F, McAnulty GB, Grossman RG, Blickman JG. Individualised developmental care for the very low birthweight preterm infant: Medical and neurofunctional effects. *JAMA* 1994; 272: 853–858.

21. Bell EF. Effect of fluid administration on the development of symptomatic patent ductus arteriosis and congestive cardiac failure in premature infants. *N Engl J Med* 1980; 302: 598.

22. Hazinski MF. Congenital heart disease in the neonate. Part I — VIII. *Neonatal Network* Feb 83–Oct 84.

23. Gil-Gibernau JJ. Ophthalmological problems in newborn infants. *Annales Nestle* 1988; 46 (1): 1–13.

24. Vanderhoof J, Zach T, Adrian T. Gastrointestinal disease. *In:* Avery GB, Fletcher MA, Macdonald MG, eds. *Neonatology: pathophysiology and management of the newborn.* 4th ed. Philadelphia: Lippincott, 1994: 614–616.

25. Henderson-Smart D. Respiratory problems of the newborn. (Unpublished notes) 1989.

26. Annand K, Hickey P. Pain and its effects in the human neonate and fetus. *N Engl J Med* 1987; 317: 1321–1329.

27. Shapiro C. Pain in the neonate: assessment and intervention. *Neonatal Network* 1989; 8: 7–21.

28. Fay MJ. The positive effects of positioning. *Neonatal Network* 1988; April: 23–28.

29. Lund C. Proceedings from National Association of Neonatal Nurses Clinical Update — Care of the extremely low birth weight infant. Hawaii: National Association of Neonatal Nurses, 1990.

30. Lund C, Kuller J, Tobin C, Lefrak L, Franck L. Evaluation of a pectin-based barrier under tape to protect neonatal skin. *J Obstet Gynaecol Neonatal Nurs* 1986; 15: 39–44.

31. Ballard RA. *Pediatric care of the ICN graduate.* Philadelphia: Saunders, 1988.

32. Bauchner H, Brown E, Peskin J. Premature graduates of the newborn intensive care unit: a guide to followup. *Pediatr Clin North Am* 1988; 35: 1207–1226.

33. Thomas D, Lindsay S. Perinatal consequences of maternal drug abuse. Sydney: Westmead Hospital, 1988.

34. Gamblian V, et al. Assessment and management of endocrine dysfunction. *In:* Kenner C, Brueggemeyer A, Gunderson LP, eds. *Comprehensive neonatal nursing: a physiologic perspective.* Philadelphia: WB Saunders, 1993: 538–540.

35. Amiel-Tison C, Ellison P. Birth asphyxia in the full term newborn: early assessment and outcome. *Dev Med Child Neurol* 1986; 28: 671–682.

36. Moore K. *The developing human.* 3rd ed. Philadelphia: Saunders, 1982.

37. Powers L, Borrington J, Gardner S, Merestein G. Pediatric surgery. *In:* Merestein GB, Gardner SL, eds. *Handbook of neonatal intensive care.* 3rd ed. St Louis: Mosby, 1993: 539.

38. Carter K, Spence K. Nursing of infants with pulmonary hypertension following repair of a diaphragmatic hernia. *The Lamp* 1984; January: 18–22.

39. Chang JHT. Neonatal surgical emergencies. Part III — congenital diaphragmatic hernia. *Perinatol-neonatol* 1979; Nov–Dec: 22–24.

40. Barr P. Newborn intensive care: a handbook for staff. Sydney: Royal Alexandra Hospital for Children, 1992: 72–82.

41. Cassani VL. Tracheal abnormalities. *Neonatal Network* 1984; Oct: 20–27.

42. Upadhyaya P. Major body wall defects. *In:* MacMahon RA, ed. *An aid to paediatric surgery.* Edinburgh: Churchill Livingstone, 1984.

43. Daberkow E, Washington R. Cardiovascular diseases and surgical interventions. *In:* Merestein GB, Gardner SL, eds. *Handbook of neonatal intensive care.* 3rd ed. St Louis: Mosby, 1993: 366–398.

44. NSW Department of Health. *Maternal and perinatal care in New South Wales.* 3rd ed. Sydney: NSW Department of Health, 1989.

45. Australian Health Ministers' Advisory Council. Superspeciality Services Subcommittee. *Guidelines for level three neonatal intensive care.* Canberra: Australian Institute of Health, 1991.

46. Ministerial Neonatal Working Party. *Neonatal services in New South Wales.* Sydney: Service Development Branch, NSW Health Department, 1990.

47. Gruden M. High frequency ventilation: an overview. *Critical Care Nurse* 1985; 5 (1): 36–40.

48. Inwood S, Finley G, Fitzhardinge P. High frequency oscillation: a new mode of ventilation for the neonate. *Neonatal Network* 1986; April: 53–58.

49. Culotta E, Koshland DE. No news is good. *New Science* 1992; 258: 1862–1865.

50. Kinsella JP, Abman SH. Inhalation nitric oxide therapy for persistent pulmonary hypertension of the newborn. *Pediatrics* 1993; 91: 997–998.

51. Spence K. Evaluation of endotracheal suction in mechanically ventilated low birth weight infants. Paper presented at 4th Annual Conference of Association of Neonatal Nurses of NSW, Kirkton Park, 1991.

52. Blackburn ST. Assessment and management of neurologic dysfunction. *In:* Kenner C, Brueggemeyer A, Gunderson LP, eds. *Comprehensive neonatal nursing: a physiologic perspective.* Philadelphia: WB Saunders, 1993: 664–665.

53. Franck L. A new method to quantitatively describe pain behaviour in infants. *Nursing Res* 1986; 35: 28–31.

54. Seigel R, Gardner S, Merestein G. Families in crisis: theoretical and practical considerations. *In:* Merestein GB, Gardner SL, eds. *Handbook of neonatal intensive care.* 3rd ed. St Louis: Mosby, 1993: 505–529.

55. Consolvo C. Siblings in the NICU. *Neonatal Network* 1987; 5 (5): 7–11.

56. Troy P, Wilkinson-Faulk D, Smith AB, Alexander D. Sibling visiting in the NICU. *Am J Nursing* 1988; Jan: 68–70.

BIBLIOGRAPHY

Beachy P, Deacon J, eds. *Core curriculum for neonatal intensive care nursing.* Philadelphia: WB Saunders, 1993.

Bellig LL. A window on the neonate's brain. *Neonatal Network* 1989; 7 (4): 13–20.

Henderson C. Overwhelmed by infant resuscitation? Remember your 'ABCDs'. *Neonatal Network* 1988; 7 (3): 35–39.

Nugent J, ed. *Acute respiratory care of the neonate: a self study course.* Petaluma, CA: Neonatal Network, 1991.

Rushton CH. The surgical neonate: principles of nursing management. *Pediatr Nursing* 1988; 14: 141–151.

Tappero EP, Honeyfield ME. *Physical assessment of the newborn: a comprehensive approach to the art of physical examination.* Petaluma, CA: NICU-INK, 1993.

Chapter 11

Care of the Infant, Child and Adolescent with Alteration to Cardiovascular Function

Carmel McQuellin

Over the past decade, considerable changes have occurred to advance cardiovascular nursing of infants, children and adolescents. Interventional cardiac procedures and advances in surgical techniques have revolutionised the care of younger infants and newborn babies with cardiac problems. These changes have imposed significant challenge for clinical nursing practice. Professional expectations encompass an ever-increasing responsibility and accountability for practice and hence specialist nursing education is mandatory.

These advances purport the need for change in the perioperative stabilisation and management of the infants. The rapid progression of the profession encompasses an ever-extending role of the nurse, due in part to the seemingly boundless achievement of biotechnology, exemplified by the highly sophisticated patient monitoring devices and the advanced life support delivery systems.

In future, even smaller, younger infants with increasingly complex lesions, once considered inoperable, will become amenable to sophisticated primary surgical corrections and palliative procedures. Though currently highly speculative, interventional cardiac procedures undertaken *in utero* may become viable treatment options for infants who may benefit from early intervention. Further, there will be increasing development of palliative procedures and heart and heart-lung transplantation, requiring more frequent support of the mechanical devices used to augment cardiac output. Currently there is a well established trend in progressive units towards technological augmentation of the child's cardiac output through the use of various myocardial support devices in the form of left and/or right ventricular assistance and to a lesser extent extracorporeal membrane oxygenation (ECMO). Heightened awareness of the legal and ethical responsibilities of care imposed by this level of technology on all members of the health care team is paramount, although the full impact of these technologies on the nursing role remains to be fully established.

This chapter reviews a multiplicity of concepts relating to the nursing care of infants, children and adolescents with acute cardiovascular dysfunction. Brief discussion of the aetiological factors of congenital heart disease (CHD) and the physiological concepts pertaining to cardiac function is included. A detailed review of these aspects is beyond the scope of this chapter, and the reader is referred to a number of excellent publications.[1-4]

The areas pertaining to cardiovascular dysfunction within paediatrics and the critically important role assumed by nursing professionals in assessment, intervention and support of the children, will be reviewed.

Aetiology of Congenital Heart Disease

Congenital cardiac malformations, the most common congenital abnormality, are known to occur in 8 per 1000 live births.[5-7] However, the incidence of cardiac abnormalities in the foetus is 5% to 8% of all pregnancies, most of which spontaneously abort due to compromised cardiac performance.[5] The total incidence of congenital heart disease (CHD) is indicated to be 10 times higher in stillborn infants than in live births.[3] Current statistical evidence reveals that congenital abnormalities of the heart and cardiovascular system account for approximately 4% of perinatal deaths in Australia.[8] The overall incidence of congenital cardiovascular malformations is 38.9 per 10 000 births, with ventricular septal defects accounting for 14.8 and transposition of the great arteries accounting for 3.9 per 10 000 births.[9]

Recent research data indicates the period associated with the greatest mortality in CHD is the first postnatal week.[10] The mortality is mostly attributed to the following lesions, which account for approximately 10% of all CHD: hypoplastic left heart; double outlet right ventricle; truncus arteriosus; and pulmonary atresia. The research suggests 86% of the infants survive the first month of life, 71% survive to the first year, and 67% will live to mid adolescence.[10]

IMPLICATIONS FOR NURSING PRACTICE

The birth of an infant with a congenital abnormality represents a crisis for parents. They may have great difficulty accepting the infant, having anticipated the birth of a healthy baby. This is especially so in some infants with CHD where the abnormality may not be immediately apparent after birth. Parents respond by grieving for the loss of their perfect infant, experiencing emotional turmoil likened to the loss of an infant or child.[11] Helplessness, sadness, anger and guilt are components of the grieving process experienced before parents reach the stage of acceptance of the infant's abnormality, following which the normal attachment processes can occur.

The role of the nurse clinician in supporting the infant and the parents is clear. Many of these infants will require ongoing management and surgery, and therefore good communication ability is an essential component in supporting the family in crisis. An ability to identify dysfunctional states (physical, behavioural and social) is paramount in seeking early referral to the appropriate support service, such as genetic counselling, social work and the clergy.[11,12]

Table 11.1 Chromosomal aberrations associated with CHD: incidence and common lesions

Syndrome	Birth incidence	CHD incidence	Cardiac lesions associated
Turner (XO)	1:2500–8000	35%	CoAO
			AS, ASD
Down (Trisomy 21)	1:800	50%	A-VC, VSD
			ASD, TET, PDA
PATOU (Trisomy 13)	1:7000	90%	ASD, VSD
			PDA
			Dextrocardia
EDWARD (Trisomy 18)	1:8000	90–99%	VSD, PDA, PS

AS = aortic valve stenosis; ASD = atrial septal defect; A-VC = atrio ventricular canal; CoAO = coarctation of aorta; IHSS = idiopathic hypertrophic subaortic stenosis; PDA = patent ductus arteriosus; PS = pulmonary valve stenosis; TA = tricuspid atresia; TET = tetralogy of fallot; TGA = transposition of the great arteries; VSD = ventricular septal defect.) Adapted from:[3,16,17]

Nursing personnel fulfil a crucial role in information giving and the education of parents. Demystifying the complexities of a congenital cardiac abnormality is often required and best achieved through informal discussion with the nurse clinician. Providing parental reassurance and reinforcement of information given during genetic counselling sessions will enhance understanding of the congenital abnormality.

Scientific research into human genetics and genetic engineering is rapidly advancing. The parents' appreciation of the concepts involving congenital abnormalities is dependent on the education provided and the accessibility of health care personnel.[13] A working knowledge of the principles of genetics and the current concepts related to cardiac dysmorphism are necessary in order to provide appropriate levels of support for parents.

Little is known of the aetiology of congenital cardiac malformation, although the extremely sensitive period of embryologic development renders days 20 to 50 as the most vulnerable period for the development of major morphologic cardiac abnormalities.[14] Various factors, including genetic and chromosomal disorders, multifactorial inheritance and exposure to certain teratogens can result in cardiac dysmorphism.[3,15] The aetiology of congenital heart disease suggests a 5% to 10% incidence attributed to gross chromosomal abnormalities, 3% to be due to genetic factors, and approximately 90% to an environmental–genetic interaction, described as multifactorial inheritance.[3,16]

GENETIC INHERITANCE AND CONGENITAL HEART DISEASE

Various chromosomal aberrations lead to syndromes having an increased incidence of CHD. Infants born with Down syndrome commonly have associated congenital cardiac anomalies. **Table 11.1** illustrates the incidence and common lesions associated with selected syndromes.

Single gene mutations which generally make up part of a syndrome have a recurrence risk of 25% for a recessive gene and 50% recurrence risk for a dominant gene.[12,16] Holt Oram, Marfan and Noonan syndromes are examples of autosomal dominant syndromes associated with CHD (see **Table 11.2**). (For detailed review of genetic abnormalities, see Chapter 8).

Table 11.2 Autosomal dominant syndromes and associated CHD[3,16,17]

Syndrome	CHD incidence	Cardiac lesions associated
Holt-Oram	70%	ASD, VSD, IHSS
Noonan	50–80%	PS, ASD, cardiomyopathy

Table 11.3 Cardiovascular teratogens: infective agents, metabolic and pharmacological agents and their association with CHD[15–18]

Agent	CHD incidence	Associated congenital cardiac abnormalities
Infectious agents		
Rubella	35%	PAS, PDA, VSD, ASD
Metabolic disturbances	3%–5%	TGA, VSD, CoAO
Maternal diabetes mellitus	30%–50%	Cardiomegaly, cardiomyopathy
Maternal PKU	15%–20%	VSD, ASD, PDA, TET
Drugs		
Alcohol	25%–30%	VSD, PDA, ASD
Dilantin	2%–3%	AS, PS, Co.Ao., PDA
Trimethadione	15%–30%	TGA, TET, HLH
Lithium	10%	Ebstein's Anomaly, TA, ASD
Amphetamines	5%	VSD, PDA, ASD, TGA
Androgen therapy	2%–4%	TGA, TET, VSD
Chemotherapy	5%?	PS, AS, VSD, ASD
Vitamin A congeners	57%	Conotruncal defect

AS = aortic valve stenosis; ASD = atrial septal defect; A-VC = atrio ventricular canal; CoAO = coarctation of aorta; HLH = hypoplastic left heart; IHSS = idiopathic hypertrophic subaortic stenosis; MI = mitral incompetence; PA = pulmonary atresia; PKU-phenylketonuria; PS = pulmonary valve stenosis; TA = tricuspid atresia; TET = tetralogy of fallot; TGA = transposition of the great arteries; VSD = ventricular septal defect.

ENVIRONMENTAL FACTORS

Links have been drawn between the use or abuse of various chemicals (such as alcohol and some anticonvulsants), and genetically predisposed foetuses with the development of structural congenital heart defects.[15] Further studies have substantiated the risk to the foetus from various maternal metabolic disturbances and the rubella virus, through their potential for potent cardiovascular teratogenic effects.[16] Maternal diabetes carries an increased risk of transmission of CHD, thought to be attributed to poor control of the ketoacidotic state during pregnancy.[15] The importance of these and other environmental factors acting as cardiovascular teratogens is highlighted in **Table 11.3**.

MULTIFACTORIAL INHERITANCE

Accounting for approximately 90% of congenital cardiac anomalies, the factors influencing multifactorial inheritance suggest an environmental trigger may act during the sensitive period for cardiac development, to induce a structural cardiac abnormality in an embryo that is genetically predisposed.[15,16]

FAMILIAL INHERITANCE

Studies detailing the recurrence risk of CHD within families clearly indicate a higher risk of transmission to an infant born of a parent with a cardiac lesion.[3,12,16] The incidence is 5% to 10%, which contrasts with the 2% to 3% risk posed to an infant by a sibling with a congenital cardiac lesion.

Introductory Physiological Concepts

CARDIAC OUTPUT DETERMINANTS

Cardiac output is a measure of the volume of blood ejected by the heart each minute. The following discussion reviews the factors that determine stroke volume and cardiac output, i.e., preload, contractility, afterload and heart rate and rhythm. An indepth appreciation of the concepts determining cardiac output, as outlined, is crucial to the intensive care nurse's ability to problem solve and intervene at an early stage by supporting the circulation of the critically ill infant or child. Dysfunctional states affecting the cardiac output and the implications to nursing will be addressed in the section Failure of Control Mechanisms.

Preload: regulation and maintenance

Preload refers to the diastolic filling pressure of the ventricle and determines the myocardial cell fibre length in end diastole.[19–22] The concept of preload is explained by the Starling law of the heart. Essentially, the law explains that the heart has an intrinsic ability to adapt to changes in venous return. The greater the stretch applied to the fibres within physiologic limits, the greater the contraction that will result.[23] Overstretching the cells, however, by excessive volume loading beyond physiologic limits will cause a decrease in the contractile ability of the cells, at which time the ventricle is said to fail.[22]

The mechanism is well illustrated with a small spring. Gently stretching the spring results in the forceful return of the coil to the original dimensions. Greater stretch produces faster and added force of recoil. Even greater stretch of the spring will eventuate in distortion of the coil with loss of recoil ability.

Haemodynamically, the assessment of right ventricular preload, which is reflected as right ventricular end-diastolic pressure, is made through direct measurement of central venous pressure or right atrial pressure. Evaluation of left ventricular-end diastolic pressure is reflected by left atrial pressure or pulmonary capillary wedge pressure. (See Haemodynamic Monitoring).

Clinical significance of preload

When preload is altered, myocardial cell fibre length is altered and a significant change to stroke volume occurs. This is exemplified in the infant or child with hypovolaemia who displays the clinical signs of low cardiac output, exhibiting an associated increase in heart rate and decrease in filling pressure. From a nursing perspective, an ability to recognise and analyse clinical findings and interpret physiologic parameters enhances ability to intervene appropriately to support the infant or child's circulation.

Physiologically, a reduction in circulating volume decreases the stretch of myocardial fibres and the cells respond with reduced contractile force. This will result in a decreased stroke volume and ultimately a decrease in cardiac output. The end result is tissue hypoperfusion with oxygen and nutrient depletion at a cellular level. Augmentation of the preload by volume loading to correct the state of hypovolaemia will increase the venous return and hence preload. Optimising the myocardial fibre stretch and improving myocardial contractility will restore cardiac output, thereby enhancing tissue perfusion.[24]

Conversely, let us consider the infant or child presenting with the clinical signs of low cardiac output in whom monitored parameters reveal both an increase in heart rate and filling pressure. In this situation the development of the low cardiac output state has resulted from abnormalities of the factors that determine cardiac output (i.e., contractility and afterload). The increase in preload causes additional tension on the ventricular muscle mass, increasing cellular metabolism and myocardial oxygen requirements without augmenting cardiac output. Manipulation to decrease the preload may be effected through the administration of diuretics and/or vasodilators or myocardial stimulants which will redistribute the volume load and reduce the ventricular end-diastolic volume or preload.[22,25]

Recognition of the variability in the pressure relationship which exists between the left and right ventricles in complex congenital cardiac malformations is essential. In many congenital cardiac lesions the normal relationship between the filling pressures of the 2 ventricles is altered. Manipulation of ventricular filling pressure in these infants and children requires careful evaluation of both left and right sided filling pressures (left and right atrial pressures). Excessive augmentation of the right-sided filling pressure, for example, may precipitate significant dysfunction of the left ventricle.

Myocardial contractility: regulation and maintenance

Contractility reflects the ability of myocardial fibres (the sarcomeres) to shorten, and is dependent on the interaction of calcium with troponin C, one of the tropomysin complexes, which are contractile regulatory proteins.[19,26,27] Contractility of myocardial fibres is dependent upon:

- the availability of calcium ions to reach the contractile protein, troponin C and
- the sensitivity of the contractile proteins to calcium.

The calcium ion is therefore the integral component for both contraction and the synchrony of that cardiac contraction, causing muscle shortening and the depolarisation of the membrane, a process referred to as 'excitation–contraction coupling'.[26]

At the time of myocardial cell depolarisation, different ions carrying different charges into and out of the cell, change the ionic permeability of the membrane.[28] Importantly, calcium enters the cell via a slow calcium channel causing a 'calcium flux,' which promotes the release of stored calcium from within the cell. The calcium released from the cell binds to troponin C and initiates cardiac contraction.[19,21,29,30] For relaxation of the myocardial cells to occur, calcium must be removed from the troponin C molecules. The calcium is then redirected; some is returned to the intracellular storage sites, the sarcoplasmic reticulum, and some is expelled to the extracellular compartment. The expulsion of the calcium requires energy input to effect the ion exchange. Adenosine triphosphate as the energy source, exchanges the intracellular ion concentration by means of the calcium–sodium exchange pump and the sodium–potassium pump mechanisms.[19,29] It becomes apparent that calcium assumes a critical role in myocardial contractility. Factors affecting the availability of calcium to the cells will therefore have a major influence on the myocardial contractile state.[30]

Other factors known to produce significant alteration to myocardial contractile force are the metabolic derangements of hypoxia, acidosis, hypoglycaemia, electrolyte imbalance and temperature instability, all of which could precipitate some degree of circulatory failure.[30,31]

Afterload: regulation and maintenance

Afterload is an expression of the force that a ventricle must overcome to eject it's contents.[19,22,31,32] There is a series of factors identified as force, velocity, length and time that determine the limits to myocardial fibre shortening and hence the volume of blood ejected by the ventricle. These factors influence the relationship at the time of ventricular fibre shortening, directly influencing end systolic volumes and consequently end-diastolic volume.[21] The normal and abnormal factors influencing afterload are therefore:

- The size of the ventricles determining the systolic wall tension and therefore the myocardial fibre shortening and the stroke volume.
- The ejection pressure, which refers to the resistance against which the ventricle must eject it's volume, i.e., the systemic vascular resistance in the case of the left ventricle and the pulmonary vascular resistance for the right ventricle.
- Mechanical obstruction to ventricular outflow, resulting in increased wall tension, an increase in myocardial oxygen requirements and an alteration to stroke volume (e.g., aortic stenosis, pulmonary stenosis).
- Vascular impedance to blood flow offered by the systemic and pulmonary arteriolar networks. The resistance offered to blood flow from the arterial and precapillary arteriolar beds, which are under the control of neural and humoral influences, are more important in infants and children. Increase in blood viscosity, which is common in neonates and infants with cyanotic congenital heart disease, results in further impedance to the blood flow.[21,32,33]

Heart rate: regulation and maintenance

Heart rate is a vital component of cardiac output, considered of greater value than stroke volume in determining the output in the neonate and very young child.[34] The factors that determine cardiac output are dependent on one another, and when alteration to one variable occurs, it rarely remains isolated to that variable. This is exemplified by an alteration to either preload or afterload, both of which ultimately influence heart rate. Further, endogenous and exogenous catecholamines influence the contractile state of the myocardium and significantly alter heart rate and rhythm. Similarly, a primary alteration of heart rate and an electrical disturbance of the conducting pathway affecting cardiac rhythm, can produce a secondary influence on the myocardial contractile state and the preload of the ventricle.[34]

A multiplicity of metabolic derangements is known to produce profound systemic effects upon the heart rate and rhythm. Electrolyte abnormalities (e.g., hyperkalaemia and hypocalcaemia), hypoxia, acidosis and hypoglycaemia impose a depressant effect on the myocardium. In addition to the metabolic abnormalities outlined, there are various drugs, central nervous system and neuromuscular problems which also evoke depressant influences on the heart. An increase in myocardial excitability will result from the electrolyte abnormalities of hypokalaemia and hypomagnesaemia.[35]

An understanding of electrocardiographic principles is important in order to identify heart rate and rhythm disturbances, interpret changes and instigate appropriate support for the child. Development of these concepts is beyond the scope of this chapter and the reader is referred to a number of excellent publications.[34,36-43]

MYOCARDIAL DEVELOPMENTAL CONSIDERATIONS

Consideration of myocardial developmental aspects in the newborn is necessary to an understanding of the differing responses that occur with manipulation of cardiac output in this group. The myocardium in the newborn infant is described as functionally immature, both structurally and biochemically.[21,29] Traditionally, the right ventricle was considered to assume the dominant role to accommodate the fetal circulation *in utero*. Current opinion, however, holds that right and left ventricular growth occur equally during the foetal period.[44] With the establishment of extrauterine circulation, the left ventricle assumes dominance over the right because of its increased haemodynamic load. The pressure and volume load imposed on the left ventricle of the newborn infant necessitate the proliferation of myocardial cells, resulting in myocyte hyperplasia and hypertrophy within that ventricle.[21] Although the myocyte development occurs in both ventricles for a 3 to 6 month period following delivery, only minimal cellular proliferation occurs in the right ventricle. Neonatal cardiac growth or cardiac enlargement is thought to be a direct result of the haemodynamic load imposed by either physiologic activity or pathological conditions (e.g., pressure/volume overload situations).[29] With the maturation of the structural development of myocardial muscle in the newborn, the contractile mass of the left ventricle increases by up to 60%, which contrasts with the 30% contractile myocardial mass in the foetus.[21] An increase in contractile force occurs with the development of the sarcoplasmic reticulum, myofibrils and the subcellular organelle, the mitochondrion.[19,21,29] The high energy yields of adenosine triphosphate required for cardiac contraction are generated from the aerobic metabolic pathway of the Krebs cycle, which takes place in the mitochondrion of the cell. Additionally, it is important to remember that sympathetic innervation within the ventricles is incomplete at the time of delivery, continuing to differentiate for several weeks.[19,32]

Clinical relevance of myocyte development

The following factors related to myocardial development hold special considerations for nursing personnel in the care of critically ill newborn infants.

- The neonate has decreased myocardial compliance due to diminished contractile mass and therefore will not respond as well as the older infant to increments in preload.[21,34,45,46]
- An elevation in systemic vascular resistance is a significant feature in the newborn infant and additional increases in afterload incur obvious limitations to myocardial performance.[21,45]
- The heart in the newborn infant functions at near maximal performance and generates a high cardiac output.[45,47] Further increases in output, as required in stress or disease states, are poorly tolerated because of the reduced myocardial contractile force in infants who have significantly elevated systemic vascular resistance.
- The incomplete sympathetic innervation in the heart in the first weeks of life enhances the influence of parasympathetic tone, predisposing the young babies to bradyarrhythmias.[21,32,45]

Failure of Control Mechanisms

The term 'heart failure' denotes an inability of the myocardium to deliver adequate cardiac output to meet the metabolic demands of the body.[45] This section addresses aspects pertaining to the aetiology and pathophysiology of cardiac failure, including neuroendocrine and metabolic influences.

AETIOLOGY OF CARDIAC FAILURE

The aetiology of cardiac failure in the paediatric patient is markedly different from that of the adult, where causes are generally attributed to coronary artery, hypertensive and valvular heart disease. Most often in infancy and childhood, heart failure is the direct result of structural cardiac lesions imposing alteration to the pressure or volume load of the ventricle. Other factors related to poor myocardial contractility can also occur. Cardiac failure in the paediatric group is therefore attributed to the following:

1. Pressure overload of the ventricles, secondary to intracardiac or extracardiac obstructive lesions. Alteration to the pressure/flow dynamics imposed by an obstructive lesion causes impedance to the ejection of blood flow from the heart; e.g., by severe semi-lunar valve stenosis (aortic or pulmonary valve stenosis) or coarctation of the aorta.
2. Volume load alterations which may cause ventricular failure, the result of a left to right shunt occurring, usually at ventricular or at great vessel level, e.g., ventricular septal defects or persistent patency of the ductus arteriosus.
3. A reduction in myocardial contractility, derived from several of the factors known to depress the contractile state, e.g.:
    *   the metabolic derangements of hypoxia, acidosis, hypoglycaemia and electrolyte imbalances;
    *   postoperative causes, secondary to anaesthetic agents or myocardial ischaemia;
    *   infective and inflammatory agents (myocarditis); and
    *   myocardial infarction, although a rare occurrence, can result from either a congenital cause (i.e., anomalous origin of left coronary arteries) or from acquired factors (as in Kawasaki disease).[48]
4. A combination of the factors involving pressure/volume alteration and myocardial dysfunction.[49]

NURSING ASSESSMENT

Optimal care for the infant or child with heart failure requires advanced clinical assessment skills by nursing personnel. The nurses' proficiency with clinical assessment provides the foundation for care and is a prerequisite to ones' ability to problem solve for the children, set goals of care and initiate supportive nursing and medical intervention with appropriate pharmacological measures at an early stage. From a nursing perspective, it is essential to consider the specific clinical features associated with myocardial failure. The cardinal features of cardiac failure in infants include tachycardia, dyspnoea, cardiomegaly and hepatomegaly. In severe failure, signs of circulatory collapse and cardiovascular shock will be detected.[50] Knowledge of the pathophysiological response of the body to myocardial failure, including the neuroendocrine and metabolic influences, enhances one's understanding of the infant or child's clinical features at presentation. The goal of care is to eliminate/minimise both the primary mechanism of the heart failure and the secondary contributing factors.

Nursing history

Obtaining a nursing history from the parents complements the clinical findings obtained in a complete nursing assessment. Parents often relate a characteristic and classical picture of cardiac failure when describing their infant's problems. They often express concern about their infants feeding pattern in that the infant feeds often, tires quickly and is unable to complete a feed. Characteristically, there is increasing irritability in an infant previously well settled. Parents relate that their infant breathes fast and always feels cool, damp or sweaty to the touch. Upon exertion (feeding or crying), beads of perspiration develop on the infant's forehead.

Tachycardia and hepatomegaly will be detected by the nursing assessment. Dependent on the severity of the failure, tachypnoea will progress to dyspnoea with associated intercostal and subcostal recession and grunting respirations. Determination of the infant's length and mass is essential, as these parameters may facilitate the detection of growth retardation related to increased metabolism and reduced caloric intake. The nursing assessment in the paediatric patient is ideally undertaken with the infant or child at rest. Evaluation of many important parameters can be made at the initial inspection without disturbing the infant. These are:

- level of consciousness
- respiratory effort and rate
- colour of the lips, nailbeds, skin
- level of activity
- alertness and the response to the environment
- position of comfort assumed by the infant or child.

CARDIOVASCULAR ASSESSMENT

A comprehensive cardiovascular nursing assessment is undertaken to determine the effectiveness of cardiac output in the infant, as depicted by the characteristic clinical features demonstrating adequate tissue perfusion — the infant will be pink in colour, warm and well perfused. To detect an alteration to the cardiac output state, it is therefore essential to determine the following.

Colour

Central cyanosis is detected through assessment of the buccal mucosa, tongue and conjunctivae, and reflects a low arterial oxygen saturation, attributed to:

- right-to-left intracardiac or extracardiac shunts
- ventilation/perfusion mismatching
- haemoglobinopathy.

Peripheral cyanosis is detected through observation of the nailbeds and earlobes, which may appear dusky to cyanosed in colour while the mucous membranes remain pink. Peripheral cyanosis with pink nailbeds may indicate a localised vasoconstriction.[51,52]

Pulse

Note the characterisation, rate and nature of the central and distal pulses, i.e., the pulses should be easily palpable and regular, not weak or bounding in nature.

Peripheral perfusion

Note the colour, capillary refill and warmth of the extremities. Pallor, a mottling appearance of the skin and cool extremities indicate circulatory inadequacy.

Blood pressure

Infants and children compensate for alteration in cardiac status by maintaining their blood pressure to a point when decompensation of their clinical condition renders them hypotensive. Changes in blood pressure in children who show signs of clinical deterioration therefore develop very late in the clinical course.

Precordial assessment

- Chest asymmetry is assessed by close inspection.
- Palpation of the chest will ascertain the presence of thrills, which are essentially cardiac murmurs that can be palpated.
- Auscultation of the precordium will detect the presence of normal and abnormal heart sounds and murmurs.
- Systemic venous engorgement is detected through the presence of liver enlargement (normally felt to have a rounded edge). Jugular venous distension is a reliable sign of venous engorgement in older children.

Respiratory status

A comprehensive cardiovascular assessment requires careful evaluation of the child's respiration. Clinical signs of tachypnoea, when associated with dyspnoea, may indicate progressing metabolic acidosis. Bradypnoea and periods of apnoea associated with other clinical signs of cardiac failure may indicate an imminent cardiac arrest, the result of hypoxic or ischaemic cerebral injury or respiratory fatigue.

Most importantly, the nursing assessment for the infant or child with cardiovascular dysfunction requires careful evaluation of:

- the effectiveness of the heart to pump;
- filling volumes and pressures;
- cardiac output; and
- mechanisms of compensation in the body.[53]

Assessing the effectiveness of the heart to pump

Features that signify a reduction in myocardial contractility are detected clinically by a reduction in arterial pulse pressure, enlargement of the heart, increases in pulmonary venous congestion and the presence of cardiac murmurs and gallop rhythms. Early signs of pulmonary congestion are detected clinically by tachypnoea. As heart failure worsens, varying degrees of dyspnoea become apparent and may include intercostal and substernal recession, grunting respirations, and nasal flaring. On auscultation, pulmonary rales and decreased air entry may be noted.[31] The detection of a murmur as an indication of significant congenital heart disease (CHD) is unreliable in the neonatal period. This feature is attributed to the alteration of intracardiac haemodynamics which occurs in the newborn with the transition from fetal to postnatal circulation (the closure of accessory vascular channels and intracardiac shunts, and the high pulmonary vascular resistance).[54,55]

A precordial bulge and chest asymmetry may indicate ventricular overactivity.[6] Heart murmurs which may be palpated are indicative of blood flow turbulence and are termed cardiac thrills.[53] Further, ventricular overactivity may produce a lift or heave, noted when the activity of the heart is abnormally forceful. Right ventricular overactivity resulting from volume overload or hypertrophy will produce a lift or heave at the lower left sternal border, whereas left ventricular overactivity is noted through the prominence of the apical impulse.[6]

Filling volumes and pressure assessment

Filling volumes and pressures are assessed by the degree of systemic venous engorgement. Liver enlargement is a reliable sign of cardiac failure from early infancy. Jugular venous distension is difficult to evaluate in the infant due to the infant's short, fat neck and inability to sit, although periorbital oedema or generalised oedema may be noted.[31] Dependent oedema and ascites are rarely seen in childhood, but may be observed as a feature in the adolescent with congestive cardiac failure.

Cardiac output assessment

Clinical assessment of cardiac output is evaluated through heart rate, blood pressure, pulse pressure, systemic vascular resistance, urine output and central nervous system signs.[53] Alteration in the level of consciousness with increased restlessness and irritability, when combined with clinical signs of low cardiac output, is indicative of decreased cerebral perfusion.[31] Sympathetic nervous system stimulation evokes potent vasoconstriction, with the skin becoming mottled, diaphoretic and cool or cold to touch. Peripheral perfusion is further assessed by the skin colour, capillary refill and the character of distal pulses. Urine output is an excellent indicator of cardiac output. Narrowing of the pulse pressure is a feature of congestive cardiac failure and shock states because of a reduction in ejection velocity.[31,53] Small, weak arterial pulsations are characteristic of elevated systemic vascular resistance. The pulses of the upper and lower limbs in infancy and childhood should be routinely palpated to assess the amplitude and quality of pulsations, thus excluding coarctation of the aorta, where discrepancies of the arterial pulsations are noted.[6] Further, a reduction in the infant's spontaneous motor activity in association with the clinical features outlined above, is indicative of an infant's low cardiac output.

PATHOPHYSIOLOGICAL RESPONSE TO CARDIAC FAILURE

A reduction in cardiac output initiates several compensatory mechanisms. The following discussion addresses the baroreceptor influences and the neuroendocrine and metabolic responses incurred by an alteration to cardiac function. Appreciation of these mechanisms of compensation will enhance the nurse's understanding of the presenting signs and the anticipated physiological response to pharmacological intervention. Myocardial failure evokes potent neuroendocrine responses which act as mechanisms of compensation for the reduction in cardiac output. Analysis of the body's responses to cardiac failure explains the classical presentation and the interventional support required to reverse the process.

Baroreceptor reflexes

The baroreceptor reflex is a rapidly acting pressure control mechanism which functions to maintain the arterial pressure following activation of sensory neurons. Sensory neurons are located in the walls of the carotid sinus, aortic arch and the low pressure regions of the atria and pulmonary arteries.[32,56,57]

In health, the baroreceptors emit signals that produce low levels of sympathetic tone, controlling the heart and peripheral vasculature and hence parasympathetic tone predominates. Initiation of the baroreceptor reflex occurs when the pressor/stretch receptors are stimulated by either hypotensive or hypertensive states. A decrease in blood pressure initiates a potent sympathetic response acting on the heart and vasculature, producing an increase in both cardiac output and systemic vascular resistance (SVR), thereby stabilising the circulation. Parasympathetic effects are inhibited at this time. By contrast, hypertension initiates the parasympathetic response, thereby reducing both heart rate and systemic vascular resistance and causing depression of sympathetic stimuli.[32] Although initiated as an acute response to the failing circulation, these pressoreceptors fail to contribute to the long-term regulation of arterial pressure.[57]

The chemoreceptors located within the carotid and aortic bodies respond to a decrease of both oxygen and carbon dioxide, and an accumulation of hydrogen ion, initiated by reduced cardiac output states. The arterial pressure is stabilised following reflex activation of the vasomotor centre, although the role played by the chemoreceptors is considered less efficacious than that of the pressoreceptors outlined above.[32,57]

Various mechanisms of compensation develop in response to cardiac failure. When the failure is unrelieved, these changes can lead to further decompensation of the cardiovascular state. Early in the course of decompensation, dilatation of the myocardial muscle mass is effective in maintaining cardiac output due to the increase in preload which provides the stimulus for increased sarcomere shortening. A combination of ventricular dilatation and increased wall stress leads to increased oxygen requirements. Eventually the increase in the ventricular end-diastolic pressure is transmitted to the systemic and pulmonary venous beds, thus promoting tissue oedema.[45]

Additional increases in sympathetic stimulation and the release of potent vasoconstrictor substances (catecholamines, vasopressin and angiotensin), promote significant increases in peripheral vascular resistance, which helps to increase the blood pressure. The workload of the left ventricle and the myocardial oxygen requirements are subsequently increased by the elevation in systemic vascular resistance, which attempts to maintain adequate cardiac output.[45]

Sympathetic nervous stimulation

Sympathetic innervation initiates the fight and flight mechanisms, which help compensate in times of extreme stress. Stimulation of the hypothalamus causes a direct increase in cardiac activity, which accelerates the heart rate and increases the contractile force of the myocardium, thereby enhancing cardiac output.[58] Perfusion to the muscles is increased, while intense vasoconstriction occurs in the skin and periphery, redirecting blood to more vital areas.[57,59]

Humoral responses

The various hormonal agents which help regulate arterial pressure through their vasoactive effects and their salt and water regulatory functions are:

Table 11.4 Major cardiovascular and respiratory effects of adrenergic stimulation of alpha and beta receptor sites[22,61,63]

Adrenergic receptor	Chemical mediator	Adrenergic stimulation of affector organ site
Beta₁	Noradrenaline	*Heart:* Rate increased Contractility increased
Beta₂	Adrenalin	*Vasculature:* vasodilation of • coronary • skeletal muscle *Lung:* bronchodilatation *Liver:* increased glycogenolysis
Alpha	Adrenalin and noradrenaline	*Vasculature:* vasoconstriction of • coronary (mild) • skin • renal • pulmonary *Sweat glands:* increased secretion

• adrenalin and noradrenaline (vasoconstrictor mechanism);
• renin angiotensin vasoconstrictor mechanism;
• vasopressin; and
• atrial naturetic peptide.

Until recently, controversy existed as to the benefit or detriment imposed on the failing circulation by sympathetic nervous stimulation in states of chronic cardiac failure. These humoral agents significantly increase the vascular resistance and induce salt and water retention and the release of potent vasoactive hormones, which help regulate cardiac output. Excessive levels of these hormones, however, initiate detrimental metabolic and biochemical effects which, when combined with an elevation in vasomotor tone, result in an increase in oxygen and energy needs, further compounding the workload of the heart.[60]

Adrenalin, noradrenaline vasoconstrictor mechanism

The chemical mediators of the alpha and beta adrenergic receptors are the hormones secreted by the adrenal medulla — adrenalin and noradrenaline.[59,61] Noradrenaline acts as the mediator for both the alpha-1 and alpha-2 adrenergic receptors and to a lesser extent the beta receptors, whereas adrenalin excites both alpha and beta receptor sites[61] (**Table 11.4**). The alpha and beta adrenergic receptors are proteins important to the regulation of calcium within the cell and are found within the sarcolemma of myocardial and vascular smooth muscle cells.[19]

Beta-1 adrenergic receptors predominate within the heart. Noradrenaline is the chemical mediator of these receptor sites and upon stimulation, results in inotropic (increased contractile force) and chronotropic (increased rate) effects on the heart.[19,22,62–64] Beta-2 adrenergic receptors are mediated by adrenalin and are located within:

• vascular smooth muscle, causing vasodilation of coronary and skeletal muscle vasculature;

- lungs, causing bronchodilation; and
- liver and muscle, causing increased glycogenolysis.[19,22,61,63]

The alpha-1 receptor sites within the ventricular myocardium are minimal.[62] Noradrenaline stimulation of postsynaptic alpha-1 adrenergic receptors (which are located within the vascular smooth muscle tissue), results in vascular constriction and hence directs the blood flow away from the skin, kidney and gastrointestinal tract. While alpha adrenergic stimulation augments systemic blood pressure and perfusion of vital tissues in states of cardiovascular collapse, stimulation of these receptor sites in congestive cardiac failure induces further haemodynamic compromise. This results in intense vasoconstriction, producing excess elevation in ventricular filling pressure and a rise in the resistance of the systemic and the pulmonary vascular beds, raising the afterload of the ventricles.[65]

Renin–angiotensin vasoconstrictor mechanism

The renin–angiotensin mechanism is also effective in re-establishing a normotensive state from one of low cardiac output. The juxtaglomerular cells of the kidney respond to the decrease in perfusion and the increased sympathetic nervous activity by secreting the enzyme renin into the circulation. The renin, reacting with angiotensinogen, forms angiotensin I. In the pulmonary vasculature, angiotensin I is converted to angiotensin II in the presence of 'angiotensin converting enzyme'.[59,66]

Angiotensin II is a potent vasoconstrictor and although rapidly inactivated in the bloodstream, causes a marked arteriolar constriction and hence an increase in SVR, thus augmenting the blood pressure. An increase in preload results from mild venous constriction, which enhances the venous return to the heart.[66,67]

The long-term augmentation of circulatory volume is further enhanced through the angiotensin mechanism. Angiotensin directly affects the kidney, resulting in the retention of salt and water, thereby increasing the circulating volume, which assists in the restoration of cardiac output.[59] Stimulation of the adrenal cortex by angiotensin causes the release of aldosterone (a corticosteroid) which increases the renal tubular reabsorption of salt. This mechanism causes an increase in the extracellular osmotic pressure, which in turn increases water reabsorption.[66,68,69]

Vasopressin (antidiuretic hormone)

Vasopressin acts to restore arterial blood pressure in both acute and chronic low cardiac output states. Vasopressin is a potent vasoconstrictor which increases systemic vascular resistance and preload by a direct action on the systemic arteriolar and venous vasculature. Released from the posterior pituitary gland, vasopressin promotes water reabsorption from the renal tubules in response to the sodium retention caused by aldosterone secretion.[59,70–72]

Atrial naturetic peptide

Atrial naturetic peptide (ANP) is a hormone released from cardiac cells, predominantly within the right atrium. It is known to influence the cardiovascular, renal and endocrine systems through its regulatory effects on fluid and electrolyte homeostasis and blood pressure.[73]

ANP is released when the atrium becomes overdistended, as in congestive cardiac failure. The peptide regulates sodium excretion, imposing a secondary influence on the excretion of water. Further, ANP inhibits the secretion of renin, aldosterone and anti-diuretic hormone. Early studies, although inconclusive, suggest ANP plays an important regulatory role in fluid overload states associated with congestive cardiac failure.[73]

Metabolic derangements: hypoxaemia and myocardial cell function

Coronary blood flow is determined by neuroendocrine, metabolic and mechanical factors. Hypoxaemia initiates vasodilation of cerebral and coronary vessels while producing a reflex vasoconstriction in less vital areas (such as the skin, kidneys). Myocardial blood flow and cellular oxygenation are essential to effective cardiac contractility. The tissue oxygenation of the myocardium is determined by both the coronary arterial perfusion and the capacity of the blood to carry oxygen.[30]

To function effectively, the myocardium requires vast amounts of energy in the form of adenosine triphosphate (ATP), obtained via aerobic metabolic pathways. When hypoxia develops, the tissues are depleted of ATP stores. The loss of available energy for myocardial contraction results in marked deterioration of cardiac muscle cell function and is attributed to the following.

- Intracellular potassium depletion and a concurrent accumulation of calcium, sodium and water caused by the loss of function of the enzyme substrates, Na-K ATPase and calcium-sensitive ATPase.
- ATP depletion which reduces the energy stores required by the ATPase enzyme responsible for myocardial contraction.
- Diminished ability of the myocardial cells to relax. For relaxation to occur, calcium must be removed from the sarcoplasmic reticulum, a process requiring energy in the form of ATP. Inadequate ATP availability results in an intracellular calcium accumulation and hence an inability of the muscle cells to relax. Coronary artery perfusion occurs in diastole, therefore reduction of the diastolic time impedes myocardial perfusion and the availability of oxygen to supply hypoxic tissues. As calcium accumulates within the mitochondria, the organelles are rendered incapable of ATP production.[30]

Clinical significance of hypoxaemia

A reduction in coronary perfusion and oxygenation poses severe, negative effects on myocardial cell function. The physiological effects of hypoxaemia are determined by the rate of depletion of ATP. The capacity to maintain ATP production in the hypoxic newborn infant is explained by the infant's high tissue glycogen stores and rate of glycolysis.[30,44] The newborn infant has relatively low energy requirements, and as such the myocardium has the ability for near complete recovery following an hypoxic event.[44] Therefore, it is postulated that glucose administration may support myocardial function through a period of hypoxia. By contrast, the introduction of inotropic agents may complicate the infant's clinical course, as these agents consume available ATP stores and augment calcium entry into the cell.

Hypoxaemia results in intracellular lactate accumulation, impeding glycolysis and the oxidative metabolic pathway. The cumulative effects of the metabolic byproducts cause distortion of cell membranes and interference with enzyme activity, resulting in further myocardial dysfunction.[30,59]

Acidosis and myocardial cell function

Acidosis of either metabolic or respiratory aetiology results in marked depression of the myocardial contractility. A decrease in blood pH stimulates the sympathetic nervous system and the adrenal cortical hormone to release adrenalin and noradrenaline. These endogenous catecholamines stimulate beta receptors to initiate compensatory inotropic effects on the myocardium. Environmental pH determines the responsiveness of the myocardium to the catecholamine. Acidosis causes decreased efficiency of catecholamines and a reduced affinity for beta adrenergic receptors, so that the catecholamines fail to improve cardiac output in the presence of acidosis.[22,59] Of additional significance, parasympathetic nervous activity is augmented in states of acidosis when the pH is less than 7.1, resulting in an increased risk of bradyarrhythmia and cardiac arrest.[59]

The following mechanisms have been postulated to explain the effects of acidosis on the myocardial contractility.

1. Acidosis promotes competition for the myocardial protein binding sites (troponin) between the excess accumulation of intracellular hydrogen ion and calcium, resulting in:
   - a decreased calcium/troponin reaction;
   - less actin/myosin reaction; and
   - reduction in myocardial contractile strength.
2. Acidosis impedes the release of calcium from the intracellular organelle (the sarcoplasmic reticulum), inhibiting the calcium/troponin reaction required for myocardial contractility.
3. The slow calcium current which controls movement of calcium ions between the intracellular compartments is restricted by a decrease in pH, influencing 'excitation–contraction coupling' and results in reduced contractility.
4. The elevation of extracellular potassium ions which accompanies acidosis will affect cardiac rhythm and myocardial contractility.[59]

Electrolyte imbalances and myocardial cell function

Ionic imbalances of calcium, potassium and sodium may precipitate significant myocardial dysfunction. The activation of vital cellular metabolic functions influencing cell membrane potentials and action potentials are reliant on an ionic balance to effect impulse conduction.

Calcium is pivotal to myocardial contractility. A deficiency of calcium ions reduces myocardial contractile strength, leading to weak, ineffective contractions which significantly reduce cardiac output. In contrast, excessive intracellular calcium induces an over-excitability of the cells and results in spastic contraction of cardiac muscle.[23]

An excess of potassium ions results in effects similar to those caused by a state of hypocalcaemia, with the cardiac muscle becoming flaccid.[74] The high serum potassium causes alteration to the muscle fibre action potential, causing the membrane resting potential to decrease which results in a decreased intensity of the ventricular conduction velocity and a widening of the QRS complex.[35] High serum potassium may reflect a low cardiac output state or impending renal failure and should be corrected.

High serum sodium concentrations cause a depressant effect on the myocardium. The exact mechanism is unexplained, although sodium competes with calcium, reducing the availability of calcium for cellular contraction.[23]

These common electrolyte problems and their effects upon cardiac function hold important implications for nursing practice. Careful assessment and interpretation of clinical, biochemical and monitored parameters ensures appropriate intervention can be undertaken before significant deterioration in cardiac function occurs.

Temperature instability and myocardial cell function

The cardiovascular response to fever results in an increase in heart rate and myocardial work, necessitating an increase in oxygen and substrate requirements.[30] Persistent tachycardia increases metabolic demand, significantly increases oxygen requirements and depletes available energy stores, precipitating myocardial depression.

In contrast, hypothermia reduces the heart rate, decreasing metabolic requirements and depressing cardiac output.[23] The increased systemic vascular resistance accompanying hypothermia reduces tissue perfusion and accentuates metabolic acidosis.[30] Infants who develop cold stress increase body heat by metabolising brown fat stores in a process termed non-shivering thermogenesis'.[33,75] The increased heat production and metabolism burdens the infant by increasing oxygen and glucose needs. The end result is hypoxaemia and hypoglycaemia, which further impede myocardial performance.[30]

Hypoglycaemia and myocardial cell function

The energy required for cardiac contraction is obtained primarily from glucose, but is also derived from fatty acid metabolism and lactate. As glucose is a major energy substrate for the myocardium, significant cardiac depression results when hypoglycaemia develops.[30,76]

Compensatory mechanisms of cardiac failure

The mechanisms of compensation for low cardiac output states are reflected by characteristic increases in preload and systemic vascular resistance, as previously discussed.

TREATMENT MODALITIES FOR RELIEF OF CARDIAC FAILURE

Implications for nursing practice

Critical assessment and evaluation of the clinical features of myocardial failure in infants and children is mandatory in order to prioritise and optimise care from a nursing perspective. The goal of care therefore aims to maximise cardiac output by:

- reducing myocardial oxygen demands, thereby improving tissue oxygenation;
- eliminating detrimental metabolic factors contributing to decreased myocardial function — hypoxia, acidosis, hypoglycaemia, electrolyte imbalances, etc;
- introducing pharmacological agents to support the myocardium, improve cardiac output and reverse the neuroendocrine responses contributing to the failure. An improved cardiac output will also tend to reverse the acidosis and electrolyte imbalances;
- providing emotional support for the infant/child and family.

Maximising cardiac output: reducing myocardial oxygen requirements

Myocardial oxygen requirements can be reduced in a number of ways. Rest is a major factor in conserving an infant's energy. Infants who develop cardiac failure rapidly deplete their energy stores as part of the neuroendocrine stress response. Inadequate oxygen and glucose substrate availability to cells depresses myocardial function. Assuring complete rest for the infant repletes energy stores and reduces oxygen demand. Available oxygen is used more effectively, thus helping to reduce the gap between supply and demand. All care is therefore planned to afford minimal disturbance to the infant, assuring adequate rest between feeds. Exertion is prevented by adopting a feeding/caring regimen specific to the infant's needs.

Older children presenting with cardiac failure generally determine their own level of activity and therefore enforced rest is rarely an issue, other than in the child with aortic stenosis. Older infants and children with severe heart failure will assume a sitting position for comfort.

Supplemental oxygen may be required to relieve hypoxaemia in infants and children with moderate to severe cardiovascular dysfunction. Humidification of the oxygen is essential. The method of administration varies and is dependent on age and the activity of the child. Appropriate methods can include nasal catheter, face mask or oxygen tent. Consideration of the fraction of inspired oxygen (FiO_2) is very important. Infants and children with significant pulmonary congestion have a ventilation/perfusion (V/Q) mismatch which affects gaseous exchange at alveolar level. Oxygen and carbon dioxide exchange is impeded. This results in both an increase in the partial pressure of carbon dioxide ($PaCO_2$), causing a rightward shift of the oxyhaemoglobin dissociation curve and a decrease in the oxygen (PaO_2) within the blood. The shift to the right signifies a reduction in the affinity of oxygen for the haemoglobin molecule.[77,78] The ramifications of myocardial hypoxia have been reviewed. Failure to reverse the process is potentially life threatening and under no circumstances is oxygen therapy withheld when required.

Caution must be observed, however, when administering oxygen to infants with a reactive pulmonary vascular bed with significant left-to-right shunts attributed to structural cardiac defects, as in babies with truncus arteriosus.[80] High concentrations of oxygen may increase the left-to-right shunt and the degree of cardiac failure in these infants, as oxygen causes pulmonary arteriolar dilatation[79] (**Table 11.5**). Dependent upon the degree of failure and the infant's response to other supportive measures and pharmacological interventions, an FiO_2 of 0.3 to 0.35 may be adequate to support these infants.

Additional supportive measures to reduce myocardial oxygen requirements

Meeting the nutritional requirements in these often cachectic infants is of great importance. In acute or severe cardiac failure, perseverance with oral feeding is inappropriate. These infants require parenteral fluid administration to provide their metabolic needs. Once an adequate response from diuretic and inotropic support is effected, small frequent feeds are reintroduced. The feeding regimen is varied to meet the infant's special needs and minimise the risk of exhaustion.[81] Caloric augmentation of feeds with polyjoule and medium-chain triglyceride oil is effective in providing the energy requirements of the infant. Fluid restriction in infants and children is poorly tolerated and problems encountered with fluid overload are managed with diuretic administration.

Temperature instability is a metabolic derangement which further increases the body's oxygen demands. Ensuring normothermia and preventing cold stress in infants will reduce myocardial oxygen needs and glucose substrate depletion. Similarly, hyperthermia should be controlled as it increases metabolic activity, resulting in both an increase in oxygen and glucose needs and the production of metabolic wastes.[30]

Table 11.5 Flow diagram depicting the vasodilatory effects imposed on the pulmonary arteriolar network by a high FiO_2 in infants with a significant left-to-right shunt

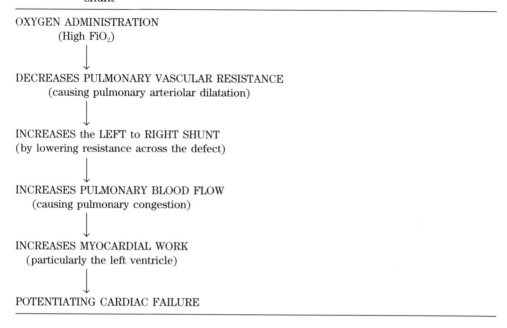

OXYGEN ADMINISTRATION
    (High FiO_2)

DECREASES PULMONARY VASCULAR RESISTANCE
    (causing pulmonary arteriolar dilatation)

INCREASES the LEFT to RIGHT SHUNT
(by lowering resistance across the defect)

INCREASES PULMONARY BLOOD FLOW
    (causing pulmonary congestion)

INCREASES MYOCARDIAL WORK
    (particularly the left ventricle)

POTENTIATING CARDIAC FAILURE

Elimination/correction of metabolic derangements

Elimination or correction of the metabolic factors known to impede myocardial performance is crucial to effective management of the infant's cardiac failure. Hypoglycaemia and electrolyte imbalances must be corrected. With adequate oxygenation and circulation restored following intervention with pharmacological preparations, metabolic acidosis will generally resolve.

Interventions to augment cardiac output

Manipulation of the haemodynamic variables which determine cardiac output is effected through the introduction of various pharmacological preparations, therapies which support the circulation and correct metabolic derangements, helping to improve tissue oxygenation. Selection of the appropriate measures to improve the cardiac output demands a sound appreciation of normal cardiovascular physiological principles and the body's response to dysfunctional states.

    Here, we concentrate on the manipulation of preload, contractility, afterload and heart rate to effect improvement in myocardial failure. Extreme caution is exercised in manipulation of these variables in the preterm and term infant who lack cardiac reserves, because of an immature myocardium.[44,45] Sympathetic innervation is incomplete at the time of birth, making the myocardium far less responsive to these drugs.[82] These infants are therefore extremely sensitive to alteration in pressure/volume dynamics and therefore have:

- limited preload reserve (i.e., reduced myocardial contractile force and shortening ability);
- a reduced ability to accommodate increments in preload; and
- limited responses from cardiotonic preparations that increase contractility.[21,45]

There are other developmental aspects pertaining to neonatal dysmaturity that impose special considerations in relation to manipulation of the circulatory variables. Immature renal function and the potential for fluid and electrolyte imbalance are important considerations. Similarly, immaturity of vasomotor function and inadequate temperature regulatory mechanisms impose special problems in the manipulation of cardiovascular status, rendering less predictable responses from interventions.[80]

Manipulation of preload and afterload: vasodilator therapy

Vasodilator drugs are commonly used in manipulation of preload and afterload, having effects on either the systemic arterioles and/or veins.[45] Vasodilator preparations improve cardiac output by:

- reducing the impedance to ventricular ejection resulting in an increase in stroke volume and a reduction in end-systolic volume (when optimal filling pressure is maintained);
- increasing venous capacitance evoking a reduction in venous return and a subsequent fall in filling pressure (i.e., promoting a decrease in end-diastolic pressure);
- reducing the filling pressure which enhances coronary artery perfusion and by improving myocardial function when the mean arterial pressure is maintained within a normal range; and
- decreasing end-diastolic volumes, thereby promoting an improvement in myocardial compliance.[21,83]

The introduction of vasodilator preparations in cardiac dysfunctional states is generally restricted to situations where there is elevation of ventricular end-diastolic pressures and systemic vascular resistance, which impose an additional workload on the failing myocardium.[25] Vasodilators are rarely effective when used in isolation, but remarkable improvement in cardiovascular status can be achieved by manipulating the other determinants of cardiac output, by optimising preload through fluid therapy and titrating inotropic support.

Acute, severe cardiac failure which develops in infancy and childhood may require the use of invasive haemodynamic monitoring as an important adjunct to clinical assessment. The haemodynamic variables which can be monitored in an infant in failure help to gauge the effectiveness of response when continuous infusion of pharmacological supports are used (i.e., inotropes such as dopamine and dobutamine and vasoactive agents like sodium nitroprusside and prostacyclin). By contrast, the infant and child with chronic cardiac failure may respond well to the administration of oral preparations. The vasodilator of choice in chronic situations is captopril, a competitive inhibitor of the angiotensin converting enzyme (ACE inhibitor)[84] (**Table 11.6**).

Diuretic therapy

Manipulation of preload results in an alteration in the ventricular end-diastolic volume, effected through change occurring within the sarcomere length.[90] Reduction in preload through the use of vasodilators (as outlined above) and diuretics, for example frusemide, reduces oedema and improves myocardial function.[68] Daily diuretic regimens of frusemide require either potassium supplementation or the addition of a potassium-sparing diuretic, (e.g., spironolactone) to prevent hypokalaemia (**Table 11.6**).

The use of frusemide for the treatment of cardiac failure in preterm infants with a patent ductus arteriosus has been shown to maintain ductal patency, the result of stimulation of prostaglandin synthesis induced by frusemide administration.[68,91] The concomitant use of frusemide with indomethacin, however, is reportedly effective in closing the ductus.[91]

Manipulation of contractility: inotropic therapy

Many different inotropes are currently available, each with specific adrenergic receptor sensitivity. The selection of the most appropriate inotrope is dependant on the underlying disease process and the clinical presentation of the infant or child.[19,30]

Inotropic preparations provide support for the failing myocardium once the primary factors of the myocardial failure are eliminated (wherever possible), and correction of the secondary factors have been instituted, i.e., oxygen carriage, metabolic derangements and augmentation of the preload and afterload.[21] A review of the inotropic preparations administered via continuous infusion is provided in the section Perioperative Cardiac Nursing: Manipulation of the Myocardial Contractile State.

Digoxin is a positive, yet weak inotropic drug used in the relief of congestive cardiac failure. The action of the drug results from inhibition of the enzyme Na–K ATPase.[19,84,91] Sodium levels become elevated in the intracellular myocardium, causing stimulation of the sodium-calcium exchange system. Calcium entry into the cell is enhanced, thereby increasing its availability for myocardial contraction, resulting in an added force of contraction.[91,92] The reduction in heart rate induced by digoxin is attributed to both a vagal effect and suppression of the sinoatrial node.[92]

Digoxin uptake is considered to be enhanced in newborn infants due to immaturity of the myocardium and therefore the inotropic effects may not significantly improve myocardial contractility.[19,84] Factors that are known to increase the sensitivity of cardiac muscle to digoxin are:

- electrolyte imbalances, particularly hypokalaemia;[93]
- hypoxaemia and ischaemia of the myocardium;
- inflammatory reactions of the heart, e.g., myocarditis; and
- simultaneous use of sympathomimetic preparations[19] (**Table 11.6**).

In summary, vasoactive preparations may be used either in isolation or in combination to effect the desired response in the child. Brief reviews of the drug receptor sites, actions and recommended doses are included in **Table 11.6**. Comprehensive reviews of all vasoactive preparations are available in other works.[19,21,91]

Emotional support: implications to nursing practice

Nursing personnel fulfil a crucial role in support of infants and children and their parents and families when confronted with illness, especially during acute and critical illness. An ability to provide optimal psychosocial care is vital, therefore relevant information must be elucidated from the parents at the time of admission. Advanced communication and counselling skills will facilitate interaction with the parents at a difficult and disquieting time. Importantly, information regarding the parents' perception of the infant's or child's illness is required. Knowledge regarding the interdependence of the family and their

Table 11.6 Drugs selected for manipulation of cardiac output in congestive cardiac failure and acute low cardiac output states: diuretics, vasodilators, inotrope/vasopressor agents

Pharmacological group	Drug mechanism/dose	Comments/ Adverse effects
Diuretics		
Frusemide	Loop of Henle (ascending limb). Inhibits sodium and potassium transport. IV: 1–2 mg/kg Oral: 2–3 mg/kg	Diuretic regimens: Second daily dose: no supplement required. Daily dose: frusemide + potassium chloride (2 mg/kg/day). Observe for: hyponatraemia; hypokalaemia; hypercalcaemia hyperuricaemia.[53,68,85]
Spironolactone	Potassium-sparing agent. Inhibits sodium, potassium and hydrogen ion exchange in distal tubule. Competitive inhibition of aldosterone. Oral: 1.5–3 mg/kg/day in 3 divided doses[53,68,85,86]	Hyperkalaemia, acidosis.
Vasodilators		
Captopril	ACE inhibitor Arteriovenous dilatation Newborn: 0.1–0.4 mg/kg/day Infant: 0.5–6.0 mg/kg/day Child: 1–1.5 mg/kg/day	Oral administration: 75% absorption 30–40% absorption with food) — Caution in renal failure.[35,47,53,69,85]
Sodium nitroprusside	Smooth muscle relaxation systemic/pulmonary arteriovenous dilatation 0.5–8 µg/kg/min	Metabolised in liver to thiocyanate, cyanide. Avoid: long-term, high-dose infusion. Consider monitoring plasma levels (thiocyanate: 5–10 mg/dl) (cyanide >200 mg/dl) Continuous monitoring of arterial pressure is essential
Nitro-glycerine	Systemic/pulmonary arteriolar dilator (primarily). 0.1–10+ µg/kg/min	Observe for hypotension Drug inactivated by polyvinyl chloride.[35,53,83]

Table 11.6 (*continued*)

Pharmacological group	Drug mechanism/dose	Comments/ Adverse effects
Tolazoline	Alpha adrenergic blocking agent. Directly affects vascular smooth muscle. Affects pulmonary and systemic vascular resistance. 1–2 mg/kg initially then, 1–2 mg/kg/hour (continuous infusion)	Observe for: hypotension; thrombocytopenia; GIT bleeding. Response variable.[35,83,86,87]
Prostaglandin E$_1$	systemic and pulmonary vasodilator 0.01–0.1 μg/kg/min	Observe for: tachycardia; headache, abdominal cramps[86,87,89]
Prostacyclin	Vascular smooth muscle relaxant	Causes disaggregation of pulmonary microthrombi.[83,88]

Inotropes

Digoxin	Inhibition of Na-K ATPase. Increases contractility by increasing calcium availability to the cells.	Therapeutic range small (1.1–2.1 ng/dL) Observe for: arrhythmia (stimulates the vagus nerve) CNS signs; GIT signs.[47,53,85]

Digitalisation (μg/kg)		Maintenance (μg/kg)
Preterm	20–25	5
Term	25	8–10
1–12 months	35	10–15
over 1 year	25–35	5–10
Adolescents	10–25	2–5

Dopamine	Sympathomimetic amine Potent inotrope/vasoactive dose related agent. *Low:* (1–5 μg/kg/min) beta$_1$ and dopaminergic agonist, increases mesenteric and renal perfusion. *Moderate:* (5–10 μg/kg/min) alpha adrenergic agonist increases SVR. *High:* (>10 μg/kg/min) alpha adrenergic effects predominate.[35,53,85,90]	Observe: tachyarrhythmia Essential for care: haemodynamic monitoring
Dobutamine	Inotrope (increases tone) synthetic catecholamine: minimal changes to heart rate beta$_1$ selective preparation (vasodilator) 2–20 μg/kg/min.[53,85,90]	High dose: — tachyarrhythmia — increases myocardial oxygen requirements

Table 11.6 (*continued*)

Pharmacological group	Drug mechanism/dose	Comments/ Adverse effects
Adrenalin	endogenous catecholamine 0.05–0.15 µg/kg/min low dose: alpha, beta$_1$ and beta$_2$ effects — alpha effects predominate at higher doses[35,53]	— increased SVR —> increases in myocardial oxygen requirements and work load
Noradrenaline	Endogenous catecholamine 0.05–1.0 µg/kg/min alpha and beta$_1$ agonist	Primary indicator: — reduced SVR/shock — observe for: — — tachyarrhythmias work and oxygen requirements — used in conjunction (phenoxybenzamine)[35]
Isoprenaline	Pure beta adrenergic agent (beta$_1$ increases heart rate and inotropy; beta$_2$ decreases SVR) — 0.05–0.1 µg/kg/min	Observe: — — tachyarrhythmia — hypotension — increases myocardial oxygen requirements[35]

support network (e.g., grandparents, extended families, significant others) enables the design of a plan for care to meet the special needs of the infant or child and family.[94,95]

Research undertaken into parental stress and paediatric intensive care units has heightened nurse's perceptions of parental stressors.[96] The research indicates the interruption to parent–child relationships imposed by acute illness and separation to be a greater stressor than the environmental effects of a paediatric intensive care facility. Further, parents of infants and children admitted to paediatric intensive care units under emergency conditions were more highly stressed by the procedures undertaken on their child when a comparison was drawn between parents of children admitted for elective surgery and children readmitted with chronic diseases.

From a nursing perspective, the study identifies the needs of parents for information and education which highlights the important role of nurses. Encouraging parents to be actively involved with their infant or child's care will help reduce the major stressor imposed by separation. Support for the parents is achieved through explanation of the child's illness and care, which helps to alleviate the stress caused by a knowledge deficit.[96] Parental adaptation to the situation and the environment is facilitated through support provided by nursing personnel. Families adopt a variety of mechanisms to cope with acute illness and intensive care. Recent research suggests the family unit is impelled to identify and develop self-coping strategies to support the infant or child and each other.[97]

In providing an optimal plan of care to support the young child who develops cardiac failure, a sound knowledge of the child's developmental stage and growth patterns is essential. A child's perception of her or his illness and response to acute hospitalisation is determined by the level of development and thus the integration of growth and development principles into the plan of care is essential.[98] Recognition of the psychological responses of children to their acute illness and management by nursing personnel allows appropriate support to be offered, which can enhance the child's adaptation to his or her illness and environment.

Perioperative Cardiac Nursing

Postoperative paediatric cardiac nursing affords a special challenge for nurses in the care of infants, children and adolescents who are often critically ill. A philosophy of care based on the pursuit and perpetuation of a standard of clinical excellence is a critical factor in determining the children's outcome.

The role of the nurse in this clinical speciality has been extended in recent times due to the advances within the profession, in paediatric cardiac surgery and in biotechnology. The outcome of the children postoperatively is in large part reliant upon the proficiency of the nurses' clinical assessment skills and the ability to analyse clinical findings and physiological parameters. Early intervention to support a failing circulation before decompensation of the infant or child's clinical state is the goal of care. In-depth understanding of intracardiac haemodynamics and physiological functioning is fundamental to nurses' critical decision making, which will aid the recovery of the infant or child.

The demands of paediatric cardiothoracic nursing involve special challenges in optimising care for the infants and children. It is well known that the various congenital cardiac lesions require considerably different approaches in management. The approach therefore to postoperative nursing care must be flexible and allow for modification when necessary. Infants and children with complex anatomical abnormalities require technically demanding surgical procedures which are often followed by a stormy and prolonged postoperative recovery. It is imperative, therefore, that precision in nursing assessment and interventional support is provided.

Critical care nursing in paediatric cardiac care assumes a heightened responsibility and accountability for clinical practice. Current trends suggest an even greater impact by the technology with the development of more highly invasive support mechanisms which will maintain the life of the critically ill infant and child following cardiovascular surgery. (**Figure 11.1**)

This section therefore aims to examine the multiplicity of factors pertaining to the perioperative nursing care of infants, children and adolescents including:

- Preoperative preparation of the infant, child, adolescent and family.
- Intraoperative considerations.
- Immediate postoperative nursing assessment and interventional support.
- The potential for complication and the implications for nursing practice.
- Postoperative progress.
- Outcomes for the infant, child and adolescent after cardiac surgery and the related nursing interventions.
- Palliative and corrective surgical procedures and implications for nursing practice.
- Principles of haemodynamic monitoring.

Importantly, the discussion emphasises the clinical nursing specialist's role in assessment, problem solving and critical decision making, which are crucial to attaining the goal of care — clinical excellence.

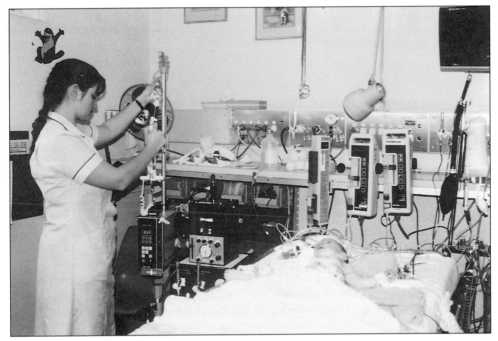

Figure 11.1 Providing care for a young infant in the acute postoperative recovery period following open-heart surgery for repair of an intracardiac problem.

PALLIATIVE CARDIAC SURGICAL PROCEDURES

Various palliative procedures are undertaken to improve cardiac states in infants and children whose condition is not amenable to surgical correction or in whom correction in infancy is not possible.[99] The various shunt procedures and the surgery for pulmonary artery banding are most often undertaken as closed-heart procedures, while the complex palliations (e.g., the Fontan procedure) require an open-heart surgical approach and the support of cardiopulmonary bypass (CPB). A review of palliative surgical procedures is included at the end of this section and includes the systemic to pulmonary artery shunt, venous to pulmonary artery shunt, atrial septectomy and pulmonary artery banding.

CORRECTIVE CARDIAC SURGICAL PROCEDURES

The relief of structural cardiac defects of congenital or acquired aetiology requires an open-heart surgical approach for repair of an intracardiac defect (e.g., ventricular septal defect, atrial septal defect and tetralogy of Fallot), whereas a closed-heart approach is used for repair of an extracardiac lesion (e.g., patent ductus arteriosus and coarctation of the aorta). Extracardiac reparative procedures generally use a surgical approach via a thoracotomy. Intracardiac repairs, however, will generally require the support of cardiopulmonary bypass via a midline sternotomy to enable the repair to be completed under optimal surgical conditions, in an essentially bloodless field with preservation of organ perfusion assured.[100]

PREOPERATIVE PREPARATION

Preparation of the infant, child or adolescent and parents at the time of cardiac surgery requires the consideration of physical, psychological, emotional and social factors. The adaptation of a child and his or her parents to a critical care environment is reliant upon careful preparation and education before surgery and therefore holds important implications for nursing personnel.

Illness and admission to a critical care facility imposes major stresses upon the family unit.[94,97,101,102] Inadequate preparation of the family can in part be detrimental to their ability to cope with the stressors of their child's surgery. Parents may be unable to develop strategies which sustain, support and strengthen the family unit. Dysfunctional patterns may develop within a family when the coping strategies fail to provide the necessary support.

Psychological and sociological considerations: implications for nursing

The initial interview on admission is crucial in determining the child and family's preparedness for the hospitalisation and surgery. The child's developmental level, perception of the operation and hospitalisation must be established. Additionally, detailed information regarding the infant or child's normal behaviours, routines and feeding regimens is required. Family ideals, wishes and needs (e.g., cultural and religious beliefs) are ascertained and will be invaluable in facilitating the child's integration into the ward and planning of care for the postoperative recovery phase.

The role nursing personnel fulfil in the preparation of the family when infants, children or adolescents require cardiac surgery is crucial. It is of the utmost importance to establish the parents' understanding of their child's hospitalisation and surgery, and to answer the child's and parent's questions, reinforcing information previously given by the cardiologist and surgeon. Expanding on information about the preoperative preparation, intraoperative considerations and the acute and ongoing recovery phase is essential. The adaptation to the critical care environment by the child and family will be optimised by the appropriate preparation. It is important that explanations are not overly technical, thereby allaying further anxiety about the surgery, yet the information must be complete, address the special needs of each family member and not conflict with information previously given.[103] Great reliance is placed on the communication and counselling ability of the nurse in the preparation for surgery of the infant, child or adolescent and family.

The information needs of the parents are multifaceted and complex. They require information about their child's emotional and behavioural responses to the surgery, the physical effects of intensive care, patterns of communication within the critical care environment and the temporary changes which can occur in the parenting role. These issues are of significant concern to parents and need to be discussed with them.

Detailed explanations regarding the infant, child or adolescent's physical preparation for the surgery is provided and includes introduction and background information on all personnel who will be involved with the surgery and recovery. It is important to provide information to the parents on the infant or child's fasting times, premedication and transfer to operating theatres. Provision of appropriate waiting room facilities for families is mandatory. All units should have a policy whereby parents are kept well informed of their infant or child's progress or problems as they arise. Reassurance is required by parents that all messages from the surgical team regarding intraoperative progress will be imparted.

To facilitate the parents' adaptation to their infant or child's surgery, detailed explanations are essential prior to the procedure. Information regarding anticipated outcomes and surgical risks, the level of respiratory support, invasive monitoring and tubes, lines, drips and drains that will be required for postoperative support should be provided. Upon the child's return to the intensive care unit, parents require further explanation about the outcome of their child's surgery, his or her clinical condition, level of consciousness, colour and pain relief. They require reinforcement of information previously given in addition to information regarding blood transfusions, support drugs and the temporary pacing aspects of their child's care. Assurance that generous pain relief will be provided and encouragement that they as parents can participate in their child's care postoperatively, is reassuring for parents and enhances their adaptation to the situation. The parents are therefore encouraged to talk to their children, hold their hands and be available for comfort and support. Ideally, the parents and the child are oriented to the critical care facility as part of the preoperative preparatory phase, if it is considered appropriate to the child's developmental level.

The requirement for adequate preoperative preparation is evident throughout the child's hospitalisation. Parents are advised that support facilities provided by nursing personnel and other health care professionals (e.g., social workers) are always available. In times of grief, the assistance of bereavement counsellors and the clergy is provided and any additional support the parents may wish should be actively sought.

Physical considerations: preoperative work-up

A comprehensive nursing and medical assessment is undertaken upon admission. The tests are undertaken routinely to establish baselines and eliminate potential problems which may influence surgical morbidity and mortality. Full blood profiles are required to exclude factors which may influence cardiac function in the postoperative phase of recovery. Infants and children with polycythaemia have increased viscosity of their blood, causing additional impedance to blood flow. A state of anaemia poses problems because of the reduction in oxygen carriage and must be excluded preoperatively. Further, the blood film can detect sepsis which may be difficult to diagnose by clinical means in sick, young infants with cardiac problems.

Monitoring of serum electrolyte, urea and creatine levels facilitates the assessment of renal function preoperatively. Establishing a baseline is vital, especially in infants where renal immaturity may present problems. Cross-matching of blood is essential for all cardiac surgical procedures. The quantity of available blood is dependent on the surgical procedure to be undertaken, the body surface area of the child and any anticipated bleeding problems.

Coagulation screening is very important in the neonate and in the older infant or child with cyanotic congenital cardiac disease because of their reduced clotting factors and platelet counts. When the red blood cell volume is elevated in children with cyanotic congenital heart disease, there is a subsequent drop in the volume of plasma which contains fibrinogen, an important constituent in blood clotting.[104] Children receiving anticoagulant therapy following valve replacements, who require additional surgery also need full coagulation screening. These children will need to cease their warfarin 3 to 4 days before surgery and are covered in the interim with continuous infusions of heparin.

Generally, prior to the surgical admission, a large number of infants and children will have undergone formal cardiac investigations to delineate specific anatomical features and physiological variables. Infants and children who are admitted for corrective and palliative procedures which do not require CPB may not require the same level of surgical work-up. The investigation and diagnostic tests undertaken are at the discretion of the cardiology and surgical team.

Routine medications (e.g., digoxin and propranolol) are withdrawn prior to CPB surgery, due to the potential for complications both intraoperatively and in the acute postoperative recovery phase caused by the long-term effects of these preparations. Digoxin is usually withheld 24 to 48 hours before the surgery to reduce the risk of intraoperative and postoperative arrhythmia, which often results from electrolyte changes resulting from CPB.[105,106] Propranolol, a beta adrenergic blocking agent used to control hypercyanotic spells in tetralogy of Fallot, is generally continued to within 24 hours of operation, then ceased due to the potential for myocardial depression. Rarely, propranolol may have to be continued up to the time of surgery.[105] Astute observation of these infants is essential, due to the risk of recurring cyanotic episodes once the blood levels of propranolol drop (see Cyanotic Congenital Heart Disease, Chapter 6). Digoxin and propranolol, however, are not usually withdrawn from infants and children in preparing for closed-heart surgical procedures.

Infants who are critically ill with severe heart failure or acute hypercyanosis will require the maintenance of various intracardiac haemodynamic and respiratory supports. The use of appropriate pharmacological preparations (i.e., inotropes and diuretics for the infant in severe heart failure or prostaglandin and sedatives) additional to mechanical ventilation for the infant with a ductal-dependent lesion, will provide the necessary support for these infants until definitive surgical therapy stabilises their cardiorespiratory status.[100]

Premedication and preparation for anaesthesia

The premedication is designed to effect a calm, relaxed, sleep inducive state before surgery. The selection of a non-cardiac-depressant anaesthetic agent is determined by the infant or child's cardiovascular status and the anaesthetist's preference. Generally, a combination of anticholinergic and analgesic or sedative–hypnotic preparations is used.[100,106]

Morphine administered in doses required for anaesthetic use (1 to 2 mg/kg) has been found to produce significant histamine release and hypotension. Reports therefore indicate a trend towards the use of other narcotic preparations.[100] Anaesthetic induction is well facilitated in an infant or child who arrives in theatre in a haemodynamically and emotionally stable state. Crying and struggling in many of these infants and children can result in an increase in their right-to-left shunt and even reversal of left-to-right shunts in some infants when pulmonary vascular resistance is significantly elevated.[107]

Controversy still exists regarding premedication of very young, sick infants[100] who often only receive atropine premedication. Atropine, an anticholinergic agent, blocks vagal tone at the time of intubation in infants who are dependant on the heart rate for maintenance of their cardiac output and reduces secretions which may precipitate aspiration or laryngospasm.[106–108]

The requirements for intraoperative monitoring are established before the infant or child arrives in theatre. The level of invasive haemodynamic monitoring is determined by the type of procedure to be undertaken (i.e., open or closed, palliative or corrective surgery), the anticipated surgical time and the potential for complication. Most infants and children for closed heart procedures require arterial pressure monitoring with or without central venous pressure monitoring. Children for CPB surgery require varying degrees of invasive haemodynamic monitoring and additional support lines. All lines other than those inserted directly at the time of surgery, e.g., left atrial, right atrial and pulmonary artery lines, are sited at the time of anaesthetic induction and include an intra-arterial line, at least 2 peripheral venous cannulae and a central venous or right atrial line with multilumen access.

Intraoperative considerations

Cardiac surgical procedures, other than the relatively straightforward procedures (e.g., ligation of a patent ductus arteriosus and closure of an atrial septal defect) generally take several hours. Following a prolonged period in the operating theatre, infants and children return to the intensive care unit in a critical condition, often hypothermic, pale and poorly perfused peripherally. This postoperative clinical status may be a consequence of the following:

- Poor preoperative status in some infants and children.
- The major insult imposed by the surgery, especially when a ventriculotomy is performed.
- The cardiodepressant action of anaesthetic agents.
- The influence of CPB upon cellular metabolism, fluid and electrolyte homeostasis, systemic and pulmonary vascular resistances and intravascular volumes.[109]

CPB is established by directing systemic venous return via an extracorporeal circuit following the cannulation of the superior and inferior vena cava or the right atrial chamber.[109] Blood flows due to gravitational force and gases are exchanged by means of a membrane oxygenator. A heat exchanger in the circuit provides for the initial cooling of the blood, to induce states of moderate or profound hypothermia which are reversed upon completion of the surgical procedure. The extracorporeal circuit (completed by the inclusion of roller pumps), redirects the oxygenated, heparinised blood via a cannula inserted in the aorta and pumps the blood at pressure to maintain optimal end-organ perfusion.

Once CPB is established, mechanical ventilation of the lungs is discontinued, although a physiological level of continuous positive airway pressure is maintained. The majority of intricate open heart repairs require a period of deep hypothermia, hypoperfusion and/or total circulatory arrest.[110] With an infant or child's nasopharyngeal temperature reduced to 18°C to 20°C, complete myocardial relaxation is achieved following aortic cross clamping and the instillation of cold cardioplegic solution into the aortic root,[105,111] The induced state of profound hypothermia reduces the body's metabolic requirements, thereby reducing oxygen consumption,[109] optimising central nervous system and myocardial protection,[100,112,113] and reducing the incidence of postoperative low cardiac output. Controversy now exists as to what constitutes a safe period of total circulatory arrest in infants, with reports indicating seizure activity in the short term and the potential for central nervous system damage in the long term, secondary to circulatory arrest.[100] Circulatory arrest times in excess of 60 minutes are suggested as unsafe, with evidence now indicating that periods of arrest in excess of 45 minute are potentially unsafe.[109,113] The aetiologic basis for cerebral damage after CPB is the result of the alteration to cerebral perfusion associated with periods of hypoperfusion, circulatory arrest or cerebral ischaemia, and the risks of embolisation, especially in children with right-to-left shunts.[114]

During CPB, infants and children are exposed to extreme fluctuations in arterial pressure, temperature, $PaCO_2$ levels and blood viscosity, all factors which determine cerebral blood flow autoregulation. Consideration of these factors and the implications they hold for the infant and child's cerebral perfusion in the intraoperative and postoperative recovery phase are important in clinical practice. The hypoperfusion that occurs during CPB may result in cerebral ischaemia, when autoregulation of cerebral blood flow is lost.[110]

Recent research highlights the extreme conditions imposed by CPB on the paediatric age group, suggesting that susceptibility to neuropsychological morbidity is greater in the young and that development of postoperative neuropsychological dysfunction increases with decreasing age. Importantly, the research concluded that temperature is a major factor in altering cerebral blood flow at the time of CPB in neonates, infants and children. The study indicated a loss of cerebral autoregulation with CPB and deep hypothermia. This contrasts markedly to a state of moderate hypothermia (25°C to 32°C), when cerebral blood flow autoregulation is preserved. Further, the researchers question the risk imposed to neonates and infants by the periods of total circulatory arrest, implying an increased risk of impairment to their cerebral perfusion.[110] Currently, the approach adopted to minimise these effects, is to maintain reduced flow rates with the CPB, using only short periods of circulatory arrest.

Current research now indicates that surgical morbidity and mortality is increased in newborn infants requiring CPB surgery using a period of profound hypothermia and circulatory arrest. These procedures initiate a severe stress response in the infant, producing detrimental endocrine and metabolic effects.[115,116] The stress response is clearly demonstrated within the newborn infant at the time of CPB surgery, profound hypothermia and circulatory arrest and is reflected in the plasma levels of catecholamines, endorphins and glucagon.[115] Further, blood sugar and lactate levels increase markedly at the time of sternotomy with additional increases noted at the time of deep hypothermia and circulatory arrest, peaking again upon completion of the surgery. The serum levels remain elevated for 12 hours. The increases in adrenalin and insulin persist within the circulation for 24 hours, with serum glucagon levels peaking by 24 hours postoperatively. The increase in catecholamine levels, especially noradrenaline, occurring with CPB is attributed to the negligible pulmonary circulation at the time of bypass. It will be recalled that noradrenaline is largely inactivated within the lungs.[109] Nurses need to appreciate these recent findings when caring for newborn infants requiring cardiac surgery. Marked improvement in the infant's clinical state can be expected when metabolic homeostasis is assured in the critical postoperative recovery phase.

The lack of myocardial reserve in the neonate and young infant and their immature physiological functioning are relative considerations in deciding for primary surgical repair as against a palliative procedure. Staged repairs, such as those performed to palliate infants prior to surgical correction, increase the risks of secondary pathological conditions which may affect the heart, lungs and central nervous system.[100]

IMMEDIATE NURSING ASSESSMENT AND SUPPORT AFTER CARDIAC SURGERY

Clinical assessment remains the fundamental component of nursing practice in the postoperative care of infants, children and adolescents, with continued nursing assessment of all body systems essential from the time of admission to the intensive care unit. The principles of assessment and interventional support remain common to all infants and children following cardiac surgical procedures, irrespective of the surgical approach

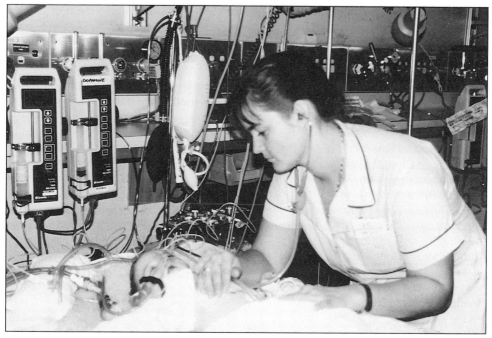

Figure 11.2 Undertaking assessment of an infant in the acute postoperative recovery period following open-heart surgery.

selected. Prioritisation of care upon the infant or child's immediate return to the critical care unit is imperative. Assessment of the general clinical state, with careful evaluation of the cardiorespiratory status is of highest priority (**Figure 11.2**).

A verbal report from the surgical and anaesthetic team will inform the intensive care staff of:

- the child's current clinical status;
- the nature and extent of the operative procedure;
- aortic cross-clamping and bypass times;
- any notable intraoperative events which may influence the recovery;
- intraoperative and post-bypass rhythm disturbances;
- the infant's response to volume loading after CPB and the filling pressure that optimises cardiac output;
- vasoactive preparations required to support circulation;
- the infant's need for ventilation and appropriate ventilatory parameters and the plan for ventilatory support; and
- the sites of invasive haemodynamic monitoring lines.[117,118]

Ideally, 2 nurses receive the infant or child into the critical care unit as part of the specialist team which settles the infant into the unit in an ordered, well planned process. The primary nurse assumes responsibility for the immediate and ongoing plan of care. The immediate nursing actions are numerous and are undertaken while maintaining continuous, careful evaluation of the clinical condition, which may be subject to change with little warning.

The priority of care is to maintain a vigilant, continuous assessment of the cardiorespiratory state while undertaking the various duties that need to be performed when receiving these infants and children into the unit. The principles of care in receiving an infant or child after cardiac surgery are the same as for any patient upon acute transfer.

Determination of the infant or child's need for ventilatory support or their suitability for extubation is generally guided by the age, the complexity of the surgery and the preoperative, intraoperative and postoperative cardiorespiratory state.[106] Generally, after closed heart and palliative procedures, the infant or child is extubated following reversal of the anaesthetic and neuromuscular blocking agents.[105,106] Oxygen delivery devices which provide appropriate humidification to gas flow are essential to adequately support the infant or child in the acute postoperative phase of recovery. Infants and young children who require careful evaluation of shunt patency are supported with mechanical ventilation until stabilised.[105] Provision of respiratory support after CPB surgery has been shown to reduce the morbidity associated with early extubation. Most centres advocate ventilation in the early phase of recovery due to the rapidly changing haemodynamic state induced by CPB and the potential for post-surgical bleeding, which could necessitate reintubation.[105] Support may therefore be required for a period of hours to several days with extubation planned once haemodynamic stability is assured.

Observance of monitored parameters

The invasive haemodynamic set-up has a high priority in post-surgical assessment. The transducers are zeroed and calibrated and attached to the computerised bedside monitoring system. Continuous displays of ECG, arterial pressure, left and right atrial pressures and at times pulmonary artery pressure are provided. Careful evaluation of monitored parameters and waveform configuration guide management when used in combination with clinical assessment (see Modalities in Haemodynamic Monitoring later in this chapter).

Estimating blood loss via percardial, retrosternal and pleural drains is important. Losses in excess of 100 mL/m^2/hour warrant screening for coagulation abnormalities and consideration for re-exploration to control surgical bleeding.

Evaluation of cardiovascular status requires awareness of various inotropic and vasodilator preparations that may be used to support the circulation. The infant or child is rewarmed before coming off CPB, but environmental influences and the transfer from theatre can precipitate a drop in body temperature. On return to the intensive care unit, the infant or child is often mildly hypothermic. Hypothermia initiates significant dysfunctional problems for myocardial contractility when not controlled. Oxygen and glucose requirements are increased and potentiate the development of hypoxia and hypoglycaemia, which further impedes myocardial function. Rewarming is therefore of high priority and is achieved with servo-controlled open-plan cribs for newborns and warming blankets and overhead radiant heaters for infants and children. Central temperature monitoring is highly desirable, other than in the neonatal period where it is not routinely practised. Problems arise with skin temperature monitoring when low cardiac output states develop. Blood flow is diverted away from the skin to more vital areas, causing skin temperature readings to be less reliable when used in isolation. Many nurses advocate the use of core/periphery temperature monitoring as a quantitative guide to cardiovascular assessment.[119] Variation in temperature of greater than 2°C is reportedly a highly reliable indication of severe cardiovascular compromise.[120]

Baseline observations of all monitored parameters including heart rate and rhythm, blood pressure, atrial pressures, temperature and urine output, are undertaken as soon as possible, once the child is settled. Blood loss and replacement is recorded carefully as are vasoactive and other infusions, ventilatory parameters and the pattern of respiration if the child is breathing spontaneously. Various diagnostic tests which guide management are attended to as soon as practicable upon the child's return from theatre and regularly during the first 24 hours of recovery (e.g., arterial blood gas levels). Serum electrolyte levels are generally estimated every 4 hours, then daily until parenteral fluids are discontinued; clotting times are sampled immediately and then as required, chest x-rays are taken immediately, at 4 hours after operation and then daily until extubation, unless indicated otherwise and an ECG is recorded immediately following surgery and then again at discharge.

Temporary epicardial pacing wires attached to the right atrium and ventricle are often inserted following CPB surgery as a precautionary manoeuvre, especially when the infant or child has demonstrated rhythm disturbances when coming off bypass.[120,121] The infant or child is considered to be at risk of rhythm disturbances following ventricular septal defect repairs and where the surgery is undertaken at atrial level, most especially in the region of the sinoatrial and atrioventricular nodes and intra-atrial pathways, (e.g., repair of an ostium primum atrial septal defect, atrio-ventricular canal defect and tetralogy of Fallot).[120] Any prolonged surgical procedure, however, predisposes the infant to arrhythmia. Continuous ECG monitoring is therefore generally maintained for a period of 36 to 48 hours postoperatively, unless rhythm disturbances demand continued, close observation for longer periods.[121]

The risk of macro and microelectrocution is an issue with all patients in critical care, especially when pacing wires are exposed and when the barrier of protection (the skin) is infiltrated with fluid-filled (often saline based) intracardiac lines. Pacing wires are insulated to the tips only and must be protected from moisture and the transmission of current leakage. Because of the potential need for urgent access, the wires are positioned to facilitate ready availability if required.

Once the infant or child is settled within the unit, the parents are encouraged to spend time with their child. The primary nurse spends time acquainting the parents with the acute situation and informs them of the need for lines, drips, drains and monitoring. It is at this time that the greatest benefit from diligent preoperative preparation is felt by parents.

The infant or child is nursed flat for the first few hours following surgery or until the cardiovascular state stabilises. Gentle repositioning each 1.5 to 2 hours is generally adequate. All basic care is attended on a 2 to 4 hourly schedule as required or as the condition permits. The goal of care is to maximise rest, therefore nursing interventions must be well planned to meet the child's needs.

RESPIRATORY ASSESSMENT AND SUPPORT

A complete respiratory assessment and evaluation of interventional support is an immediate priority of care. The majority of infants and children following CPB and a number following simple and more complex palliative procedures, especially in the neonatal period, will require respiratory support for a period, ranging from hours to several days postoperatively.[105,120] The necessity for ventilation is dependent upon the infant or child's cardiovascular status, the type of operative procedure undertaken and anticipated problems which may influence recovery. A gentle transition from the anaesthetised state following more complex surgical procedures is preferred. Reversal of the anaesthetic and relaxant agents is therefore not undertaken.[100]

The mode of ventilation which will best support the infant or child in relieving the workload of breathing is selected, commonly adopting a time-cycled, pressure-limited approach to ventilation. The parameters are set to include tidal volume, peak and positive end expiratory pressure limits, ventilation rate, inspiratory and expiratory ratio and oxygen level. Alarm limits are set and a thorough clinical assessment is undertaken to evaluate the adequacy of the selected pattern of ventilation in meeting the infant or child's particular needs. Pulmonary function and acid base status are further evaluated through arterial blood gas analysis. A chest x-ray is required to detect fluid or air collection, collapse or consolidation. Additional non-invasive, continuous monitoring of the cardiorespiratory status is achieved through devices which record levels of end-tidal carbon dioxide, transcapillary oxygen and carbon dioxide and oxygen saturations, which are obtained via pulse oxymetry.[120,122,123]

Complex surgical procedures may necessitate extended periods of ventilatory support with a need for additional analgesic cover and sedation used in conjunction with full muscle relaxation. Optimal ventilatory management in these infants and children is imperative, as even mild oxygen derangements may have a profound influence on cardiac performance.[100]

Less complex surgical procedures performed in infancy and childhood, (e.g., ligation of a patent ductus arteriosus and closure of atrial septal defect) rarely require ventilatory support, however, an oxygen-enriched, well humidified environment is essential. Once haemodynamic stability is assured, elective extubation is undertaken following reversal of the anaesthetic and muscle relaxant. Arterial blood gas sampling in children with arterial lines and pulse oxymetry is a feature of continuous clinical assessment of the cardiorespiratory state.

Once the infant is extubated, the pattern of respiration should be assessed, observing for any signs of respiratory fatigue or compromise, such as tachypnoea associated with agitation or irritability. The increased work of breathing associated with respiratory distress is manifest by intercostal or substernal recession, grunting respirations, the use of accessory muscles of respiration and nasal flaring. In respiratory distress a reduction in functional residual capacity and lung compliance and a ventilation/perfusion mismatch will culminate in a state of hypercarbia, acidosis and hypoxaemia. Irritability in an infant necessitates a full clinical assessment to determine the cause and eliminate a state of hypoxia before analgesia and sedation are increased. The need for careful assessment of the respiratory status cannot be overemphasised and if the child is unable to cope effectively, early intervention with intubation and ventilation will prevent him or her from becoming too tired and developing cardiorespiratory failure. The clinical nurse has a most important responsibility in identifying the early signs of respiratory compromise, and alerting the medical staff, thereby facilitating the infant's reintubation at an appropriate time.

CARDIOVASCULAR ASSESSMENT AND SUPPORT

Continuous assessment of the cardiovascular state is imperative and includes assessment of clinical cardiovascular variables and the comprehensive monitoring of multiple haemodynamic parameters. Used in combination, these data accurately guide postoperative interventional support.

The clinical assessment will include evaluation of the child's colour, tissue perfusion and skin temperature, urine output and level of responsiveness. The goal of care is to optimise cardiac output, which will be demonstrated in an infant or child who is alert, pink, warm and well perfused, with strong peripheral pulses, brisk capillary refill and passing adequate volumes of urine. Evaluation of the monitored parameters includes ECG assessment of rhythm and rate and all other vital signs, including arterial pressure, left and right atrial pressures or central venous pressure and pulmonary artery pressure. Computerised monitoring allows for the continuous display of all monitored parameters and trend recordings at desired intervals, which in essence negates the need to maintain written records of the pressure variables.

Manipulation of cardiac output variables is guided by direct monitoring of intracardiac and intravascular parameters and cardiac output, the results of systemic and pulmonary vascular resistance and the clinical evaluation of cardiovascular status (see Haemodynamic Monitoring). Cardiac output is optimised by maintaining adequate filling pressure, evaluated by measurement of left and/or right atrial pressure. Optimal filling pressures postoperatively are determined by the underlying intracardiac and extracardiac anatomy, the preoperative haemodynamic status, the contractile state of the myocardium, the systemic and pulmonary vascular resistances and residual abnormalities.

Manipulation of the preload variables can be achieved with either crystaloid or colloid infusions, the selection of which remains somewhat controversial.[124] Experience has shown that preload manipulation is best achieved through the selection of blood and other colloid infusions, the final determinant being the infant or child's haematocrit level. Ventricular filling pressures are further manipulated through the secondary influences of vasoactive preparations.

Advanced clinical assessment skills, an ability to problem solve and intervene early are the keys to providing excellence in care for these children. Evaluation of blood loss via chest drains is also important in a complete cardiovascular assessment. It is generally accepted that increases in ventricular filling pressure are achieved with a transfusion of whole blood, pump blood or packed cells when the haematocrit is less than 40%, whereas fresh frozen plasma (FFP) or 5% albumin are the colloids of choice when the haematocrit is greater than 40%.[125] Due to the increased bleeding tendencies in infants and children with cyanotic congenital heart disease, FFP is the colloid of choice for volume expansion as it provides the necessary clotting factors. While losses need to be replaced, bleeding may necessitate early re-exploration of the chest. The possibility of tamponade should always be kept in mind, especially when bleeding suddenly stops or slows down, and the cardiovascular status deteriorates.

During extracorporeal circulation, there is generally an accumulation of fluids and crystaloids in the extravascular compartment. Maintenance intravenous fluid regimens are therefore initially reduced upon return to the unit until the dynamic changes with the circulation subside and cardiovascular stability is achieved, generally within 2 to 4 hours. When cardiovascular instability is prolonged, however, crystaloid replacement is instituted. Fluid regimens are severely restricted and take into account all infusion fluids (all intravenous maintenance fluids, vasoactive supports, analgesia and muscle relaxation including flush fluids given via the transducer). Extreme care must be exercised in delivery of all support infusions to ensure the accuracy of delivery is maintained, astute awareness of the doses per kilogram per minute are observed and that minimal volumes are infused.

PAIN ASSESSMENT AND RELIEF

Postoperative pain, distress and agitation can impose significant physiological compromise in critically ill infants and young children, evoked by the neuroendocrine response to stress.[125] Pain assessment and relief is therefore one of the most important aspects of care for infants, children and adolescents in the postoperative recovery period. Generous analgesic support through the administration of continuous infusion of opioid preparations, (e.g., morphine or fentanyl) or the combined use of an opioid and benzodiazapine, as with morphine and midazolam will provide effective pain relief and sedation. Both approaches ensure an effective approach to pain relief for the ventilated patient in all age groups, from the newborn infant to the adolescent.

Continuous opioid analgesic infusions are advocated because of their safe and immediate effectiveness in providing pain relief and the ease of titration in reaching the desired clinical responses in all age ranges.[126] Continuous infusions eliminate the need for regular painful intramuscular injections which fail to provide a constant pain-free state, given the cyclic peaks and troughs that occur with intermittent narcotic administration, which only further increases anxiety in the children.

Dosage regimens are the subject of continuous debate, as analgesic infusion rates require careful titration to the infant or child's individual clinical responses. Titration of the infusion is undertaken to ensure adequacy of drug plasma levels which will effectively alleviate pain, yet not induce central nervous system and respiratory depression in spontaneously breathing infants, children and adolescents. When respiratory support is provided through mechanical ventilation, the dosage regimens are more flexible and generous. Caution is advised in the selection of opioids and the infusion doses for analgesic cover in very young infants who are breathing spontaneously and in newborn infants who demonstrate problems with apnoea.[126] Careful observation of their respiratory status is essential and the ready availability of respiratory support is advised due to the decreased opioid clearance in infants, which can be attributed to hepatic and renal immaturity.[126,127] Studies have indicated that infants beyond the age of 3 to 6 months are no more prone than adults to opioid-induced respiratory depression.[126]

Once weaning and withdrawal from respiratory support is contemplated, titration of the infusion is undertaken to reduce the infusion doses. Careful clinical observation of the infant or child is imperative at this time to ensure the infusion doses alleviate pain but avoid somnolence and depression of the respiration.[126]

Misconceptions abound regarding pain assessment in the paediatric patient and hold major implications for pain management in children. Traditionally, health care personnel have underestimated pain levels in children, resulting in an overwhelming reluctance to administer appropriate pain relief.[128–132] Heightened awareness of pharmacokinetics, improved assessment abilities and documentation of the safe use of these preparations in neonates, infants and children has bought about more frequent and effective pain relief. Evidence now substantiates the presence of pathways for nociception from peripheral receptor sites in the preterm infant. These findings have altered health care professionals' perceptions of the pain experienced by the newborn infant.[125]

Various pain rating scales have been advocated for use with children and adolescents to quantitatively define their level of pain, thus helping alleviate the difficulty with nurses' perception of their level of pain.[128,130,132] All scales require presurgical preparation and the selection of a scale which is developmentally appropriate to the child or adolescent. Use of one scale throughout the postoperative recovery period will provide consistency and minimise confusion.[130]

From a clinical assessment perspective, various physiological and behavioural variables can be used to guide pain assessment in infants and young children.[129,131-133] Sympathetic nervous system stimulation increases the heart rate, blood pressure, respiratory rate and palmar diaphoresis. Pain is inferred when these signs are present, when combined with decreases in transcutaneous oxygen levels and oxygen saturations and when linked with hormonal and biochemical responses and certain behavioural patterns displayed by infants and children.[131,134]

Studies have indicated that certain behaviours, facial expression, crying and body movements are indicative of pain when used in parallel with the physiological findings outlined, and measured levels of serum cortisol and endorphin.[131,134] This has been further substantiated by the stress response in the neonate to CPB surgery and deep hypothermic circulatory arrest, which produces an overwhelming release of catecholamines, endorphins and glucagon.[115] Recognition of these clinical features and the use of proven assessment tools will facilitate recognition of pain levels and optimise pain relief, a priority of nursing care for infants and children.

POSTOPERATIVE PROBLEMS: IMPLICATIONS FOR NURSING

Complications following cardiac surgery in infancy, childhood and adolescence include states of low cardiac output, haemorrhage, arrhythmia and less commonly, infection. The postoperative problems often remain isolated to a single body system, however multisystem complications are common and may become intensified by neuroendocrine, metabolic and haematological influences. The most significant problem to arise in the paediatric age group following cardiac surgery in both open and closed heart procedures is development of a low cardiac output state with associated renal, neurological and pulmonary complications, which will ultimately progress to multiple organ failure.

Postoperative low cardiac output

Essentially, the critical reduction in cardiac output attributed to a multiplicity of factors of cardiac malfunction results in an impaired perfusion of vital tissues. Once a low cardiac output state becomes established, it is extremely difficult to reverse the process and stabilise the infant or child's circulation. The damage that may have developed from the poor tissue perfusion generally results in a further reduction in cardiac function, leading to acute renal failure, neurological sequelae and significant pulmonary problems.

The clinical signs of low cardiac output are:

- increasing restlessness or irritability;
- decreased urine output;
- deterioration in peripheral perfusion demonstrated by colour (pink to pale to grey), warmth (warm to cool to cold), pulses (strong to weak to absent) and capillary refill (brisk to sluggish).

These signs are a reliable index of decreased cardiac output,[31,33,63,119] with hypotension being an unreliable and late sign of shock. Astute observation should interpret these clinical signs at an early stage. Nursing assessment of the early signs of increasing irritability in an infant previously well settled, when associated with subtle changes in skin colour, perfusion and urine output, may be the first step in averting a disaster. The above clinical signs warn of impending disaster, often hours before a low cardiac output state becomes obvious through changed blood pressure and heart rate recordings.

It is possible, therefore, for an infant to exhibit clinical signs of a low cardiac output state despite apparently good haemodynamic parameters as demonstrated by arterial, central venous and right atrial pressures. Interpretation of the warning signs of reduced output at an early stage through astute nursing observation can prevent the establishment of a low cardiac output state through the early institution of appropriate treatment.

To appreciate the problems related to postoperative low cardiac output, consideration of the factors that determine cardiac output (i.e., preload, contractility, afterload and heart rate) is warranted. Manipulation of these factors should be aimed at providing the optimal cardiac output.

Manipulation of preload

Cardiac output is the product of the heart rate times the stroke volume. The preload of the heart is reflected by the left and right atrial pressures, which are used as guides for volume loading and which reflect end-diastolic pressure (the filling pressure) of the ventricle.[31,120] The filling pressures are raised by transfusion of blood or other colloid, which will optimise myocardial stretch. Recent nursing research has supported the hypothesis that use of colloid requires less loading and is more effective than crystaloid in maintaining haemodynamic stability.[124] Difficulty remains within paediatrics regarding the specification of optimal filling pressure. This is exemplified in children following closure of an atrial septal defect, who have excellent myocardial compliance. They generally exhibit all the clinical signs of a good cardiac output, requiring a low filling pressure (right, atrial pressure [RAP]), often ranging between 3 and 5 mmHg.

In contrast, a child following correction of tetralogy of Fallot will require a significantly higher right atrial pressure, perhaps to a value of 10 to 15 mmHg, to effect a satisfactory cardiac output. This increased RAP reflects the non-compliance of a stiff, hypertrophied, right ventricular muscle mass, exposed to the surgical insult from a ventriculotomy.[120] The right ventricle therefore becomes increasingly non-compliant due to local tissue damage and oedema imposed by the surgery and the effects of CPB, as outlined previously. Careful observation of both LAP and RAP is extremely valuable as elevation of the LAP may indicate that factors other than preload require adjustment. Overfilling of the heart by increasing preload beyond a physiological limit can precipitate myocardial failure and pulmonary oedema.

Caution must be exercised in the manipulation of preload, be it through volume loading to increase preload or through pharmacological manipulation with vasoactive substances and diuretics to decrease preload. Optimising myocardial fibre stretch to increase cardiac output is the goal of therapy. The nursing role in clinical assessment of children during this manipulation is crucial. Excess fluid loading will result in added stress through the increase in myocardial cell wall tension which in turn increases oxygen requirements. Depleting the circulating volume with pharmacological preparations may impede cardiac performance by decreasing preload. The sympathetic nervous system response to decreased preload will increase heart rate, thus further increasing oxygen requirements which may ultimately affect coronary artery perfusion and blood pressure.

Manipulation of the myocardial contractile state

When cardiac output remains low in spite of optimisation of preload, manipulation of other variables known to effect the circulation are instituted. Improvement in myocardial contractility is effected with inotropic support (e.g., dopamine, dobutamine) and the relief of increased systemic vascular resistance (SVR) achieved with vasodilator preparations, such as sodium nitroprusside.[33,63,105]

The reduced myocardial contractility may be the result of the infant or child's pre-operative condition, any intraoperative events or postoperative changes. A poor pre-operative condition with pre-existing congestive cardiac failure and myocardial damage may significantly compromise the infant or child in the acute postoperative phase of recovery. Similarly, intraoperative problems e.g., hypoxia, hypotension, intramyocardial haemorrhage and inadequate myocardial protection resulting in myocardial infarction, can significantly impede myocardial contractile performance.[135] A reduction in contractility may result from a residual or recurrent defect or from oedema of the myocardium, however, it is often the product of potent metabolic and neuroendocrine influence.

Improvement in myocardial contractility is reliant upon elimination of any abnormal metabolic and neuroendocrine factors.[33] Hypoxia, metabolic acidosis, hypoglycaemia and hypothermia must be corrected and electrolyte homeostasis established if improvement in the myocardial contractile state is to be effective with the introduction of inotropic agents.[21] Selection of the appropriate sympathomimetic agent is determined by the desired therapeutic response. Appreciation of the adrenergic receptor sites and drug specificity, therefore enables selection of the most appropriate pharmacological preparation.[25,82]

Special challenges present when attempting to support the circulation in the newborn infant due to the immaturity of the heart and the physiological functioning of the body's regulatory mechanisms. As temperature control, fluid and electrolyte homeostasis, vasomotor and renal regulation and liver function are incompletely developed, the pharmacological effects of vasoactive preparations are less precise.

Dopamine, a natural precursor of adrenalin and noradrenaline, has positive inotropic effects that activate dopaminergic, alpha and beta responses, dependent on dosage. Low rates of infusion provide a dopaminergic dose (less than 4 µg/kg/minute) and improves coronary, cerebral, renal and splanchnic perfusion.[21] Moderate doses (in excess of 5 and less than 10 µg/kg/minute) stimulate beta adrenergic receptors to produce inotropic and mild chronotropic effects. High-dose dopamine infusions (in excess of 10 µg/kg/minute) induce potent alpha adrenergic responses that increase SVR and cause renal vascular constriction.[19,21,32,33,63,85,105] The ability of dopamine to increase cardiac output is reliant upon endogenous noradrenaline availability. Gestational age and exposure to factors known to be potent stressors to the neonate, determine noradrenaline availability. Dopamine is reportedly less effective in the preterm asphyxiated infant. Hypoxia and acidosis increase pulmonary vascular resistance, which is further exacerbated by dopamine.[82]

Dobutamine is a synthetic inotropic preparation that primarily effects beta-1 receptors, increasing contractile strength and tone thus increasing the cardiac output and renal perfusion.[19,85] The stimulation of beta-2 and alpha adrenergic receptors that results from the use of dobutamine is minimal.[21,33,63,82,105]

Isoprenaline is a beta adrenergic agent which increases cardiac output due to the potent chronotropic and inotropic effects. Absence of alpha adrenergic effects of isoprenaline results in decreased systemic vascular resistance, which may reduce coronary artery perfusion, when arterial pressure decreases. Isoprenaline has arrhythmogenic properties related to beta adrenergic stimulation which increase myocardial oxygen requirements and may significantly decrease cardiac output at a critical time.[19,21] It has been useful in establishing an increase in cardiac output in infants and children after cardiac surgery, where bradyarrhythmias develop. Further, isoprenaline relaxes the pulmonary vasculature when infused via the pulmonary artery in infants with increased pulmonary vascular resistance where an additional increase in heart rate does not preclude use.

Careful evaluation of the clinical response to inotropic preparations and dosage titrations is maintained by nursing personnel. Continuous assessment for potential problems is effected by interpretation of clinical and monitored parameters which reflect cardiovascular status. **Table 11.6** provides a summary of the various inotropic agents, their mechanisms of action, recommended doses and adverse effects.

Manipulation of afterload

Afterload manipulation is one of the first determinants of cardiac output that should be adjusted due to the marked increase in systemic vascular resistance (SVR) which follows CPB surgery. The majority of infants and children will require vasodilation therapy to decrease the peripheral vascular resistance, thereby reducing the workload of the heart and thus the myocardial oxygen requirements.

When low cardiac output states develop in infants and children, the reversal of this state requires the manipulation of afterload. SVR increases in response to sympathetic nervous system and neuroendocrine stimulation, the mechanisms of compensation to improve cardiac output (see Failure of Control Mechanisms). The elevation in SVR causes an increase in afterload, resulting in an additional workload for the ventricle, an increase in myocardial oxygen requirements and a reduction in stroke volume. Various pharmacological preparations may be used to reduce the elevation in SVR. The drugs for afterload reduction include sodium nitroprusside, phenoxybenzamine, nitroglycerine, hydralazine and phentolamine with the use of isoprenaline and tolazoline in certain specific situations, where a decrease in pulmonary vascular resistance (PVR) is required (**Table 11.6**). Relief of the increased SVR results in a decrease in ventricular end-diastolic pressure. As the ventricles empty more effectively, oxygen requirements are reduced and cardiac output improves, as long as optimal preload is maintained. The arteriolar dilatation reduces the hydrostatic pressure in the capillaries, facilitating movement of fluid back into the intravascular space. This in effect will precipitate a decrease in colloid osmotic pressure and serum protein levels and a reduction in blood viscosity and haematocrit.[22]

Extreme caution in the manipulation of the afterload is essential when a low cardiac output state becomes established in an infant or child, given that manipulation of 2 or more of the determinants of cardiac output will generally be essential. Ensuring adequate circulatory volume is of primary importance if further decompensation is to be avoided. Infants and children with inadequate circulating volume who maintain a degree of cardiac output due to increased SVR will decompensate rapidly if vasodilator preparations are employed without appropriate volume replacement. Adequately supporting the circulation in low cardiac output states with vasopressors, ensures the maintenance of mean arterial pressure, which is crucial for protection of cerebral, cardiac and renal perfusion.

Manipulation of heart rate and rhythm

Disturbances of cardiac rhythm or rate are important factors that can compromise cardiac output, especially in the acute phase of the child's recovery. Manipulation of the heart rate and rhythm are commonly undertaken postoperatively, to improve stroke volume and hence cardiac output. The well-being of infants and children is reliant upon nursing personnel to interpret acute and significant changes in the heart rate and rhythm, assuring early detection of ECG disturbances and initiation of treatment which can prevent a deterioration in the clinical condition. The arrhythmogenic problems that are encountered in the paediatric age group can be linked to:

- hypoxaemia and acid base abnormalities;
- electrolyte imbalances;
- surgical trauma;
- anaesthetic agents;
- endogenous and exogenous catecholamines;
- pharmacological agents; and
- mechanical factors (e.g., intracardiac catheters).[120,136]

Postoperative bradycardia is the product of electrical conduction system disturbances or injury induced by varying metabolic derangements, pharmacological preparations or the iatrogenic influences of surgery. Transient arrhythmogenic problems may result from localised tissue oedema of the conducting pathways, which can in turn result in incomplete or complete heart block. Permanent disruption to conduction resulting from surgically induced trauma of electrical conduction pathways is a rare complication.[41,137]

The aims of management are to exclude the factors which predispose to bradyarrhythmia and control any haemodynamic compromise resulting from the disturbance. Dependent upon the structural cardiac defect and the surgical procedure undertaken, various rhythm disturbances result. Commonly, infants and children experience atrial, junctional and, to a lesser extent, ventricular disturbances where isolated escape beats may be the only manifestation.[138] Dependent upon the site of impulse initiation and the haemodynamic consequences of the arrhythmia, temporary pacing is initiated to optimise cardiac output with atrial, ventricular or atrioventricular (A-V) sequential pacing.

Atrial and A-V sequential pacing produces the best haemodynamic effects in the infant or child who requires temporary pacing as atrial augmentation of ventricular filling is maintained. In the absence of atrial pacing wires, ventricular pacing will be effective in maintaining an appropriate heart rate when the underlying heart rate and rhythm has failed to meet metabolic needs.

Pharmacological intervention is used with caution to control bradyarrhythmias in children who are haemodynamically compromised and who are without pacing wires. Preparations like atropine sulphate, which increase sinoatrial node discharge and enhance conduction across the A-V node, can be used for 1st and 2nd degree A-V block. Isoprenaline is a pure beta adrenergic agonist and is effective in increasing heart rate and contractility in a small number of infants where systemic and pulmonary vasodilation is also desirable.[30,33]

Tachycardia in infants and children after bypass surgery will almost certainly reduce cardiac output. Before intervention is initiated, exclusion of the possible precipitating factors (e.g., hypovolaemia, hypoxaemia, acidosis, hypercarbia, pyrexia, catecholamine excess and pericardial tamponade) should be undertaken. With the above problems excluded, various treatment options are available to reverse acute tachyarrhythmias. The tachycardiac disturbances commonly seen in children are atrial and junctional in origin. Ventricular tachycardia is rarely seen in children following cardiac surgery.[137]

Pharmacological agents like digitalis are commonly used in supraventricular tachycardia (SVT). Other agents like sotolol and amiodorone could be useful in situations where digitalis is ineffective or contraindicated. Overdrive atrial pacing may be effective in terminating SVT in the acute postoperative period,[34,121,139] where the introduction of pharmacological agents to reverse a resistant SVT may be life threatening.[140] Electrical cardioversion may also be effective in terminating SVT, which imposes critical haemodynamic compromise.[121,34]

Lignocaine is a treatment option for ventricular tachycardia when cardiac output is maintained. Where ventricular tachycardia produces a critical reduction in cardiovascular status and level of consciousness, the definitive treatment is defibrillation and the institution of basic and advanced life support procedures.[34] Caution must be exercised with the administration of digitalis in the acute setting for control of tachyarrhythmias.

Mechanical support of the failing circulation

Biotechnology now provides various sophisticated modalities of mechanical support for the failing circulation in infancy and childhood. This is exemplified by the development of left ventricular assistance devices, extracorporeal membrane oxygenation (ECMO) and the intra-aortic balloon pump (IABP), which was previously the support device used exclusively for the adult cardiac patient in cardiogenic shock.[122,141]

Several types of pumps are now available which assist the circulation during the acute phase of recovery.[142] These pumps draw blood from the right or left atrium of the heart and pump the blood back into the circulation, either into the aorta or the pulmonary circulation. In situations where the primary problem is a compromised left ventricle, mechanical augmentation of the failing circulation can be undertaken. The left ventricle can be assisted to support the child by drawing the blood from the left atrium and pumping it into the aorta (without an oxygenator in the circuit), a procedure that can be life saving (**Figure 11.3**).

There are several other mechanical assist devices which can be used to tide a child over a crisis. Until recent years ECMO has been used exclusively for support of the circulation during open heart surgery. Its use is now extended to neonatal and paediatric critical care settings where it has been used successfully to provide respiratory support and mechanical support of the circulation in a variety of acute, life-threatening and essentially reversible clinical problems. Currently, in some centres there is continued interest in the use of ECMO, a highly sophisticated support system for a very small number of infants and young children with acute, yet reversible cardiorespiratory dysfunction; children with myocardial depression following cardiac surgery.[10,142]

ECMO is effective in reducing the myocardial workload by supporting the failing circulation and resting the heart in infants with reactive pulmonary hypertensive disease states attributed to CHD, for example in those infants with transposition of the great arteries where there is a large ventricular septal defect,[143] truncus arteriosus and total anomalous pulmonary venous return. Venous blood flow is diverted via a large-bore cannula from the internal jugular vein to the ECMO circuit, where oxygen and carbon dioxide are exchanged via a membrane oxygenator, heated and pumped back into the body by way of a roller pump mechanism into either the arterial or venous circulations, effecting either partial or complete bypass.[10] Generally, when ECMO is used for postoperative cardiac support, a venoarterial circuit is used[58] (**Figure 11.4**). The use of the

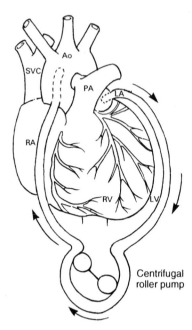

Figure 11.3 Mechanical augmentation of the failing circulation: diagrammatic representation of left ventricular assistance whereby arterial blood is withdrawn
from the left atrium and pumped back into the systemic circulation at the
level of the aorta.

membrane oxygenator will optimise recovery of the pulmonary vascular bed at a critical
time in the postoperative recovery phase in infants with reversible cardiac failure and
labile pulmonary hypertensive disease who are not responding to more conventional
support measures.[143] Recent success with this support device in the postoperative period
has effectively lowered mortality.[53,112,143,144] Inherent in this technological support for infants and children is an extension of the nursing role without previous parallel and with
implications for clinical practice of enormous proportion.

The IABP is a device which supports the failing circulation by producing a
counterpulsation effect within the aorta, causing forward displacement of blood volume,
an increase in tissue perfusion, relief of left ventricular afterload and a decrease in
myocardial oxygen consumption (**Figure 11.5**). With the current availability of catheters
and balloons designed for use in children less than 13 kg bodyweight, there is potential
for effective circulatory assistance in postoperative low cardiac output states. Early results with this support device in children of varying ages are, however, disappointing.[141]

RENAL SYSTEM CONSIDERATIONS

Acute renal failure (ARF) is a serious complication which reportedly develops in 8% to
10% of infants following CPB surgery when there is an acute reduction in cardiac output.
The incidence of ARF is reportedly highest in the neonatal period and is attributed to
renal immaturity.[121]

Many factors contribute to the development of postoperative ARF in infants and

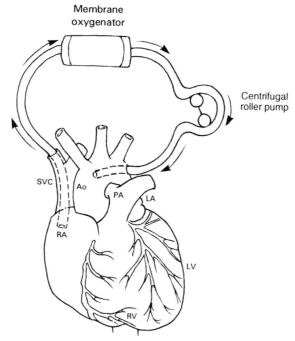

Figure 11.4 Mechanical augmentation of the failing circulation: diagrammatic representation of extra corporeal membrane oxygenation (ECMO) whereby venous blood is diverted from the right side of the heart, passed through a membrane oxygenator and with the assistance of a roller pump device, is pumped back into either the arterial (as depicted) or venous circulation.

children. Renal dysfunction that occurs in the preoperative period in the infant with cardiac failure and a low cardiac output or in the child with cyanotic congenital heart disease are clearly linked with postoperative ARF.[120,121] The necessity to carefully evaluate renal function preoperatively is therefore evident.

Intraoperative factors are also closely linked with renal dysfunction. A reduction in renal perfusion associated with a low cardiac output state, may result at any stage intraoperatively or postoperatively. Renal hypoperfusion may therefore result from aortic cross-clamping, from states of hypovolaemia or from decreased myocardial contractile force, where periods of hypotension impose ischaemic damage to renal tissue.[24,145] Other intraoperative factors contributing to the development of ARF are microemboli and haemolysis, the result of red blood cell destruction, which increases with the duration of CPB time.[121]

Urinary output is a highly reliable index of cardiac output and therefore careful monitoring of exact volumes is practised. In infants, children and adolescents urine volumes of less than 0.5 mL/kg/hour constitute oliguria. Similarly, oliguria exists in the newborn infant when the volume decreases to less than 1 mL/kg hour.[125,146]

Intervention to reverse ARF is guided by clinical assessment parameters, such as cardiovascular stability and acid base status. Serum electrolyte levels and osmolarity, creatinine and urea levels in addition to urinary electrolytes and osmolarity are closely

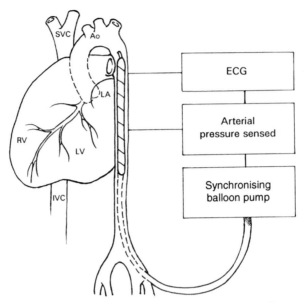

Figure 11.5 Mechanical augmentation of the failing circulation: diagrammatic representation of intra-aortic balloon counterpulsation.

monitored for abnormality. Preload augmentation, afterload reduction and manipulation
of the myocardial contractile state will improve cardiac output, increase renal perfusion and
may protect the infant from further compromise where acute renal failure is suspected.[121,145]

A trial dose of frusemide is administered and repeated at higher dose ranges if the
infant is unresponsive. A fluid challenge, if appropriate to the hydration status of the
infant, attempts to differentiate prerenal from intrinsic ARF. A rapid response to treatment is observed in infants with prerenal failure, whereas persistent oliguria suggests
intrinsic ARF following the above treatment modalities.[145]

Failure to control the fluid overload state and electrolyte imbalances, especially
hyperkalaemia and acid base derangements associated with ARF requires, peritoneal
dialysis. Early intervention with dialysis is the key to successful support in the critically
ill infant or child after CPB.[120] See Chapter 12 for a review of the principles of assessment
and care of children in ARF.

NEUROLOGICAL CONSIDERATIONS

The potential for neurological complications is considerable following cardiac surgery, in
particular CPB surgery where periods of deep hypothermia and total circulatory arrest
are required. Current practice with improved surgical support techniques and postoperative care offers better protection against these iatrogenic influences which can effect
neurological outcomes.

Intraoperative factors pertaining to CPB, deep hypothermia and total circulatory arrest have been discussed. The neurological outcome is further complicated intraoperatively
by periods of hypoxia, hypotension, prolongation of the extracorporeal circulation time
and the risks of air or particulate embolisation.[109]

Additionally, pre-existing conditions and various postoperative factors are strongly implicated in the establishment of neurological dysfunctional states that produce transient dysfunction or cerebral infarction from impaired tissue perfusion. The contributing factors, additional to those outlined above, include:

- states of low cardiac output and extreme hypotension;
- acidosis;
- hypoglycaemia;
- hypocalcaemia;
- hyperpyrexia;
- cerebral oedema from fluid and electrolyte imbalances;
- thrombosis in children with severe polycythemia; and
- intracerebral haemorrhaging in infants and children with clotting defects.

Reports of seizure activity in infants and children after CPB varies, with a suggested incidence between 4% and 10% in the immediate postoperative period. Researchers conclude, however, that the seizures are not indicative of permanent neurological damage. A variability in the results of developmental assessments in children following prolonged circulatory arrest times, suggests central nervous system dysfunction at a subclinical level.[100,109]

Neonates and infants are prone to serious hypoglycaemia, particularly in times of stress which may result in severe cerebral damage. Hypoglycaemia is also a common cause of twitching in these infants, and if uncorrected may progress to convulsions.

Implications for nursing practice

From a nursing perspective, awareness of the potential for central nervous system complications and astute observation of neurological parameters is vital as soon as practicable after surgery. Regular assessment of the infant or child's level of consciousness, pupillary and gross motor responses is undertaken. When muscle relaxants are used to facilitate the child's recovery, neurological assessment is difficult and enhances the need to evaluate closely pupillary response and physiological parameters that may signify a problem. Close monitoring of acid-base status, tissue oxygenation, serum electrolyte and glucose levels will minimise the potential for neurological sequelae from metabolic derangements.[121]

Caution is further exercised in the care of infants and children who have right-to-left intracardiac shunts with the potential for embolisation into the systemic and cerebral circulations. The possibility of air embolism in infants with a mixing of circulations should be kept in mind, and all injections and infusions should be carefully monitored to avoid any small amount of air entry into the systemic circulation which may cause cerebral embolisation.

RESPIRATORY CONSIDERATIONS

Infants and children may be confronted with a variety of pulmonary problems after heart surgery, including pulmonary parenchymal disease, where there may be collapse, consolidation or infection. Regular chest physiotherapy will help to reduce complications associated with cardiothoracic surgery, both in those who are spontaneously breathing and those who require prolonged periods of respiratory support.[120] After thoracotomy infants and children require chest physiotherapy and encouragement to breath deeply. Analgesic cover to minimise postoperative pain will prevent splinting of their chest wall and facilitate chest expansion and coughing to clear secretions.

After CPB surgery, there are additional contributing factors which complicate the respiratory state, e.g., low cardiac output, pulmonary hypertensive disease and pulmonary oedema. Prolongation of CPB and periods of low cardiac output are associated with endothelial damage of the pulmonary capillary walls, which causes pulmonary oedema and ventilation/perfusion mismatch.[120]

Pulmonary hypertension

Many young babies presenting for cardiac surgery have persistently elevated pulmonary artery pressure, while many others have elevated but labile pulmonary vascular resistance (PVR). While infants with labile, reversible PVR are accepted for surgical repair, older infants with severely elevated and irreversible PVR pose a difficult management problem unless heart–lung transplantation is considered.

The acute postoperative recovery for infants with pulmonary hypertension represents a significant therapeutic problem as paroxysmal episodes of pulmonary hypertension (pulmonary hypertensive crisis) may develop. When pulmonary artery pressure reaches suprasystemic levels, cardiac output falls and the clinical condition deteriorates rapidly. The pulmonary blood flow decreases significantly with the increased PVR, thereby impeding alveolar gas exchange. The oxygen saturation falls despite maximal increases in FiO_2 and there is a subsequent rise in $PaCO_2$.

Infants considered at high risk from a highly reactive pulmonary vascular bed include those with truncus arteriosus, total anomalous pulmonary venous return, transposition of the great arteries with ventricular septal defects (VSD), complete atrioventricular canal defects and large VSDs.[143,147,148] Postoperatively these infants may maintain excellent haemodynamic stability until a sudden stimulus evokes a potent, rapid and potentially devastating deterioration of the cardiovascular state due to sudden increases in the PVR leading to severe pulmonary arteriolar hypertension.

The pulmonary precapillary arteriolar bed evokes a potent vasoconstrictor response to hypoxia, hypercarbia and acidosis, as well as environmental and physical stimulation.[149] The goal of treatment is multifaceted and aims to prevent the development of a pulmonary hypertensive state. Minimisation of noxious stimuli is achieved by optimising ventilation to enhance oxygen carriage and the elimination of carbon dioxide, thus facilitating improved tissue perfusion and acid base balance. Maintaining a mild respiratory alkalosis with a $PaCO_2$ less than 25 mmHg and providing an FiO_2 of greater than 0.9 will dilate the pulmonary vascular bed.[87] Stimulation incurred with physical handling is minimised and infants are given liberal doses of narcotics, with continuous infusions of fentanyl or morphine and midazolam. Muscle relaxation assists in stabilising the pattern of ventilation and may need to be continued until weaning from the ventilator is attempted.

The stabilisation of intracardiac haemodynamics and circulation in infants is achieved with various vasoactive preparations which provide inotropic support and vasodilatation. No vasodilator preparations selectively reduce PVR. Most in use also produce undesired responses for the systemic circulation,[87] Tolazoline and phenoxybenzamine are alpha adrenergic receptor blockers and therefore have potent vasodilator properties, although their use is limited in the relief of postoperative pulmonary hypertension. Current trends support the infusion of prostacyclin, a non-selective vasodilator, for relief of pulmonary hypertension,[87] and more recently the inhalation of nitric oxide which has emerged as a new treatment approach.[143]

In spite of the best efforts to minimise stimuli, support the circulation and control ventilation, some infants will develop labile episodes of increased PVR. Alterations in monitored parameters which indicate an imminent crisis include tachycardia and unfavourable changes in pulmonary and systemic pressures, hypercarbia, hypoxia and acidosis, at which time prompt intervention is mandatory.

Management involves symptomatic and supportive treatment and eradication of the factors instrumental in the crisis. Arterial blood gases will guide the infant's treatment, which includes:

- hyperventilation with an FiO_2 of 1.0;
- narcotic and muscle relaxant bolus;
- exclusion of mechanical factors which may have been instrumental in the pulmonary hypertensive episode, e.g., airway obstruction, pneumothorax; and
- consideration of additional support medications: vasodilators, calcium gluconate, sodium bicarbonate.

Implications for nursing practice

Astute clinical assessment of these infants is imperative. Before initiating any routine care or procedures, the nurse must be cognisant with every aspect of management. In recognising the potential response from external stimulation when the PVR is increased, minimisation of all disturbances to the infant is strictly observed. This includes minimisation of all non-essential routine care and any other stimuli which may precipitate an elevation in pulmonary artery pressure. Careful respiratory evaluation is a priority of care and gentle chest physiotherapy is at times required. All oral, nasopharyngeal and endotracheal suction is minimised as is the instillation of sodium chloride into the endotracheal tube. Higher doses of narcotic and muscle relaxation agents are imperative preceding any of the high-risk procedures.

The postoperative nursing care of these infants often poses a challenge as the circumstances are so variable and situations so unpredictable. It is therefore essential that ideal conditions be maintained in the delivery of critical care nursing to these infants. The level and efficiency of nursing care in the postoperative period contributes and may even determine the outcome of these desperately ill infants who pose this therapeutic challenge.

Chylothorax

Chylothorax seen in the postoperative setting is often the result of direct thoracic duct injury. In more complex situations, however, it is the result of very high systemic venous congestion, as seen following the Glenn shunt and the Fontan procedure combined with trauma to the thoracic duct or small lymph channels within the mediastinum.[120,121]

HAEMATOLOGICAL CONSIDERATIONS

Haematological problems constitute a major area for consideration in postoperative care. Haemorrhage is a serious complication which may result in the development of a low cardiac output state when it is not recognised and controlled appropriately. Factors which contribute to bleeding tendencies are the result of ineffective surgical haemostasis and coagulation abnormalities. These abnormalities may be both pathological and iatrogenic, as in incomplete heparin reversal or excessive use of protamine sulphate. Further, children who have had previous surgery are predisposed to risks of bleeding postoperatively because of adhesions.[150]

CPB usually results in haemodilution, which results in a deficiency of clotting factors. When haemodilution is combined with heparinisation and the potential for excess administration of protamine sulphate, bleeding problems tend to intensify. A decrease in platelet numbers results from haemodilution. It is the process of extracorporeal membrane oxygenation that causes destruction to the platelets, which is further intensified by the suction devices used during CPB surgery.[125,150] These factors will temporarily impair haemostasis and thus children become prone to bleeding in the immediate postoperative phase.[150]

Coagulopathy in the neonate results from a reduction in clotting factors produced by the liver. In contrast, children with cyanotic CHD develop polycythemia in response to an hypoxic stimulus which increases erythropoiesis.[104,106] Polycythaemia is in part responsible for coagulopathy because of the reduced plasma levels of clotting factors. Increased fibrinolysis and platelet dysfunction are additional factors which potentiate the coagulation problem.[104,106,135] Extensive mediastinal collateral networks develop in these children in response to the progressive hypoxaemia and further increase bleeding tendencies.[138]

Hypervolaemia may develop from an increase in red cell volumes. When the haematocrit is greater than 70% blood viscosity increases, which impedes the peripheral circulation and the perfusion of vital tissue. Thrombosis and infarction of pulmonary and cerebral vascular beds have been reported with progressive metabolic acidosis resulting from decreased tissue perfusion.[104,106]

Infants and children with profound cyanosis who have significant polycythemia, require strict attention to preoperative hydration and may require a partial volume exchange (red cell phoresis) with fresh frozen plasma during or after surgery. Following this procedure, reports indicate that platelet abnormalities improve with the return of normal platelet function within 3 days.[106]

Pericardial tamponade

The most devastating complication of bleeding is pericardial tamponade, which also constitutes another cause of postoperative low cardiac output. In the acute postoperative period, an accumulation of blood in the pericardial space will result in compression of the underlying myocardial muscle mass, impedance to diastolic filling of the ventricles and a reduction in cardiac output. The potential for tamponade exists in all open-heart surgical patients. It may even develop upon removal of transthoracic monitoring lines. As a precautionary measure in children who require long-term anticoagulation, treatment is withheld until all intracardiac lines, chest drains and epicardial pacing wires are removed. In more chronic states of congestive cardiac failure, the development of a significant pericardial fluid accumulation may prompt the same complication, though large volumes are required to cause tamponade in this situation.[151]

Clinically, infants and children display all the signs of low cardiac output as previously discussed. Caution is exercised in the infant or child who suddenly ceases to lose blood via the chest drains, where previously the loss has been consistent.[120] Heart sounds become muffled and monitored parameters reveal an increase in heart rate and a changing relationship between the right and left atrial pressure, with both increasing to a point where the pressure may equalise.[121,135,151] A decrease in pulse pressure and a fall in arterial pressure signifies very late findings of severe cardiogenic shock.[152]

Confirmation of tamponade is provided through echocardiographic assessment. Diagnosis requires prompt evacuation of the pericardial fluid accumulation to relieve the compression on the myocardium. Ideally, the relief of the tamponade is performed under controlled surgical conditions in the operating theatre, the child's condition permitting the transfer. Urgent relief of the pressure build-up may be effected through the release of blood clots obstructing flow through the drains or by emergency evacuation of the tamponade following chest reopening.[31,121]

Cardiac arrest is the inevitable result of pericardial tamponade when intervention is inappropriately delayed. Cardiac tamponade is a potentially preventable complication as the recognition of the early warning signs of low cardiac output and the initiation of early treatment will prevent complete cardiovascular collapse.

Nursing personnel fulfil a critical role in preventing the development of potentially devastating complications like tamponade. Astute assessment of clinical and monitored parameters, sound understanding of physiological and pathophysiological concepts pertaining to cardiovascular function will facilitate accurate interpretation of clinical findings. Advanced problem solving skills will ensure appropriate initiation of treatment, thereby reducing the morbidity and mortality associated with this complication.

POSTPERICARDIOTOMY SYNDROME

Postpericardiotomy syndrome is a complication which can be seen in any infant, child or adolescent where the pericardium has been entered at the time of CPB surgery.[31,137,153] Evidence suggests an autoimmune aetiology as the most likely factor to explain the complexity of symptoms associated with the syndrome, although an aetiology of viral origin has also been postulated. It is suggested that an antibody reaction results from damage of blood or autologous tissue in the pericardial space. The finding of high anti-heart antibody, which correlates with clinical findings, supports this theory.[137,153] The literature further indicates that the autoimmune response may be triggered by a viral illness, with studies finding a conclusive rise in antiviral antibody in these patients.[137,153]

Clinically, children present with pain, fever, malaise and lethargy associated with a pericardial friction rub. Diagnosis is confirmed with an echocardiogram, ECG and chest x-ray. Management is aimed at providing rest and reducing the inflammation, fever and pain, primarily with aspirin or non-steroidal anti-inflammatory agents or, less commonly, with the use of corticosteroids.[121,153] When a pericardial effusion develops in these children, it causes haemodynamic compromise and a pericardial tap will be undertaken to relieve the clinical signs.

INFECTIVE CONSIDERATIONS

Infants and children are at significant risk of nosocomial infection after heart surgery. Factors which contribute to their high risk are determined in large part by their preoperative condition, the number of invasive monitoring lines required for support, and their duration of placement in potentially immunocompromised infants who are critically ill at the time of their surgery. Similarly, those who are chronically hypoxic, in cardiac failure or who are malnourished before their surgery have increased infection risks.[120]

Prophylactic antibiotic cover is recommended from the time of anaesthetic induction to cover the surgery and the acute postoperative recovery phase until all invasive lines and drains are removed.[121,137] The risks of infection are increased when prosthetic material is used for surgical repair, e.g., the teflon material used to fashion conduits for shunt procedures and the patch material for closure of intracardiac defects.[121]

The organisms commonly found to be responsible for infection in the paediatric group are staphylococci and Gram-negative organisms. Statistically, evidence suggests the actual occurrence of infection is negligible, a tribute to the meticulous care provided by all health care personnel.[120,121] Screening preoperatively for detection of hepatitis B surface antigen in high-risk groups reduces the risk of intraoperative and postoperative infection spread.[137]

POSTOPERATIVE PROGRESS

Stabilisation of the infant or child's clinical condition generally occurs within the first 24 to 48 hours, dependent upon the preoperative status and the intricacy of the surgery. A comprehensive assessment of cardiorespiratory and neurological status will ascertain the infant or child's preparedness for weaning from vasoactive preparations and ventilatory support, and will detect any abnormal factors which may influence or impede successful support withdrawal. Following completion of the gentle weaning process, the invasive monitoring lines are removed slowly. The direct intrathoracic lines are removed very cautiously one at a time, as the potential for arrhythmia and haemorrhage is well recognised. Exclusion of a pericardial accumulation of blood following withdrawal of these lines is essential. Chest drains are removed under generous narcotic cover, once all drainage has subsided.

All other invasive devices (e.g., the arterial line and urinary catheter) are removed as soon as practicable. Bowel sounds are assessed to exclude paralytic ileus before the nasogastric tube is removed. Within approximately 4 hours of extubation, oral fluids are reintroduced as tolerated. Narcotic analgesia may be required for an additional period and is then replaced by regular oral analgesic medication. Gentle ambulation and the reintroduction of the diet are then encouraged.

SURGICAL OUTCOMES

Most children who undergo open-heart repairs are discharged within approximately 5 to 6 days. Those who required additional support of their cardiorespiratory state are generally discharged home within 7 to 10 days of surgery. The procedures that required only minimal dissection and short anaesthetic time, e.g., ligation of a patent ductus arteriosus, necessitate hospitalisation for only a few days. Children recover rapidly from their surgery, which is facilitated by appropriate presurgical preparation and an honest approach that keeps them well informed of their progress.

Nursing personnel fulfil a vital role in preparing children and parents for discharge. Instruction is given regarding medication if required, diet, level of activity, wound care and the necessity for medical follow-up.[154]

Essentially, all forms of CHD are now amenable to surgical correction, sophisticated palliation or therapeutic intervention, with some procedures soon to be performed *in utero*. Perioperative morbidity and mortality has been linked to the child's clinical state at the time of surgery, highlighting the need to exclude current illness that may complicate the acute recovery phase and influence outcome.[100]

Current surgical techniques and support devices have revolutionised care of the infant and child with cardiovascular disease, and have significantly reduced long-term morbidity and mortality. It is postulated that an increasing incidence of arrhythmia in the paediatric group results secondary to complex cardiac surgical procedures and the improvement that has occurred in the children's survival rates.[139] Children who sustain a poor haemodynamic result have an increased risk of sudden death. Similarly, children who demonstrate severe exercise intolerance, are symptomatic and have an enlarged heart on chest x-ray and who experience arrhythmias are at a higher risk of sudden collapse and death. Retrospective studies show a link with arrhythmia development and haemodynamic compromise in children postoperatively the year preceding collapse. In children following tetralogy of Fallot repair and in infants following the Mustard and Senning procedures for transposition of the great arteries, there is a higher incidence of sudden death postoperatively with mortality listed at 4% to 10% and 2% to 8% respectively.[155]

The contribution of nursing

The present and future level of biotechnology holds major implications for the nursing profession providing more highly invasive support mechanisms to monitor infants, children and adolescents with cardiac problems. To remain progressive in this technological age, nurses must strive to project the future needs in the care of the children.

Currently, the data provided by technology enhances the ability to identify and interpret trends in a child's clinical profile. The nurse assumes responsibility for the early interpretation of altered variables, both clinically and mechanically derived, however subtle, through astute and continued clinical assessment of the infant or child. To prevent decompensation in a critical and sometimes irreversible state, appropriate intervention and evaluation of clinical responses to the various cardiovascular and respiratory treatment modalities is required.

As an integral member of a multidisciplinary team, the nurse is responsible for the delivery of specialist care which requires precision, at times under pressure. The demand for detailed monitoring of physiological variables and the need for accurate analysis of data, heightens the nurse's need for proficiency and confidence in her or his clinical assessment skills, analytical ability, critical decision making and the need to be conversant with the state-of-the-art computerised technology. The importance of the nursing assessment cannot be overemphasised as it remains the foundation for attaining a standard of clinical excellence for infants and children, a goal to which nurses continually strive. The holistic approach to care is achieved by the nurse who provides the human element to support the frightened infant or child and distressed or anxious parents.

PALLIATIVE CARDIAC SURGICAL PROCEDURES

The following discussion is included to provide brief insight into the various simple and more sophisticated palliative cardiac surgical procedures undertaken in childhood. These techniques are used when corrective surgery is not possible due to the complexity of the children's cardiac anomalies or when there is compromise of the cardiac performance in the infant or child rendering corrective surgery inadvisable at the time of presentation.

Systemic-to-pulmonary artery shunts

Systemic-to-pulmonary artery shunts are an effective form of palliation for many neonates and infants who experience a significant reduction in pulmonary blood flow due to cyanotic congenital heart disease, e.g., pulmonary atresia with or without ventricular septal defect, severe tetralogy of Fallot and single ventricle with pulmonary stenosis and tricuspid atresia.[99,120]

A variety of shunt procedures may be performed directing systemic arterial blood to the pulmonary artery, e.g., the Blalock-Taussig procedure (classical and modified), and a venous shunt such as the Glenn shunt, the Waterston's shunt and the Pott's shunt. The aim of these procedures is to augment the blood supply to the oligaemic pulmonary circulation.

Blalock-Taussig procedure (modified)

The classical Blalock-Taussig shunt, uses either the left or right subclavian arteries to effect an end-to-side anastomosis to the pulmonary artery. It is, however, the modified approach which is currently the more commonly adopted procedure. This approach uses a synthetic graft of gortex material and is anastomosed side to side between the subclavian and the pulmonary arteries. The pulmonary arterial supply is thus enhanced in infants and children with complex cyanotic lesions and associated pulmonary oligaemia. A right-sided anastomosis is favoured in children with ultimately correctable lesions, because of the ease of shunt removal at the time of surgical correction.

A recent study indicates a trend toward the classical shunt for neonates and infants with complex CHD. The study suggested patency of the classical shunts was maintained for a significantly longer period than with the synthetic grafts, prompting consideration of routine antithrombotic treatment for infants and children where the synthetic grafts are used.[156]

Glenn procedure

Most recently, this form of shunt procedure has increased in acceptance as an effective and long-lasting systemic to pulmonary artery shunt procedure. The anastomosis of the right pulmonary artery to the superior vena cava enhances the pulmonary artery blood flow. It is now commonly undertaken as the first stage to a more sophisticated palliation with the Fontan procedure described below.

Waterston's and Pott's shunts

Both the Waterston's and Pott's shunts are forms of aortopulmonary shunts. The Waterston's shunt creates a side-to-side anastomosis between the ascending aorta and the right pulmonary artery. The Pott's shunt effects a side-to-side anastomosis between the descending aorta and the left pulmonary artery.[99,120]

In recent years the Waterston's and the Pott's shunts have both lost favour due to the potential for complication associated with their use. The size of these shunts is reportedly difficult to confine and may result in an overly generous pulmonary blood flow which may rapidly lead to the development of pulmonary hypertension, which is often irreversible.[120] Additionally, there is difficulty with removal of the shunts at the time of corrective surgery.

Implications for nursing practice

A variety of complications may arise in infants following palliative shunt procedures. The greatest problem which requires reoperation is shunt occlusion, which results from early thrombosis.[120] Recent studies suggest a 13% to 16% operative mortality.[99,156] Other complications that may occur relate to the following:

- Cardiac failure when the shunt is too large.
- Tissue hypoperfusion of the affected limb when significant arterial blood flow is diverted following the classical Blalock-Taussig procedure.
- Local nerve damage due to surgical trauma.
- Decreased bone and muscle mass development, which results from interference with limb perfusion following the Blalock-Taussig procedure.[120]

From a nursing perspective, appreciation of the potential for complication following shunt procedures is essential. Recognition of early signs of shunt occlusion, cardiac failure and local tissue perfusion problems can facilitate early intervention, thereby preventing major complications.

Fontan procedure

The Fontan procedure is a highly sophisticated palliation currently having a widening application to many varied, yet complex congenital heart lesions.[157,158] Though having undergone many modifications since the original operation, the underlying principle of the procedure is to direct all systemic venous return from the right atrium or vena cava to the pulmonary artery, thus bypassing the right ventricle. Today, the Fontan procedure is almost always a cavopulmonary rather than the atriopulmonary anastomosis.[159,160]

Originally developed for palliation of tricuspid atresia, the current modifications to the procedure enable its successful application to many complex lesions where there is effectively only one ventricle (e.g., double inlet left ventricle). The success of the Fontan procedure is determined by several factors with pulmonary vascular resistance (PVR) being of utmost importance. Increases in PVR will impede systemic venous return, increase venous pressure and result in pleural effusion and ascites postoperatively. Further, the left ventricular function must be near normal and there can be no anatomical obstruction to blood flow pathways within the heart.[160,161]

Certain anatomical features, such as severe hypoplasia of the pulmonary artery, are considered a contraindication to surgical palliation with the Fontan procedure. It is considered that the inherently high PVR of early infancy excludes the young infant from surgical consideration.[160]

Potential for complication following a Fontan procedure includes significant postoperative problems due to compromise to the pulmonary blood flow, inadequate cardiac output and residual postoperative shunts.[160] Addressing the factors which may compromise the early postoperative phase of recovery is imperative for survival. Following the Fontan procedure, the systemic venous pressure is the force which drives blood flow through the pulmonary circuit. The venous pressure within the circuit must be kept high for adequate pulmonary blood flow, but lower than the plasma oncotic pressure to avoid fluid extravasation.[162]

A number of postoperative complications may arise as a result of maintaining continually high venous pressures. Pleural and pericardial effusions commonly occur and are attributed to both the high venous pressures and the general inflammatory response which follows the surgery. The effusions often become chylous in nature and may respond to a low-fat, medium-chain triglyceride diet together with continuous drainage of the pleural effusion. In situations where effusions persist, thoracic duct ligation may be required. When pericardial effusions persist, a surgical procedure to insert a pericardial window may be essential.[160]

Other problems infants and children may experience following Fontan procedures are ascites, liver failure and cerebral oedema, secondary to the high systemic venous pressures, thus causing systemic venous engorgement. Early extubation of these children is advocated as a safe and theoretically beneficial procedure, given that it reduces the complications caused by ventilation-induced elevation in venous pressures.[162] Spontaneous respiration reduces the mean intrathoracic pressure, whereas positive pressure ventilation increases it.

Results of surgery following the Fontan procedure: The operative mortality is highly variable and is dependent on the child's age, anatomy, myocardial function and pulmonary vascular resistance. The perioperative mortality ranges from 5% to 30%, with a 10% late mortality within 5 years of palliation[28,158] Recent follow-up data indicate that stress postoperatively induces an abnormal haemodynamic response and a decrease in exercise tolerance, deleteriously affecting the pulmonary circulation.[163]

Other associated risks with the Fontan procedure are atrial arrhythmias and atrial thrombosis, secondary to chronic atrial dilatation. These features have the potential to be eliminated with further modification to the procedure, recently described as a total cavopulmonary connection.[157] A recent study suggests the Fontan procedure provides medium to long-term benefit to the children with tricuspid atresia, as the repair enhances their left ventricular function, significantly improving their chance of survival.[164]

Atrial septectomy

The Blalock Hanlon atrial septectomy, now rarely performed, is a surgical palliation whereby the atrial septum is excised in infants who require atrial decompression and mixing of their systemic and venous circulations to sustain their life (e.g., mitral atresia). The procedure is effective in improving oxygenation in a very small group of infants not responsive to the interventional catheterisation procedures of balloon atrial septostomy.[99]

Pulmonary artery banding

The procedure of pulmonary artery banding offers an effective palliation in a small number of infants with high pulmonary blood flow in whom primary surgical correction in infancy is not possible or appropriate. The procedure restricts large left-to-right shunts, thus controlling heart failure and reducing pulmonary artery pressure (e.g., complicated VSD, single ventricle, truncus arteriosus and atrioventricular septal defect). In the past, pulmonary artery banding was adopted as a first stage in a corrective procedure in many infants with a large VSD. Problems arose, however, due to distortion of the pulmonary arteries at the site of the banding, which increased the risk of definitive repair resulting in a significant incidence of residual pulmonary artery stenosis.[165]

Current trends in palliative surgery: implications to nursing

Marked improvement may be seen in the clinical condition of infants with complex CHD, from the various palliative procedures outlined. Current surgical practice, however, favours early surgical repair where feasible. This contrasts with the staged repairs of the past when a palliation was followed by a secondary repair. This trend is the product of current sophisticated surgical techniques and the intraoperative and postoperative management now available.[161,166] It has, however, imposed special considerations for nurses in the care of younger infants with increasingly complex lesions. These infants now require extended periods of nursing support and are reliant upon more intensive pharmacological and technical assistance. From a nursing perspective, the principles of perioperative assessment and care are common to both open and closed heart surgical procedures performed in infancy and childhood.

Heart transplantation

Heart transplantation now provides an effective palliative treatment for infants and young children with end-stage cardiac disease due to structural lesions (e.g., hypoplasia of the left heart and cardiomyopathy of viral or idiopathic aetiology).[158,167–170] Heart and lung transplantations are undertaken in a small number of infants and children with severe pulmonary hypertensive disease resulting from structural cardiac defects or irreversible pulmonary disease (e.g., cystic fibrosis).[168,170,171]

Statistically, the hospital survival rate following heart transplantation is between 81% and 89%,[168,171] with 62% actuarial survival at 2 years.[172] The evidence regarding long-term survival in children following heart transplantation is conflicting, with complications ranging from coronary atherosclerosis, immunosuppression-induced malignancy and renal toxicity from cyclosporin.[168]

The survival in children following heart and lung transplantation is 60%, although the numbers of children so far transplanted remains small.[170] The 5-year survival following heart and lung transplantation is only 20%.[168] Susceptibility to severe pulmonary infection is a major factor determining outcome in these immunosupressed patients, especially when the infective agent is cytomegalovirus or other viral, bacterial or protozoan agents.[168,170] The potential for accelerated atherosclerosis still remains a major problem in the long-term prognosis of these infants.

Ethical considerations regarding organ donation to effect palliation and improve quality of life in these infants and children, albeit temporarily, raises highly complex issues, discussion of which are beyond the scope of this chapter. There is a trend for wider acceptance of this form of treatment. Improvement in immunosuppression therapy, whereby the potential side effects are further minimised, will help establish transplantation as a viable treatment option for a very small number of infants and children with irreversible cardiac and cardiopulmonary disease.

Modalities in Haemodynamic Monitoring

Today, the responsibilities of the nurse in the care of infants and children with cardiovascular dysfunction necessitates a sound understanding of the intracardiac haemodynamics associated with the various structural anomalies. Currently, the data provided by technology enhances the nurses' ability to identify and interpret trends in a child's clinical profile. Nurses assume responsibility for the early interpretation of altered variables, however subtle, through astute and continued clinical assessment of the infant and child, thus preventing decompensation to a critical and sometimes irreversible state.

The rapid progress in biotechnology now provides highly sophisticated computerised monitoring systems, by both non-invasive and invasive means, which enhance clinical assessment. Extreme accuracy and precision in the monitoring of a variety of physiological parameters is now attainable.[173,174] Nursing responsibility in care of these infants and children requires the development of advanced clinical assessment and analytical skills. Clinical findings are analysed and the information integrated in conjunction with the intracardiac and other monitored parameters. The nurse's ability to identify early trends in a child's clinical profile through the interpretation of altered clinical signs and haemodynamic variables facilitates intervention at an early stage which can arrest and prevent the development of problems. Often the changes detected by the nurse are subtle, yet they signify a very important and early alteration in a child's clinical status and therefore astute and continuous monitoring by the nurse responsible for care is required. Understanding of a child's clinical condition and a highly developed problem solving ability, which will facilitate critical decision making, is mandatory for paediatric cardiac nurse specialists.

Computerisation in critical care has imposed special considerations for nursing personnel. The capacity for detailed monitoring of physiological variables and the sophistication of data analysis heightens nurses' need for proficiency and confidence in their clinical assessment skills, analytical ability and the need to be conversant with the computer technology. Computerised facilities now provide simultaneous and continuous displays of multiple, monitored parameters with most equipment capable of trend identification. These functions provide the nurse with clear documentation of stability or change in a child's clinical profile. As critical care nurses place great reliance on the invasive haemodynamic monitoring technology as a guide to early intervention, cognisance of the limitations of monitoring is essential. The technology on which cardiac care services rely increases the responsibility and accountability for professional practice. With the wide acceptance of invasive monitoring as an aid to assessment and the various treatment modalities comes an increasing need for nurses to appreciate fully the medicolegal implications for their practice.

THE PERIOPERATIVE PERIOD

In the acute postoperative phase of an infant or child's recovery, the nurse will assess changes in a child's clinical state and interpret the physiological parameters. The haemodynamic data yields important information on variables determining cardiac output which are commonly monitored in postsurgical assessment (i.e., preload, afterload, contractility and heart rate and rhythm). Dependent on the complexity of the surgical repair or palliation, infants and children return to the intensive care unit with varying degrees of invasive monitoring lines, intra-arterial, central venous and transthoracic right and left atrial lines. Direct pulmonary artery monitoring is generally required in infants with reactive pulmonary vascular resistance states which may pose a problem postoperatively. This monitoring facilitates their acute management and aids recovery through early, accurate intervention.

The availability of computerised monitoring for the measurement of physiological variables enables determination of cardiac output using either the Fick principle, thermodilution or dye dilution studies.[120,144,175–180] Additionally, precise determination of myocardial function and residual postoperative intracardiac shunts can be assessed.[181]

ASSESSMENT OF CARDIAC OUTPUT

Cardiac output is the product of the heart rate times the stroke volume and yields results measured in litres per minute.

Direct comparisons of cardiac output results are not possible between infants, children and adolescents due to differences in body surface areas. For this reason, assessment of cardiac index provides a reliable indication of myocardial function, making possible a comparison of cardiac output states.[178] Determination of cardiac index (CI) is reached by dividing cardiac output (CO) by body surface area (BSA), as shown in the following equation CI = CO/BSA.[182–184]

Body surface area is readily determined by plotting the body weight and length or height on a Dubois body surface chart. The point of intersection of the 2 parameters determines the BSA in square metres.[180,185]

The normal values for the cardiac index range between 3.5 and 4.5 L/min/m^2 for all children.[33] A decrease to less than 2.2 L/min/m^2 will result in a significant alteration in tissue perfusion.[174,178] Prompt nursing assessment of all parameters, both clinically and mechanically derived, is required, as early intervention may reverse or prevent the establishment of a low cardiac output state.

ASSESSMENT OF SYSTEMIC AND PULMONARY VASCULAR RESISTANCE

Assessment of vascular resistance of both the systemic and pulmonary circulation is readily undertaken as a guide to therapeutic intervention with either vasodilator or vasopressor agents.[185]

Systemic vascular resistance

Systemic vascular resistance (SVR) measures the impedance to blood flow afforded by the systemic arteriolar circuit. When the calculated value is high, significant vasoconstriction is present leading to increased myocardial work and a subsequent increase in oxygen and glucose requirements. In contrast, decreased readings imply a generalised vasodilation as seen following pharmacological manipulation with vasodilator preparations or in distributive shock states (e.g., sepsis, especially in Gram-negative septicaemia) or in anaphylaxis.[185]

Calculation of SVR requires calculation of mean arterial pressure (MAP), and measurement of right atrial pressure (RAP) or central venous pressure (CVP) and cardiac output (CO), using the following formula:[174,185,186]

$$\frac{MAP - CVP}{CO} \times 80 = SVR \text{ (dyne/sec/cm}^{-5}) \text{ (physical resistance)}$$

$$\frac{2 \text{ (Diastolic BP)} + \text{Systolic BP}}{3} = MAP$$

Approximate derived values for systemic vascular resistance in infants and children are included in **Table 11.7**.

Comparison of results of SVR between infants and children of different sizes is made

Table 11.7 Approximate values of systemic and pulmonary vascular resistance in infants and children recorded[182,186]

	Vascular resistance (dyne/sec/cm^{-5})
Systemic	
Neonate	800–1200
Older infant	1200–1600
Child	1600–2400
Pulmonary	
Neonate	640–800
Infant to adult	80–240

possible by deriving the value of the systemic vascular resistance index (SVRI). To calculate the SVRI, divide the SVR by body surface area (BSA) as shown, to record a value in dyne/sec/cm^{-5}/m^{2}:[140]

$$SVR/BSA = SVRI \text{ (dyne/sec/cm}^{-5}/\text{m}^{2})$$

Pulmonary vascular resistance

Calculation of pulmonary vascular resistance (PVR) indicates the impedance offered by the pulmonary circuit to right ventricular ejection.[178] Many structural congenital cardiac defects impose significant volume and pressure loading on the pulmonary circulation, resulting in severe increases in PVR, exemplified by ventricular septal defects. The calculation of PVR requires measurement of mean pulmonary artery pressure (MPAP), pulmonary capillary wedge pressure (PCWP) and cardiac output (CO) using the following formula:[186]

$$\frac{MPAP - PCWP}{CO} \times 80 = PVR \text{ (dyne/sec/cm}^{-5})$$

A table of the derived values for pulmonary vascular resistance in infants and children is included in **Table 11.7**.

To enable a comparison of results between infants and children, the PVR score is divided by the BSA to yield the pulmonary vascular resistance index (PVRI) as shown:[144,186]

$$PVR/BSA = PVRI \text{ (dyne/sec/cm}^{-5}/\text{m}^{2})$$

The value of PVRI is therefore recorded in dyne/sec/cm^{-5}/m^{2}. These calculations are used at the time of cardiac catheterisation to determine the suitability of the infant or child for surgical correction. In the acute postoperative period, the PVRI may be used to determine the need for pharmacological interventions to reduce the persistent or recurring increase in PVR.

WAVEFORM CHARACTERISTICS

Great vessels and intracardiac chambers

A sound understanding of normal intracardiac and extracardiac haemodynamics is necessary in order to interpret early and often subtle changes in an infant or child's clinical

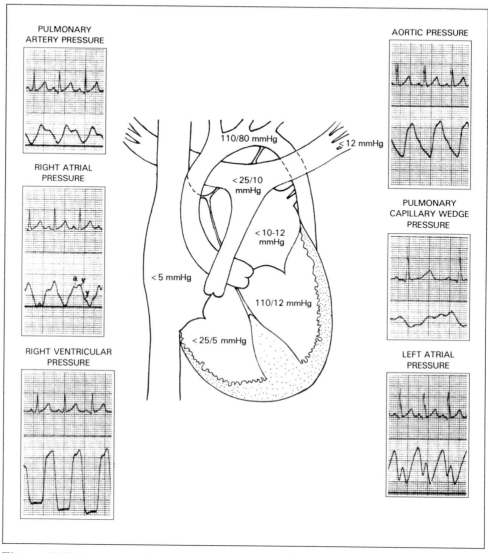

Figure 11.6 Normal atrial and ventricular pressure wave conformations, shown in correlation with the electrocardiographic representation of sinus rhythm.

condition. Recognition of characteristic waveforms and an appreciation of normal pressure ranges within the great vessels and intracardiac chambers is therefore essential to the nurse's problem solving and critical decision making ability (**Figure 11.6**).

Atrial pressure waves: the 'a', 'c' and 'v' waves

The atrial chambers, referred to as the low-pressure chambers of the heart, produce 3 characteristic pressure elevations during the cardiac cycle; the 'a', 'c', and 'v' waves. Examination of an atrial pressure trace in conjunction with an electrocardiographic representation will show that the first pressure elevation, the 'a' wave, corresponds to atrial contraction[187] (**Figure 11.6**).

The second positive deflection, the 'c' wave is produced as the ventricles begin to contract. The pressure within each ventricular chamber continues to peak until the increased ventricular pressure causes a bulging of the atrioventricular valves (A-V valves) towards the atrium.[197] Additionally, the myocardial fibres of the atrium are stretched as the ventricle begins to contract. Both these factors contribute to the 'c' wave, however, it may not always be clearly observed when it notches upon the preceding 'a' wave.

The third positive deflection, the 'v' wave is produced towards the end of ventricular contraction, as the blood in the atrium builds up against a closed A-V valve. Once the ventricle relaxes and the pressure reduces to less than atrial pressure, the A-V valves open and the blood from the atria passively fills the ventricle. It is the opening of the A-V valves which corresponds to the steep decline of the 'v' wave, the 'y' descent.[187]

Clinical relevance of the 'a' and 'v' wave

Measurement of the pressure variation in the atrial chambers must include observation of the characteristic undulating waveform which signifies line patency and hence ensures more accurate interpretation of the physiological variables. Accurate evaluation of the haemodynamic data is essential as treatment is instigated in response to the results of clinical and monitored parameters.

Nurses may observe an unusual prominence of the 'a' and 'v' waves in certain congenital cardiac defects. Giant 'a' waves may be observed in children with:

- atrioventricular valvular stenosis, i.e., tricuspid or mitral valve stenosis;
- arrhythmic disturbances, e.g., atrioventricular dissociation;
- ventricular pacing (when the atrium contracts against a closed atrioventricular valve).

Giant 'v' waves, known as cannon waves, can be observed when there is atrioventricular valve incompetence, i.e., tricuspid or mitral incompetence.[181,185,188]

Characteristic pressure fluctuations or swings are observed in conjunction with respiratory excursions. Spontaneous inspiration produces a decrease in intrathoracic pressure causing a concomitant decrease in intravascular and intracardiac pressures. This results in a fall in central venous pressure, right atrial, pulmonary artery, pulmonary capillary wedge and left atrial pressures.[177]

Central venous pressure

Measurement of central venous pressure (CVP) provides: a direct assessment of the filling pressure of the right heart; and an indirect assessment of right ventricular function. The normal pressure range is 0 to 9 mmHg (3 to 12 cm/H_2O).

CVP recordings taken in isolation, although yielding valuable information, cannot be considered as important as a child's response to interventional measures which are demonstrated through an assessment of CVP trend profiles.

Atrial pressure characteristics: right atrial pressure

Right atrial pressure (RAP) indirectly represents right ventricular end-diastolic pressure (RVEDP). Therefore, as indicated for CVP measurement, the RAP reflects preload or filling pressure of the right heart and right ventricular function (as RAP indirectly represents the end-diastolic filling pressure of the right ventricle in the absence of obstructive valvular lesions). When monitoring intra-atrial pressure, the mean pressure in the atrium is recorded during each cycle. The normal pressure range is 0 to 5 mmHg.[177,189]

RAP may be measured via percutaneous or direct intracardiac transthoracic lines. Low RAP will be observed in states of hypovolaemia.[185] Effective myocardial performance is demonstrated by clinical assessment signs signifying a good cardiac output, combined with RAP values in the lower range of normal. This contrasts with the situation of right ventricular failure when elevation of RAP is evident.

Left atrial pressure

Left atrial pressure (LAP) indirectly represents left ventricular end-diastolic pressure (LVEDP) when there is absence of mitral valve disease, i.e., incompetence or stenosis of the mitral valve. LAP therefore reflects the preload or filling pressure of the left heart and indicates the function of the left ventricle. The normal mean pressure range is 5 to 12 mmHg.[189,190]

As left ventricular function deteriorates in certain pressure or volume overload states, the LVEDP will rise with a concomitant rise in LAP.

Right ventricular pressure

The normal pressure range is 15 to 25 mmHg (systolic) and 0 to 5 mmHg (diastolic).[177,189]

Right ventricular pressure (RVP) is not routinely monitored. Characteristic right ventricular waves and pressures may be observed when a right atrial catheter migrates into the right ventricle or when a pulmonary artery line slips back into the right ventricle. RVEDP indirectly represents RAP in infants and children with normal function of the tricuspid valve.[33,190] A catheter which is floating in the right ventricle could cause irritation of the ventricle and produce ventricular arrhythmias.

Elevation of RVP is observed in infants and children with: right ventricular outflow obstruction (e.g., pulmonary valve stenosis, tetralogy of Fallot); pulmonary hypertension related to a moderate to large shunt, as in ventricular septal defect or patent ductus arteriosus; and constrictive pericarditis or pericardial tamponade.[188,190]

Pulmonary artery pressure

The normal pressure range is 15 to 25 mmHg (systolic) and 8 to 10 mmHg (diastolic).[177,189]

Pulmonary artery pressure (PAP) assesses the dynamics of the pulmonary arteriolar circuit. Elevation of PAP is observed in infants and children with: increased pulmonary blood flow (e.g., ventricular septal defect, patent ductus arteriosus); increased pulmonary vascular resistance; and increased pulmonary venous pressure (e.g., mitral stenosis, left ventricular failure).[190]

Pulmonary capillary wedge pressure

The normal pressure range is less than 12 mmHg.[177,189]

Pulmonary capillary wedge pressure (PCWP) indirectly represents LAP, which indirectly represents LVEDP in infants and children with normal pulmonary vascular resistance and normal function of their mitral valve.[188,190]

INVASIVE MONITORING DEVICES: POTENTIAL FOR COMPLICATION

With the widespread acceptance, availability and use of invasive haemodynamic monitoring techniques and procedures, there is an inherent potential for an overwhelming array of complications to arise. Potentially devastating complications may arise with the use of percutaneous and transthoracic intracardiac devices. Problems range from infection, haemorrhage, thrombosis, embolism of air or particulate matter, arrhythmias, micro or macro electrocution, pneumothorax and haemothorax. Additional complications are associated with the use of right heart flotation catheters which measure pulmonary artery and pulmonary capillary wedge pressure. Problems encountered with their use, additional to those previously outlined include perforation, especially rupture of the pulmonary artery branches, pulmonary infarction, valvular damage and thrombocytopenia.[144,173,180–182,188,191–194]

Arterial pressure monitoring

Direct intra-arterial pressure monitoring enables accurate, continuous assessment of systolic, diastolic and mean blood pressure. In addition, arterial pressure monitoring provides access for blood sampling for arterial blood gases, electrolytes and other blood profiles. There are, however, certain blood tests for which samples should not be routinely taken from the lines (e.g., coagulation screens). The simultaneous display of the electrocardiogram and the arterial waveform may facilitate early interpretation of arrhythmias as alterations in pulse pressure and the characteristic arterial waveform become apparent.

The rapid upstroke of the arterial waveform (the anacrotic limb) corresponds to the ejection of left ventricular volume at the time of systole. As the left ventricular pressure falls rapidly in diastole, a pressure gradient develops between the aorta and left ventricle. The momentum of blood flowing back towards the aortic valve causes the snap closure of the aortic valve which is represented as the dicrotic notch on the pressure wave[84,144,195] (**Figure 11.7**). The second, yet small positive pressure wave, is representative of the momentary back-flow of blood which continues on to the aortic valve.[84]

Factors affecting pulse pressure

A number of factors influence the pulse pressure and therefore the characteristic arterial waveform. The stroke volume, compliance of the arterial tree and to a lesser extent, the character of systolic ejection are the factors which determine pulse pressure.[84] There are several mechanisms which alter pulse pressure.

- An increase in heart rate causing a decrease in stroke volume.
- A decrease in systemic vascular resistance causing an increase in venous return and hence an increase in preload, resulting in an increase in stroke volume.
- An increase in preload from rapid volume loading, causing a concomitant increase in stroke volume and an increase in pulse pressure.

Pulse pressure may be further augmented with the introduction of inotropic preparations which boost myocardial performance and the use of vasoactive preparations which manipulate increases in systemic vascular resistance. An increase in venous return to the heart and an increase in stroke volume will result.

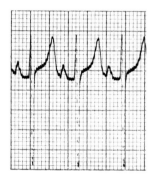

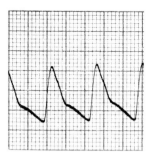

Figure 11.7 Arterial pressure waveform showing characteristic features seen in conjunction with electrocardiographic representation of normal sinus rhythm.

Arterial pressure wave conformations in CHD

Variation of the pressure wave may be noted in infants and children with structural congenital heart defects. Direct arterial pressure monitoring in an infant or child with persistent patency of the ductus arteriosus, aortic valve incompetence or truncus arteriosus will show a characteristic wide pulse pressure. In infants with a patency of the ductus arteriosus there is a rapid aortic run-off of blood into the pulmonary artery following the ejection of blood from the left ventricle, causing a decrease in diastolic pressure. Palpation of the pulses in these infants reveals a pulsation which is collapsing in nature, indicative of the rapid aortic run-off. Similarly, the child with aortic incompetence has a degree of aortic run-off when the aortic valve fails to close effectively at end ventricular systole.[84]

A child with valvular or subvalvular aortic stenosis will have a narrow pulse pressure, slower upstroke of the arterial pressure wave, with a sustained peak and a slurring of the dicrotic notch. These features are due to the obstruction to blood flow and hence the prolongation of ejection time.[196]

ARTERIAL LINES

Site selection

The selection of the site for insertion of a direct intra-arterial catheter is of major importance. Arterial cannulation is established following confirmation of an alternative arterial supply to distal tissue, as demonstrated with radial artery cannulation and the application of the Allen's test.[178,195] This reduces the risk of inadequate tissue perfusion to the limb, secondary to embolus, thrombosis or vasospasm.[192] Access to the site causing least disturbance to the infant or child and a site that is easily secured and free from contamination are important criteria for site selection.[178] The radial artery is therefore the preferred site for cannulation, although the dorsalis pedis and posterior tibial arteries can be used.[182,194]

The need for careful site selection, as peripheral as possible, cannot be overemphasised. When the above criteria are observed, the risk of iatrogenic complication from arterial thrombosis is minimised. The potential for complication and long-term sequelae from the use of invasive devices increases with the duration of monitoring.

Selection of brachial and femoral arteries is associated with increased risks for vascular and nerve damage and the potential for hypoperfusion to the limbs. In addition, the contamination risk associated with femoral cannulation lends credence for alternate site selection. Temporal cannulation is not practised due to the risk of retrograde embolisation into the cerebral circulation. Cerebral ischaemia or infarction may result and are associated with the flushing of air and particulate material.[100,178] Similarly, umbilical artery lines are avoided in newborn infants with decreased blood flow in the descending aorta exemplified by coarctation of the aorta and aortic arch interruption because of the increased risks for necrotising enterocolitis.[100]

Nursing considerations

The following care and observations are essential to optimise management for an infant or child with an arterial line:

- Observe strict asepsis in all sampling from the line and minimise risk of contamination of lines by changing all manometer lines each 48 to 72 hours.
- Firmly secure the cannula and manometer lines, and comfortably support the limb to minimise nerve damage and eliminate the potential for catheter dislodgment and haemorrhage.
- Ensure cannula connections are visible, Luer-locked at all times and clearly labelled or colour coded for ease of identification.
- Observe distal and local perfusion of limb. Any discolouration or blanching which occurs with flushing of the line and signs of mottling, redness or swelling requires: immediate investigation to eliminate the cause; immediate removal of cannula; and documentation of the findings.
- Ensure continued patency of the arterial lines with heparinised infusions, always aspirating a line before flushing to prevent air or particulate matter from entering the arterial circulation. Avoid hand flushing of the lines at all costs in order to minimise the risks of retrograde embolisation.
- Ensure continuous heparinised flushing of the line is maintained until cannula removal, thereby eliminating the risk of thrombus formation at the catheter tip and subsequent embolisation upon withdrawal.
- Upon removal of the cannula, firm application of pressure to the site is required for a period of 5 to 10 minutes to prevent bleeding.[144,195]

PRESSURE TRANSDUCERS

Pressure transducers are the essential component to all monitoring systems in that they convert one form of energy, mechanical energy, to another form which produces an electrical signal. The determination of intravascular pressures is facilitated by the movement of the transducer diaphragm. In response to a force applied to the diaphragm, movement proportional to the degree of force is amplified and recorded on the pressure monitoring device.[194,197,198]

ZEROING AND CALIBRATION OF MONITORING EQUIPMENT

The anatomical landmark selected as a reference point for zeroing of monitoring equipment is the phlebostatic axis, at the level of the right atrium.[177,144,199] Uniformity in site selection for regular rezeroing and calibration of equipment is essential. This will eliminate inaccuracies with patient assessment and subsequent inappropriate interventional support attributed to technical inaccuracy.

IMPLICATIONS FOR NURSING PRACTICE

Appreciation of the potential for complication and an ability to problem solve and make critical decisions can prevent significant complications which may arise from invasive monitoring. Continuous invasive haemodynamic monitoring may be associated with various problems, either artifactual in aetiology or attributed to a variety of mechanical problems which can arise at the site of the transducer or the lines, or alternately may signify problems with catheter placement or dislodgment. The problems encountered with invasive haemodynamic monitoring include:

* dampening of pressure wave amplitude;
* overshoot of wave form conformation;
* catheter whip or fling;
* inaccuracies with zeroing and calibration.

Dampening of pressure wave amplitude results when kinetic energy is absorbed or dissipated within the fluid-filled monitoring system, causing the amplitude of the normal wave oscillations to fade.[178] The loss of wave clarity may be due to:

* compressible air or particulate matter in the monitoring system;
* mechanical obstruction of the catheter due to occlusion, kinking or compression;
* establishment of a low cardiac output state.

The immediate nursing intervention requires:

* assessment of the infant or child's circulation, general condition and perfusion of the affected limb;
* the isolation and removal of the causative factors.

An increase in pressure may be seen with the upstroke of the arterial pressure wave in systole, because of an artificial phenomenon causing overshoot of the pressure, resulting in false, high systolic readings. Similarly, this phenomenon may also be seen in diastole, as the pressure overshoots the baseline, giving falsely low diastolic pressures. This problem is attributed to resonance and is described as a 'tendency of physical systems to vibrate at a natural frequency'.[194] The problems of resonance and damping may be overcome by close monitoring of the mean arterial pressure, which is ascribed as being essentially unaffected by the artefact. Minimising the factors which predispose to artefact on the pressure wave necessitates the selection of narrow bore, non-pliable, rigid manometer tubing, ideally less than 120 cm in length.

Catheter whip or fling occurs when a fine catheter lying within a high-flow, high-pressure vessel causes excessive catheter movement. This may result in spurious recordings of pressures and wave conformations attributed to artefact and is a significant problem in pulmonary artery monitoring systems.[144,194,195,200]

The nurse must remain cognisant of the potential for complication associated with the use of invasive monitoring now so commonplace in paediatric critical care settings. The benefits to be gained for the infant or child must always be considered against the risk of complication resulting from the use of the various invasive devices.[201] The potential for complication is reduced with careful site selection for catheters, restriction in the duration of catheter use and precision in catheter insertion and monitoring techniques.[48]

Critical care nursing with the current and future projected level of biotechnology, imposes heightened responsibility and accountability for the nurse and results in an inevitable increase in professional liability.[173] The educational requirements imposed on the clinical nurse specialist by this level of biotechnology are complex. Highly individualised orientation and in-service programs are required[202] to facilitate acquisition of clinical assessment skills, the ability to analyse the clinical findings and interpret physiological parameters which enhance our ability to assess, plan, implement and evaluate care for the infants and children.

ACKNOWLEDGMENTS

I gratefully acknowledge the continued support provided by my colleagues in developing this chapter and I wish to thank Ms L Houston for her comments in the early stages of development. Most especially, I wish to extend my very special thanks to my nursing colleagues Ms V. Leveaux and Mr B. O'Connor, and medical colleagues Dr R. Hawker and Dr J. Tharion for their support, and their highly valued assistance in critiquing the cardiovascular component of this book throughout its development.

REFERENCES

1. Adams FH, Emmanoulides GC, Riemenschneider TA, eds. *Moss' heart disease in infants, children and adolescents.* 4th ed. Baltimore: Williams and Wilkins, 1989.
2. Guyton A. *Textbook of medical physiology.* 8th ed. Philadelphia: Saunders, 1991.
3. Hoffman JIE. Congenital heart disease: incidence and inheritance. *Pediatr Clin North Am* 1990; 37: 25–43.
4. Marieb EN. *Human anatomy and physiology.* Redwood City, CA: Benjamin Cummings, 1992.
5. Oberhaensli I, Extermann P, Friedli B, Beguin F. Ultrasound screening for congenital cardiac malformations in the foetus: its importance for peri and postnatal care. *Pediatr Radiol* 1989; 19: 94–99.
6. Sholler GF. Paediatric cardiology in general practice. *Mod Med Aust* 1989; June: 49–57.
7. Veille JC, Mahowald MB, Sivakoff M. Ethical dilemmas in fetal echocardiography. *Obstet Gynaecol* 1989; 73 (part 1): 710–714.
8. Australian Bureau of Statistics. Perinatal deaths: foetal and neonatal deaths by sex of child and main cause or condition in foetus/infant and mother, Australia, 1990. *Perinatal deaths in Australia.* Table 6, 7–8. Canberra: ABS, 1990.

9. Australian Institute of Health. The health status of Australians. *In: Australia's Health 1990.* Canberra: AGPS, 1990: 7–40.

10. Reich O. Natural history of congenital heart disease: Central European experience. Third world congress of pediatric cardiology, Bangkok. [Abstract S 19.2, 14] November/December, 1989.

11. Lynch ME. Congenital defects: parental issues and nursing supports. *J Perinatal Neonatal Nursing* 1989; 2 (4): 53–59.

12. Osband BA. Multifactorial inheritance: implications for perinatal and neonatal nurses. *J Perinatal Neonatal Nursing* 1989; 2 (4): 43–52.

13. Farrell CD. Genetic counselling: the emerging reality. *J Perinatal Neonatal Nursing* 1989; 2 (4): 21–33.

14. Moore KL. The cardiovascular system. *In:* Moore KL. *The developing human: clinically oriented embryology.* 4th ed. Philadelphia: Saunders, 1988: 286–333.

15. Moore KL. The causes of human congenital malformations. *In:* Moore KL. *The developing human: clinically oriented embryology.* 4th ed. Philadelphia: Saunders, 1988: 131–158.

16. Nora JJ. Etiologic aspects of heart disease. *In:* Adam FH, Emmanoulides GC, Riemenschneider TA, eds. *Moss' heart disease in infants, children and adolescents.* 4th ed. Baltimore: Williams and Wilkins, 1989: 15–23.

17. Lin AE. Congenital heart defects in malformation syndromes. *Clinics in Perinatology,* 1990; 17: 641–673.

18. Seaver LH, Hoyme HE. Teratology in pediatric practice. *Pediatric Clinics of North America,* 1992; 39: 111–134.

19. Driscoll DJ. Use of inotropic and chronotropic agents in neonates. *Clin Perinatol* 1987; 14: 931–949.

20. Josker J, Maciejewski M, Cousins M. Advanced case studies in haemodynamic monitoring — Post operative cardiovascular patients. *Crit Care Nursing Clin North Am* 1994; 6 (1): 187–197.

21. Keeley SR, Bohn DJ. The use of inotropic and afterload-reducing agents in neonates. *Clin Perinatol* 1988; 15: 467–489.

22. Rice V. Shock management Part 11; pharmacologic intervention. *Crit Care Nurse* 1985; 5 (1): 42–57.

23. Guyton A. Heart muscle; the heart as a pump. *In:* Guyton A. *Textbook of medical physiology.* 8th ed. Philadelphia: Saunders, 1991: 98–110.

24. Kallen RJ, Lonergan JM. Fluid resuscitation of acute hypovolaemic hypoperfusion states. *Pediatr Clin North Am* 1990; 37: 287–294.

25. Schulkind ML. Management of pediatric shock. *Topics Emergency Med* 1988; 9 (4): 53–69.

26. Lucchesi BR. Role of calcium on excitation – contraction coupling in cardiac and vascular smooth muscle. *Circulation* 1989; 80 (Suppl 4): 1–13.

27. Zelis R, Moore R. Recent insight into the calcium channels. *Circulation* 1989; 80 (Suppl 4): 14–16.

28. Garson A. *Depolarisation and repolarisation: cellular electrophysiology.* Philadelphia: Lea and Febiger, 1983: 9–18.

29. Fisher DJ, Towbin J. Maturation of the heart. *Clin Perinatol* 1988; 15: 421–446.

30. Perkin RM, Anas NG. Nonsurgical contractile manipulation of the failing circulation. *In:* Swedlow DB, Raphaely RC, eds. *Cardiovascular problems in pediatric critical care. Clinics in critical care medicine.* Vol 10. New York: Churchill Livingstone, 1986: 229–256.

31. Slota MC. Assessment of systemic perfusion in the child. *Crit Care Nurse* 1987; 7 (4): 69–73.

32. Perloff WF. Physiology of the heart and circulation. *In:* Swedlow DB, Raphaely RC, eds. *Cardiovascular problems in pediatric critical care. Clinics in critical care medicine.* Vol 10. New York: Churchill Livingstone, 1986: 1–85.

33. Hazinski MF. Shock in the pediatric patient. *Crit Care Nursing Clin North Am* 1990; 2: 309–324.

34. Wetzel RC, Stiff JL, Rogers MC. Heart rate and rhythm as determinants of cardiac output. *In:* Swedlow DB, Raphaely RC, eds. *Cardiovascular problems in pediatric critical care. Clinics in critical care medicine.* Vol 10. New York: Churchill Livingstone, 1986: 257–278.

35. Garson A. Effects of alterations on the electrocardiogram. *In:* Garson A. *The electrocardiogram in infants and children: a systematic approach.* Philadelphia: Lea and Febiger, 1983: 170–194.

36. Curley M. Cardiac dysrhythmias. *In:* Keeley SJ, ed. *Pediatric emergency nursing.* California: Appleton and Lange, 1988: 253–275.

37. Fuller R. Cardiac function and the neonatal EKG: Part 1, introduction to neonatal EKGs. *Neonatal Network* 1989; 7 (4): 47–51.

38. Fuller R. Cardiac function and the neonatal EKG: Part 2, bradycardia. *Neonatal Network* 1989; 7 (6): 61–63.

39. Fuller R. Cardiac function and the neonatal EKG: Part 3, tachycardia. *Neonatal Network* 1989; 7 (6): 65–67.

40. Fuller R. Cardiac function and the neonatal EKG: Part 4, chamber enlargement and axis deviation. *Neonatal Network* 1989; 8 (1): 77–81.

41. Fuller R. Cardiac function and the neonatal EKG: Part 5, EKGs and common disorders. *Neonatal Network* 1989; 8 (2): 41–43.

42. Garson A. *The electrocardiogram in infants and children: a systematic approach.* Philadelphia: Lea and Febiger, 1983.

43. Kombol P. Dysrhythmias in infancy. *Neonatal Network* 1988; April: 41–52.

44. Friedman WF. Neonatal cardiac function. *In:* Yacoub M, ed. *1987 Annual of cardiac surgery.* London: Gower Academic Journals, 1987 15–19.

45. Friedman WF, George BL. New concepts and drugs in the treatment of congestive heart failure. *Pediatr Clin North Am* 1984; 31: 1197–1227.

46. Kulik LA, Hickey PA, Lawrence PR. Pharmacologic interventions for the neonate with compromised cardiac function. *J Perinatal Neonatal Nursing* 1991; 5 (2): 71–83.

47. Kuipers JRG. Myocardial function in the newborn. Third world congress of pediatric cardiology, Bangkok. [Abstract P2, 3.] November/December, 1989.

48. Baker A. Acquired heart disease in infants and children. *Crit Care Nursing Clin North Am* 1994; 6: 175–186.

49. Talner NS. Heart failure. *In:* Adams FH, Emmanoulides GC, Riemenschneider TA, eds. *Moss' heart disease in infants, children and adolescents.* 4th ed. Baltimore: Williams and Wilkins, 1989: 890–911.

50. Savedra M, Eland JN, Tesler M. Pain management. *In:* Craft MJ, Denehy JA, eds. *Nursing interventions for infants and children.* Philadelphia: Saunders, 1990: 304–325.

51. Flynn PA, Engle MA, Ehlers KH. Cardiac issues in the pediatric emergency room. *Pediatr Clin North Am* 1992; 39: 955–983.

52. Scheiber RA. Noninvasive recognition and assessment of the failing circulation. *In:* Swedlow DB, Raphaely RC, eds. *Cardiovascular problems in pediatric critical care, clinics in critical care medicine.* Vol. 10. New York: Churchill Livingstone, 1986: 87–127.

53. Kohr LM, O'Brien P. Current management of congestive heart failure in infants and children. *Nursing Clin North Am* 1995; 30 (2): 261–290.

54. McNamara DG. Value and limitations of auscultation in the management of congenital heart disease. *Pediatr Clin North Am* 1990; 37: 93–113.

55. Monett ZI, Moynihan PJ. Cardiovascular assessment of the neonatal heart. *J Perinatal Neonatal Nursing* 1991; 5 (2): 50–59.

56. Cohn JN. Abnormalities of peripheral sympathetic nervous system control in congestive heart failure. *Circulation* 1990; 82 (Suppl 2): 59–67.

57. Guyton A. Nervous regulation of the circulation, and rapid control of arterial pressure. *In:* Guyton A. *Textbook of medical physiology.* 8th ed. Philadelphia: Saunders, 1991: 194–204.

58. Walsh RA. Sympathetic control of diastolic function in congestive heart failure. *Circulation* 1990; 82 (Suppl 2): 52–58.

59. Lister G, Fahey JT. Shock. *In:* Adams FH, Emmanoulides GC, Riemenschneider TA, eds. *Moss' heart disease in infants, children and adolescents.* 4th ed. Baltimore: Williams and Wilkins, 1989: 911–925.

60. Packer M. Role of the sympathetic nervous system in chronic heart failure. *Circulation* 1990; 82 (Suppl 2): 1–6.

61. Guyton A. The autonomic nervous system; the adrenal medulla. *In:* Guyton A. *Textbook of medical physiology.* 8th ed. Philadelphia: Saunders, 1991: 667–678.

62. Bristow MR, Hershberger RE, Port JD, Gilbert EM, Sandoval A, Rasmussen R, Cates AE, Feldman AM. Beta adrenergic pathways in non failing human ventricular myocardium. *Circulation* 1990; 82 (Suppl 1): 12–25.

63. Rimar JM. Shock in infants and children; assessment and treatment. *Am J Maternal Child Nursing* 1988; 13 (2): 98–105.

64. Mutnick AH, Felitt S. Cardiac drugs and chronotropic agents. *Nursing 87* 1987; 17 (10): 58–61.

65. Leier CV, Binkley PF, Cody RJ. Alpha adrenergic component of the sympathetic nervous system in congestive heart failure. *Circulation* 1990; 82 (Suppl 1): 68–76.

66. Guyton A. Dominant role of the kidneys in long-term regulation of arterial pressure and in hypertension: The integrated system for pressure control. *In:* Guyton A. *Textbook of medical physiology.* 8th ed. Philadelphia: Saunders, 1991: 205–222.

67. Kennedy GT. Captopril in the treatment of congestive cardiac failure. *Crit Care Nurse* 1990; 10 (2): 39–46.

68. Guignard JP, Gouyon JB. Body fluid homeostasis in the newborn infant with congestive heart failure: effects of diuretics. *Clin Perinatol* 1988; 15: 447–466.

69. McCance KL, Richardson SJ. Structure and function of the cardiovascular and lymphatic systems. *In:* McCance KL, Huether SE, eds. *Pathophysiology: the biological basis for disease in adults and children.* St Louis: Mosby, 1990: 859–915.

70. Guyton A. Local control of blood flow by the tissues, and humoral regulation. *In:* Guyton A. *Textbook of medical physiology.* 8th ed. Philadelphia: Saunders, 1991: 185–193.

71. Guyton A. Renal and associated mechanisms for controlling extracellular fluid osmolality and sodium concentration. *In:* Guyton A. *Textbook of medical physiology.* 8th ed. Philadelphia: Saunders, 1991: 308–319.

72. Guyton A. The pituitary hormones and their control by the hypothalamus. *In:* Guyton A. *Textbook of medical physiology.* 8th ed. Philadelphia: Saunders, 1991: 819–830.

73. Cosgrove JA. Atrial naturetic peptide: a new cardiac hormone. *Heart Lung* 1989; 18: 461–465.

74. Rice V. The role of potassium in health and disease, *Crit Care Nurse* 1982; 4 (3): 54–73.

75. Merenstein GB, Gardner SL, Woods Blake W. Heat balance. *In:* Merenstein GB, Gardner SL, eds. *Handbook of neonatal intensive care.* St Louis: Mosby, 1989: 111–125.

76. Lees MH, King DH. Heart disease in the newborn. *In:* Adams FH, Emmanoulides GC, Riemenschneider TA, eds. *Moss' heart disease in infants, children and adolescents.* 4th ed. Baltimore: Williams and Wilkins, 1989: 842–855.

77. Chatburn RL, Carlo WA. Assessment of neonatal gas exchange. *In:* Carlo WA, Chatburn RL, eds. *Neonatal respiratory care.* 2nd ed. Chicago: Year Book Medical, 1988: 40–60.

78. West JB. Gas transport to the periphery. *In:* West JB. *Respiratory physiology: the essentials.* 4th ed. Baltimore: Williams and Wilkins, 1990: 69–85.

79. Teitel D. Care of the infant with heart disease. *In:* Ballard RA, ed. *Pediatric care of the ICN graduate.* Philadelphia: Saunders, 1988: 226–239.

80. Hastrieter AR. Preface to cardiovascular disease in the neonate. *Clin Perinatol* 1988; 15 (3): xi–xii.

81. Gadish HS, Gonzales JL, Hayes JS. Factors affecting nurses' decisions to administer pediatric pain medication postoperatively. *J Pediatr Nursing* 1988; 3: 383–390.

82. Crockett M, Tappero E. Dopamine and dobutamine: neonatal indications and implications. *Neonatal Network* 1989; 7 (5): 13–19.

83. Steward DF. Afterload; non surgical manipulation of the failing circulation. *In:* Swedlow DB,

Raphaely RC, eds. *Cardiovascular problems in pediatric critical care, clinics in critical care medicine*, Vol. 10. New York: Churchill Livingstone, 1986: 221–228.

84. Guyton A. Vascular distensibility and functions of the arterial and venous systems. *In:* Guyton A. *Textbook of medical physiology*. 8th ed. Philadelphia: Saunders, 1991: 159–169.

85. McNeil JJ, Sloman JG. Cardiovascular diseases. *In:* Speight TM, ed. *Avery's drug treatment: principles and practice of clinical pharmacology and therapeutics*. 3rd ed. Auckland: Adis Press, 1987: 591–675.

86. Hurwitz RA. Drugs and doses in pediatrics. *In:* Adams FH, Emmanoulides GC, Riemenschneider TA, eds. *Moss' heart disease in infants, children and adolescents*. 4th ed. Baltimore: Williams and Wilkins, 1989: 1038–1048.

87. Hammerman C, Yousefzadeh D, Jung-Hwon C, Kim-chi Bui. Persistent pulmonary hypertension of the newborn. *Clin Perinatol* 1989; 16: 137–156.

88. Drinkwater DC, Laks H. Principles of pediatric heart surgery. *In:* Adams FH, Emmanoulides GC, Riemenschneider TA, eds. *Moss' heart disease in infants, children and adolescents*. 4th ed. Baltimore: Williams and Wilkins, 1989: 1032–1036.

89. Budney J, Anderson-Drevs K. Intravenous inotropic agents: dopamine, dobutamine and amrinone. *Crit Care Nurse* 1990; 10 (2): 54–62.

90. Raphaely RC, Browning RA. The role of preload in the manipulation of the failing circulation. *In:* Swedlow DB, Raphaely RC, eds. *Cardiovascular problems in pediatric critical care, clinics in critical care medicine*, Vol 10. New York: Churchill Livingstone, 1986: 205–220.

91. Chemtob S, Kaplan BS, Sherbotie JR, Aranda JV. Pharmacology of diuretics in the newborn. *Pediatr Clin North Am* 1989; 36: 1231–1250.

92. Hastrieter AR, John EG, van der Horst RL. Digitalis, digitalis antibodies, digitalis-like immunoreactive substances, and homeostasis: a review. *Clin Perinatol* 1988; 15: 491–521.

93. Daly PA, Sole MJ. Myocardial catecholamine and pathophysiology of heart failure. *Circulation* 1990; 82 (Suppl 1): 35–43.

94. Jacono J, Hicks G, Antonioni C, O'Brien K, Rasi M. Comparison of perceived needs of family members between registered nurses and family members of critically ill patients in intensive care and neonatal intensive care units. *Heart Lung* 1990; 19: 72–78.

95. Moore AC. Crisis intervention: a care plan for families of hospitalised children. *Pediatr Nursing* 1989; 15: 234–236.

96. Carter MC, Miles MS, Hall Buford T, Stephenson Hassanein RP. Parental stress in intensive care units. *Dimensions Crit Care Nursing* 1985; 4: 180–188.

97. Philichi LM. Family adaptation during a pediatric intensive care hospitalisation. *J Pediatr Nursing* 1989; 4: 268–276.

98. Gillis AJ. Nurses knowledge of growth and development principles in meeting psychosocial needs of hospitalised children. *J Pediatr Nursing* 1990; 5 (2): 78–87.

99. del Nido PJ, Williams WG, Coles JG, Trusler GA, Freedom RM. Closed heart surgery for congenital heart disease in infancy. *Clin Perinatol* 1988; 15: 681–697.

100. Jonas RA, Lang P. Open repair of cardiac defects in neonates and young infants. *Clin Perinatol* 1988; 15: 659–679.

101. Carter JH, Hancock J. Caring for children: how to ease them through surgery. *Nursing 88* 1988; 18 (10): 46–50.

102. Hickey PA, Rykerson S. Caring for the parents of critically ill infants and children. *Crit Care Nursing Clin North Am* 1992; 4: 565–571.

103. Rushton CH. Strategies for family centred care in the critical care setting. *Pediatr Nursing* 1990; 16: 195–199.

104. O'Brien SW, Konsler GK. Alleviating children's postoperative pain. *Am J Maternal Child Nursing* 1988; 13: 183–186.

105. Lell WA, Reves JG, Samuelson PN. Anaesthesia for cardiovascular surgery. *In:* Kirklin JW, Barratt-Boyes BG. *Cardiac surgery: morphology, diagnostic criteria, natural history, techniques, results, and indications*. New York: John Wiley and Sons 1986; 109–138.

106. Moore R. Anesthesia considerations for patients undergoing palliative or reparative operations for congenital heart disease. *In:* Swedlow DB, Raphaely RC, eds. *Cardiovascular problems in pediatric critical care.* Clinics in critical care medicine, Vol 10. New York: Churchill Livingstone 1986; 169–204.

107. Radnay PA. Anaesthetic management of surgery requiring cardiopulmonary bypass. *In:* Radnay PA, ed. *International anaesthesiology clinics; anaesthetic considerations for pediatric cardiac surgery.* 1980; 18: 95–122.

108. Simpson JC. Anaesthesia for infants undergoing cardiac surgery. *In:* Yacoub M, ed. *1988 Annual of cardiac surgery.* London: Gower Academic Journals 1988: 16–21.

109. Kirklin JW, Barratt-Boyes BG. Hypothermia, circulatory arrest and cardiopulmonary bypass. *In:* Kirklin JW, Barratt-Boyes BG. *Cardiac surgery: morphology, diagnostic criteria, natural history, techniques, results, and indications.* New York: Churchill Livingstone, 1993: 61–128.

110. Greeley WJ, Ungerleider RM, Kern FH, Brusino FG, Smith LR, Reves JG. Effects of cardiopulmonary bypass on cerebral blood flow in neonates, infants and children. *Circulation* 1989; 80 (Suppl 1): 209–215.

111. Kirklin JW, Barrett-Boyes BG. Myocardial protection during cardiac surgery with cardiopulmonary bypass. *In:* Kirklin JW, Barratt-Boyes BG. *Cardiac surgery: morphology, diagnostic criteria, natural history, techniques, results, and indications.* New York: John Wiley and Sons, 1986: 83–108.

112. Ilbawi MN. Current status for congenital heart diseases. *Clin Perinatol* 1989; 16: 157–176.

113. Walsh AZ, Forbes Morrow D, Jonas RA. Neurological and developmental outcomes following cardiac surgery. *Nursing Clin North Am* 1995; 30 (2): 347–364.

114. Taylor KM. Brain damage during cardiac surgery. *In:* Yacoub M, ed. *1987 Annual of cardiac surgery.* London: Gower Academic Journals, 1987: 36–39.

115. Anand KJS. Neonatal stress responses to anaesthesia and surgery. *Clin Perinatol* 1990; 17: 207–214.

116. John E, Klavdianou M, Vidyasagar D. Electrolyte problems in neonatal surgical patients. *Clin Perinatol* 1989; 16: 219–232.

117. Mason CB, Davis JE. Cardiac surgery. *In:* Mason CB, Davis JE, eds. *Cardiovascular critical care.* New York: Van Nostrand Reinhold, 1987: 378–439.

118. Rotondi P. Intensive care unit management in the post operative cardiac surgery patient. *Crit Care Q* 1986; 9 (2): 49–63.

119. Fagan MJ. Relationship between nurses' assessments of perfusion and toe temperature in pediatric patients with cardiovascular diseases. *Heart Lung* 1988; 17: 157–165.

120. Schleien CL, Setzer NA, McLaughlin GE, Rogers MC. Post operative management of the cardic surgical patient. *In:* Rogers MC, ed. *Textbook of pediatric intensive care.* 2nd ed. Baltimore: Williams and Wilkins, 1992: 467–531.

121. Kirklin JW, Barratt-Boyes BG. Postoperative care. *In:* Kirklin JW, Barrat-Boyes BG. 2nd ed. *Cardiac surgery: morphology, diagnostic criteria, natural history, techniques, results, and indications.* New York: Churchill Livingstone: 1993: 195–248.

122. Carroll P. Clinical application of pulse oximetry. *Pediatric Nursing* 1993; 19: 150–151.

123. Curley MAQ, Thompson JE. End tidal Co2 monitoring in critically ill infants and children. *Pediatric Nursing* 1990; 16: 397–403.

124. Ley SJ, Miller K, Skou P, Preisig P. Crystalloid versus colloid fluid therapy after cardiac surgery. *Heart Lung* 1990; 19: 31–40.

125. Frank LS. Issues regarding the use of analgesia and sedation in critically ill neonates. Clinical issues in critical care nursing. *Am Assoc Crit Care Nurses* 1991; 2: 709–719.

126. Berde CB. Pediatric postoperative pain management. *Pediatr Clin North Am* 1989; 36: 921–940.

127. Koren G, Butt W, Chinyanga H, Soldin S, Yok-Kwang Tan, Pope K. Post operative morphine infusions in newborn infants: assessment of disposition characteristics and safety. *J Paediatr* 1986; 27: 963–967.

128. Beyer JE, Wells N. The assessment of pain in children. *Pediatr Clin North Am* 1989; 36: 837–854.

129. Broome ME, Slack JF. Relieving pain in children. *Am J Maternal Child Nursing* 1990; 15: 159–162.

130. Ellis JA. Using pain scales to prevent undermedication. *Am J Maternal Child Nursing* 1988; 13: 180–182.

131. Johnston CC, Stevens B. Pain assessment in newborns. *J Perinatal Neonatal Nursing* 1990; 4: 41–52.

132. Wong D. Pain assessment in children. International paediatric nursing 'down under' conference paper. Sydney, May 1990: 78–94.

133. Roop Moyer SM, Howe CJ. Pediatric pain intervention in the PACU. *Crit Care Nursing Clin North Am* 1991; 3: 49–57.

134. Porter F. Pain in the newborn. *Clin Perinatol* 1989; 16: 549–564.

135. Craig J. The postoperative cardiac infant: physiologic basis for neonatal nursing interventions. *J Perinatal Neonatal Nursing* 1991; 5 (2): 60–70.

136. Garson A. Arrhythmias. *In:* Garson A. *The electrocardiogram in infants and children: a systematic approach.* Philadelphia: Lea and Febiger, 1983: 195–375.

137. Engle MA. Postoperative problems. *In:* Adams FH, Emmanoulides GC, Riemenschneider TA, eds. *Moss' heart disease in infants, children and adolescents.* 4th ed. Baltimore: Williams and Wilkins, 1989: 964–972.

138. Zeigler VL. Postoperative rhythm disturbances. *Crit Car Nursing Clin North Am* 1994; 6: 227–235.

139. Boisvert JT, Reidy SJ, Lulu J. Overview of Pediatric arrhthmias. *Nursing Clin North Am* 1995; 30 (2): 365–379.

140. Case CL, Crawford FA, Gillette PC. Surgical treatment of dysrhythmias in infants and children. *Pediatr Clin North Am* 1990; 37: 79–92.

141. Anella J, McClosky A, Vieweg C. Nursing dynamics of paediatric intra-aortic balloon pumping. *Crit Care Nurse* 1990; 10 (4): 24–37.

142. Jain L, Vidyasagar D. Iatrogenic disorders in modern neonatology. *Clin Perinatol* 1989; 16: 255–273.

143. Rykerson S, Thompson J, Wessel DL. Inhalation of nitric oxide: an innovative therapy for treatment of increased pulmonary vascular resistance. *Nursing Clin North Am* 1995; 30 (2): 381–390.

144. Webster H. Bioinstrumentation: principles and techniques. *In:* Hazinski MF. *Nursing care of the critically ill child.* 1992: 929–1028.

145. Schaffer SE, Norman ME. Renal function and renal failure in the newborn. *Clin Perinatol* 1989; 16: 199–218.

146. Hazinski MF. Postoperative care of the critically ill child. *Crit Care Nursing Clin North Am* 1990; 2: 599–610.

147. Friedman WF, Heiferman MF. Clinical problem of postoperative pulmonary vascular disease. *Am J Cardiol* 1982; 50: 631–635.

148. Rabinovitch M. Pulmonary hypertension. *In:* Adams FH, Emmanoulides GC, Riemenschneider TA eds. *Moss' heart disease in infants, children and adolescents.* 4th ed. Baltimore: Williams and Wilkins, 1989: 856–886.

149. Henry GW. Perioperative management of the child with pulmonary hypertension and congenital heart disease. *In:* Harned HS, ed. *Pediatric pulmonary heart disease.* Boston: Little Brown, 1990: 355–375.

150. Hunt BJ, Banner NR. Recent advances in the management of haemorrhage during cardiac surgery. *In:* Yacoub M, ed. *1988 Annual of cardiac surgery.* London: Gower Academic Journals, 1988: 9–14.

151. Yates A. The pericardium: cardiac tamponade. *Br J Hosp Med* 1979; January: 13–16.

152. Barbiere CC. Cardiac tamponade: diagnosis and emergency intervention. *Crit Care Nurse* 1990; 10 (4): 20–22.

153. Kronick-Mest C. Postpericardiotomy syndrome: etiology manifestations and interventions. *Heart Lung* 1989; 18: 192–197.

154. O'Brien P, Boisvert JT. Discharge planning for children with heart disease. *Crit Care Nursing Clin North Am* 1989; 1: 297–305.

155. Denfield SW, Garson A. Sudden death in children and young adults. *Pediatr Clin North Am* 1990; 37: 215–231.

156. Lee WS, Cartmill TB, Nunn G, Hawker RE. Blalock and goretex shunts in the palliation of cyanotic congenital heart disease. Third World Congress of Pediatric Cardiology, Bangkok, November/December 1989. [Abstract F 470] 114.

157. de Leval MR, Kilner P, Gewilling M, Bull C. Total cavopulmonary connection: a logical alternative to atriopulmonary connection for complex Fontan operations. Third World Congress of Pediatric Cardiology, Bangkok, November/December 1989. [Abstract S2.3] 7.

158. Zahka KG, Spector M, Hanisch D. Hypoplastic left heart syndrome, transplantation, or compassionate care. *Clin Perinatol* 1993; 20 (1): 145–154.

159. McAvoy MR, Fitzgerald E. Reducing multisystem failure after Fontan procedure. *Dimensions Crit Care Nursing* 1988; 7 (3): 150–159.

160. Sade RM, Fyfe DA. Tricuspid atresia: current concepts in diagnosis and treatment. *Pediatr Clin North Am* 1990; 37: 151–169.

161. Norwood WI, Pigott JD. Recent advances in cardiac surgery. *Pediatr Clin North Am* 1985; 32: 1117–1123.

162. Schuller JL, Sebel PS, Bovill JG, Marcelletti C. Early extubation after Fontan operation. *Br J Anaesthesia* 1980; 52: 999–1004.

163. Fontan F, Kirklin JW, Fernandez G, Costa F, Nattel DC, Tritto F, Blackstone EH. Outcome after a 'perfect' Fontan operation. *Circulation* 1990; 81: 1520–1536.

164. Gewllig MH, Lundstrom UR, Deanfield JE, Bull C, Franklin RC, Graham TP, Wyse RK. Impact of Fontan operation on left ventricular size and contractility in tricuspid atresia. *Circulation* 1990; 81: 118–127.

165. Callow LB. Nursing implications of interventional device placement in pediatric cardiology and pediatric cardiac surgery. *Crit Care Nursing Clin North Am* 1994; 6: 133–151.

166. Cohen DM. Surgical management of congenital heart disease in the 1990's. *Am J Dis Child* 1992; 146: 1447–1452.

167. Bailey NA, Lay P, Loma Linda University infant heart transplant group. New horizons: infant cardiac transplantation. *Heart Lung* 1989; 18: 172–178.

168. Cameron DE, Reitz BA. Heart and heart-lung transplantation. *In:* Adams FH, Emmanoulides GC, Riemenschneider TA, eds. *Moss' heart disease in infants, children and adolescents.* 4th ed. Baltimore: Williams and Wilkins, 1989: 973–983.

169. Johnston J. Cardiac transplantation in early infancy. *Crit Care Nursing Clin North Am* 1992; 4: 521–525.

170. Jones S. Paediatric heart and lung transplantation: postoperative nursing care. International Paediatric Nursing Down Under, Conference Proceedings, Sydney, May 1990: 178–186.

171. Yacoub M, Haghani A, Miyamura H, Sono J. Heart-lung transplantation. *Japan J Surg* 1990; 20: 247–251.

172. O'Brien P, Hanley FL. New directions in pediatric heart transplantation. *Critical Care Nursing Clin North Am* 1992; 4: 193–203.

173. Sinclair V. High technology in critical care; implications for nursing role and practice. *Focus Crit Care* 1988; 15 (4): 36–41.

174. Urban N. Integrating hemodynamic parameters with clinical decision making. *Crit Care Nurse* 1986; 6 (2): 48–61.

175. Berne RM, Levy MN. The cardiac pump. *In:* Cardiovascular physiology. 5th ed. St Louis: Mosby, 1986: 50–75.

176. Daily EK, Schroder JS. Cardiac output measurements. *In:* Daily EK, Schroder JS. *Techniques in bedside hemodynamic monitoring.* 4th ed. St Louis: Mosby, 1989: 179–199.

177. Schermer L. Physiologic and technical variables effecting hemodynamic measurements. *Crit Care Nurse* 1988; 8 (2): 33–40.

178. Swedlow DB, Cohen DE. Invasive assessment of the failing circulation. *In:* Swedlow DB, Raphaely RC, eds. *Cardiovascular problems in pediatric critical care. Clinics in critical care medicine Vol 10.* New York: Churchill Livingstone, 1986: 129–168.

179. Vincent RN, Elixson EM. Hemodynamic monitoring. *Crit Care Q* 1986; 9 (2): 40–48.

180. Yacone LA. Monitoring cardiac output. *In:* Darovic GO, ed. *Hemodynamic monitoring; invasive and non invasive clinical application.* Philadelphia: Saunders, 1987: 185–199.

181. Elixson EM. Hemodynamic monitoring modalities in pediatric cardiac surgical patients. *Crit Care Nursing Clin North Am* 1989; 1: 263–273.

182. Hazinski MF. Hemodynamic monitoring in children. *In:* Daily EK, Schroder JS. *Techniques in bedside hemodynamic monitoring.* 4th ed. St Louis: Mosby, 1989: 247–315.

183. Hazinski MF. Cardiovascular disorders. *In:* Hazinski MF. *Nursing care of the critically ill child.* 2nd ed. St Louis: Mosby Year Book, 1992: 117–394.

184. Rimar JM. Recognising shock syndromes in infants and children. *Am J Maternal Child Nursing* 1988; 13 (2): 32–37.

185. Darovic GO. Pulmonary artery pressure monitoring. *In:* Darovic GO. *Hemodynamic monitoring: invasive and non invasive clinical application.* Philadelphia: Saunders, 1987: 137–183.

186. Freed MD. Invasive diagnostic and therapeutic techniques. *In:* Adams FH, Emmanoulides GC, Riemenschneider TA, eds. *Moss' heart disease in infants, children and adolescents.* 4th ed. Baltimore: Williams and Wilkins, 1989: 130–147.

187. Darovic GO. Cardiovascular anatomy and physiology. *In:* Darovic GO. *Hemodynamic monitoring: invasive and non invasive clinical application.* Philadelphia: Saunders, 1987: 33–63.

188. Daily EK, Schroder JS. Central venous and pulmonary arterial pressure monitoring. *In:* Daily EK, Schroder JS. *Techniques in bedside hemodynamic monitoring.* 4th ed. St Louis: Mosby, 1989: 88–150.

189. Seifert Hultgren M. Pulmonary management of children after cardiac surgery. *Crit Care Nurse* 1991; 11 (3): 55–69.

190. Siok H Chew. Nursing critically ill children requiring ECMO; an Australian experience. International Paediatric Nursing Down Under, Conference Proceedings, Sydney, May 1990: 175–178.

191. Kyff JV. Invasive haemodynamic monitoring Part 1: Using the pulmonary artery catheter. *J Post Anaes Nursing* 1989; 4: 287–295.

192. Macpherson TA, Shen-Schwarz S, Valdes-Napena M. Prevention and reduction of iatrogenic disorders in the newborn. *In:* Guthrie RD, ed. *Neonatal intensive care: clinics in critical care medicine.* New York: Churchill Livingstone, 1988: 271–312.

193. Masters S. Complications of pulmonary artery catheters. *Crit Care Nurse* 1990; 9 (9): 82–91.

194. Tabata B, Kirsch JR, Rogers MC. Diagnostic tests and technology for pediatric intensive care. *In:* Rogers MC, ed. *Textbook of pediatric intensive care.* Baltimore: Williams and Wilkins, 1987: 1401–1431.

195. Van Riper S, Van Riper J. Arterial pressure monitoring. *In:* Darovic GO, ed. *Hemodynamic monitoring; invasive and non invasive clinical application.* Philadelphia: Saunders, 1987: 95–114.

196. Daily EK, Schroder JS. Monitoring signs and symptoms. *In:* Daily EK, Schroder JS. *Techniques in bedside hemodynamic monitoring.* 4th ed. St Louis: Mosby, 1989: 13–33.

197. Daily EK, Schroder JS. Principles and hazards of monitoring equipment. *In:* Daily EK, Schroder JS. *Techniques in bedside hemodynamic monitoring.* 4th ed. St Louis: Mosby, 1989: 34–56.

198. Van Riper J, Van Riper S. Fluid filled monitoring systems. *In:* Darovic GO, ed. *Hemodynamic monitoring; invasive and non invasive clinical application.* Philadelphia: Saunders, 1987: 83–94.

199. Yacone LA. Monitoring central venous pressure. *In:* Darovic GO, ed. *Hemodynamic monitoring; invasive and non invasive clinical application.* Philadelphia: Saunders, 1987: 115–135.

200. Daily EK, Schroder JS. Intra arterial pressure monitoring. *In:* Daily EK, Schroder JS. *Techniques in bedside hemodynamic monitoring.* 4th ed. St Louis: Mosby, 1989: 151–178.

201. Headrick CL. Hemodynamic monitoring of the critically ill neonate. *J Perinatal Neonatal Nursing* 1992; 5 (4): 58–67.

202. Clohesy JM. Introducing new technology: biomedical engineers and staff nurse involvement. *Crit Care Nursing Q* 1987; 9 (4): 64–69.

Chapter 12

Nursing Care of the Critically Ill Infant, Child and Adolescent

Marilyn Cruickshank and Tina Kendrick

This chapter focuses on the infant, child and adolescent who require intensive care. This encompasses children who have sustained a life-threatening event or infection (e.g., severe head injury or septicaemia) and those who are at risk of developing a life-threatening event, (e.g., respiratory failure, cardiac arrhythmia or metabolic disturbance). These children all require a higher level of monitoring and nursing care than is readily available in a ward setting, and the care of critically ill infants, children and adolescents is frequently carried out in specialised paediatric intensive care units (PICUs) and high dependency units.[1]

Paediatric cardiopulmonary resuscitation and hypovolaemic shock are addressed first. A review of monitoring and standard care performed in PICUs follows and finally we focus in greater detail on specific disease and illness processes which paediatric patients commonly cared for in the intensive care setting may experience.

Cardiopulmonary Resuscitation

Sudden cardiac arrest in children is rare — there are usually observable stages of deterioration. Ventilator assistance and other action can prevent progression to cardiac arrest.

PATIENTS AT RISK OF CARDIAC ARREST

It is important to identify patients who may be at risk of cardiac arrest so that appropriate monitoring and treatment may be instigated. They include children:

- with unstable cardiovascular conditions, such as haemorrhage, hypotension, arrhythmia, congestive cardiac failure;
- who develop rapidly progressive pulmonary disease such as asthma, severe pneumonia, respiratory distress syndrome;
- in the immediate postoperative period due to the effects of general anaesthetic and heavy sedation, which may significantly alter a child's ability to respond appropriately to a variety of physiological stimuli;

- with an artificial airway, as their respiratory status depends directly on airway patency;
- with deteriorating neurological status, such as coma, with insufficient reflexes to protect their airway or sufficient respiratory drive to sustain adequate ventilation.

There are a number of stressful procedures which may precipitate cardiac arrest in high-risk patients. These include:

- endotracheal suctioning, which may cause hypoxia, atelectasis, reflex bradycardia;
- chest physiotherapy, which may mobilise excessive secretions and block the airway;
- withdrawal of respiratory support or inspired oxygen;
- administration of sedatives (e.g., narcotics, barbiturates, cough suppressants), which may decrease respiratory drive;
- procedures associated with valsalva manoeuvres (e.g., holding for a lumbar puncture);
- procedures associated with vagal stimulation causing bradycardia, (e.g., passing a nasogastric tube or airway manipulation).

CAUSES OF CARDIAC ARREST IN CHILDREN

The most common cause of cardiac arrest in children is hypoxia and it is therefore important to recognise the signs and symptoms of hypoxia in children.[2] Hypoxia may result from respiratory obstruction, lung disease, respiratory depression or increased pulmonary shunting. The signs and symptoms of hypoxia include poor peripheral perfusion, tachycardia followed by bradycardia, change in respiratory pattern, apnoea, restlessness, cyanosis and decreased response to stimuli. Other causes of cardiorespiratory arrest in children include progressive hypotension (caused by bleeding, dehydration), electrolyte imbalance (e.g., hypocalcaemia, hyperkalaemia in renal failure), postoperative complications, and cardiac disease such as cardiomyopathy and arrhythmia due to congenital cardiac lesions or tricyclic poisoning.[3] However, cardiac arrest is not the only condition in the paediatric sphere that requires resuscitation. Many conditions short of cardiac arrest, such as shock, require active intervention. The signs of shock in children are subtle — hypotension in children is a relatively late sign.

DIAGNOSIS OF CARDIOPULMONARY ARREST

The diagnosis of cardiac arrest is made in a child who is unconscious, apnoeic, with no palpable central pulses. The child may be mottled or pale, with cool, clammy skin.

Other signs of increased sympathetic activity are tachycardia, irritability, hyperventilation, cool extremities, poor peripheral perfusion, weak pulses, oliguria and metabolic acidosis. The causes may be as diverse as hypovolaemia, cardiac or toxic shock.

HELP

Help should be summoned immediately by the person who discovers the arrest. It is important that this person does not leave the child unless it is absolutely necessary, so that they are able to commence resuscitation immediately.

Box 12.1 Priorities for initiating resuscitation.

1. If respiratory failure is present, open airway, oxygenate and commence ventilation.
2. If shock is evident, ensure equipment is available for vascular access and infusion of volume expansion or vasoactive infusion or both.
3. If cardiopulmonary failure is present, oxygenate and commence ventilation then, reassess for shock/respiratory failure.

ASSESSMENT OF THE CRITICALLY ILL INFANT AND CHILD

Box 12.2 Management of cardiac arrest.

A Airway
B Breathing
C Circulation

D Drugs
E ECG
F Fibrillation/fluids

A. Assess airway

Decide if:

- the child can maintain the airway without assistance;
- the child can maintain the airway with standard interventions such as positioning, suctioning or requires insertion of artificial airway and/or rebreathing bag;
- the airway can only be maintained by intubation.

B. Assess breathing

- Is the work of breathing normal, increased, decreased or absent?
- Check air entry. Does the chest rise? Are there breath sounds?
- Determine the rate of breathing.
- Assess the child's colour.

Box 12.3 Airway and breathing management.

Position the child to have access to the airway and upper chest, protecting the head and neck by moving it as a unit.

1. Open the airway to lift soft tissues and tongue from the posterior pharynx.
   Infants: place one hand under the shoulder blades and lift while pressing down with the other hand on the forehead to place the head in a 'sniffing position.' Do not hyperextend the neck as the cartilage is unable to give firm support to the trachea in infants and young children.
   Older children: place the hand under the neck and support the head tilting backwards.

Box 12.3 (*continued*)

2. Check for signs of breathing.
    *   Observe for chest movement.
    *   Auscultate chest.
    *   Listen for breath sounds over mouth and nose.
    *   Suction mouth and pharynx, or turn head to one side and clear mouth with finger.

Box 12.4 Ventilation management.

Institute artificial ventilation if there is no spontaneous breathing or gasping.
1. Maintain head tilt.
2. Seal airway by pinching nose or covering infant's mouth and nose with your mouth.
3. Give 2 slow breaths while observing chest movement; check for a central pulse.
4. Switch to rebreathing bag and 100% oxygen as soon as possible.
5. Be certain to maintain head tilt and tight mask fit.
6. Insert oral airway if required to maintain airway patency.
7. Frequency of ventilation:
    *   infants   20–24 breaths/minute
    *   child   16–20 breaths/minute
    *   older child   12–16 breaths/minute

C. Assess circulation

*   Determine efficiency of circulation — skin perfusion, capillary refill, extremity temperature. Is the skin colour pink, pale, blue, or mottled?
*   Assess central nervous system perfusion. Does the child recognise parents, no recognition, withdraws from pain, postures to pain, no response to pain? Is there evidence of cranial nerve dysfunction?
*   Are peripheral pulses strong, weak, or absent? If weak or absent, begin cardiac compression.
*   Assess heart rate, blood pressure, stroke volume, vascular resistance.

Box 12.5 Circulation management.

Check for circulation: (Central pulse — carotid, femoral)

If there is no central pulse, institute artificial circulation:
*   Place child on a firm surface
*   Locate the ends of the sternum
*   Place hand/fingers on end third of sternum

Box 12.5 (*continued*)

- Depress sternum in a perpendicular direction to avoid damage to the ribs, stomach, spleen or liver.

Compressions

	Frequency (per minute)	Depth
Infant	120	1–1.5 cm
Child	100	1.5–2.5 cm
Older child	80	2.5–3 cm

Only pause cardiac compression for:
- 5 seconds to check pulse/pupils
- 15 seconds to move patient
- 15 seconds to intubate patient.

Apply pressure for approximately 50% of the cycle to allow for adequate filling of the heart during the upstroke — this gives greater cardiac output and results in better peripheral perfusion. The cycle should be rhythmical and not jerky. The effectiveness of compression is best evaluated by the presence of a central pulse. For infants the ratio is always 5 compressions to 1 breath regardless, of whether there are 1 or 2 operators. For older children and adolescents, the ratio for 1 operator is 15 compressions to 2 breaths.

D. Drugs

Box 12.6 Major drugs.

- Oxygen
- Adrenaline
- Atropine
- Sodium bicarbonate
- Calcium gluconate/chloride

When drawing up drugs for arrest, remember:
- Draw up all drugs into 10 mL syringe.
- Label or stick ampoule to syringe.
- Draw up 10 mL normal saline to flush line between drugs.
- Keep all syringes full in preparation for another 'round'.

Oxygen

Oxygen is the most important drug in the arrest situation. Remember, lack of oxygen not only stops the motor but wrecks the machinery! Do not preclude the use of 100% oxygen in the emergency situation — oxygen toxicity should only be considered during prolonged ventilation. The oxygen concentration after resuscitation should be determined by arterial blood gas results.[4]

Adrenaline

Adrenaline is a potent beta stimulator with some alpha receptor stimulation. It has both *inotropic* (increases cardiac contractility) and *chronotropic* (increases heart rate) effects and thus increases both stroke volume and coronary blood flow.

Adrenaline initiates cardiac rhythm in cardiac arrest by its stimulating effect on the sinoatrial node cells. It lessens the degree of heart block, since conduction in the AV node, His bundles, Purkinje fibres and ventricles improves.

Preparation: 1:10 000 10 mL ampoule.

Administration: IVI, IV infusion, Intracardiac, ETT if no IV line.

Dose: 25 µg/kg of body weight (i.e., 0.25 mL/kg).

Sodium bicarbonate

Sodium bicarbonate is used to correct metabolic acidosis due to arrest.

Preparation: 10 mL ampoule of 8.4% solution; 100 mL bottle of 8.4% solution (8.4% = 1 mEq/mL).

Dose: 1 mEq/kg/2 minutes arrest, then 1 mEq/kg every 5 minutes arrest thereafter.

Calcium (gluconate or chloride)

Calcium increases the tone and contractility of the myocardium in cardiac arrest.

Preparation: Gluconate — 10 mL ampoule of 10% solution; Chloride — 100 mg/mL.

Dose: Gluconate — 0.2 mL/kg; Chloride — 20–40 mg/kg.

Atropine

Atropine blocks the vagal nerve (parasympathetic) and increases sinoatrial discharge rate in sinus bradycardia.

Preparation: 400 µg/mL.

Dose: 20 µg/kg. Draw up 400 mg ampoule and dilute to 10 mL with normal saline = 40 µg/mL.

E. ECG trace

ECG trace must be established as soon as possible following arrest, to establish the rhythm disturbance causing arrest, so that appropriate treatment may be given. *Note:* Although the ECG may show electrical activity, perhaps even at a normal rate, cardiac output is determined by both rate and blood pressure. Cardiac output, therefore, may be insufficient to perfuse the heart and brain, thus cardiac massage must be initiated.

F. (i) Fibrillation

- Use DC shock — 1 joule/kg initially, then *double* progressively if no response.
- Use only enough paste to cover the paddle electrodes.

- Don't place paddles too close together. One should be placed to the right of the upper sternum below the clavicle. The second paddle should be placed to the left of the left nipple.[2]
- On reversion to sinus rhythm, continue external cardiac massage (ECM) until spontaneous cardiac output is adequate.

(ii) Fluids

- Type of fluid is based on electrolyte results.
- Use colloid if the patient is hypovolaemic or in shock.

Care of the Shocked Infant and Child

DEFINITION

Shock is a physiological state of severe tissue hypoperfusion resulting in cell dysfunction and, if untreated, cell death.[2]

Three types of shock have been described: hypovolaemic shock, cardiogenic shock and septic (or distributive) shock. Hypovolaemic shock is the most common form of shock seen in children and is the most easily treated. It is related to the loss of circulating blood volume through events such as trauma, gastrointestinal tract bleeding, burns, peritonitis, diarrhoea and osmotic diuresis.[5] Fluid losses may be hidden in circumstances such as in intraperitoneal fluid accumulation and profoundly vasodilated states. Septic shock results from the release of endotoxins causing vasodilatation and capillary leak, resulting in hypovolaemia and direct myocardial depression. Cardiogenic shock is rare in the paediatric patient, is seen mainly after open heart surgery and severe myocarditis or untreated shock[6] and is discussed in Chapter 11.

PATHOPHYSIOLOGY

Shock is commonly associated with low cardiac output, but may be present with high cardiac output if distribution of cardiac output is inappropriate or if there are excessive oxygen requirements. Cardiac output is the product of heart rate and stroke volume. Stroke volume is determined by preload, afterload and intrinsic myocardial contractility. When cardiac output falls, blood flow is preserved to the heart and brain at the expense of other organs. In compensation, heart rate increases and blood flow is decreased in the gastrointestinal tract and renal beds, producing the clinical signs of shock — tachycardia, pallor, cool skin and reduced urine output. The child is initially able to compensate effectively. Thus the early signs of increased sympathetic activity are subtle: unexplained tachycardia; cool, pale extremities; hyperventilation; and irritability. As decompensation supervenes, tachypnoea, metabolic acidosis, oliguria and somnolence occur and the child may become obtunded, hypotensive and apnoeic. Hypotension is a relatively late and dangerous sign. Shock syndromes develop over time — blood pressure will frequently not fall until blood loss equals 20% to 25% of circulating blood volume.[2]

Acute circulatory insufficiency will respond to volume expansion if treated promptly — don't wait for hypotension to occur before restoring blood volume. Those children who do not respond to volume alone will require invasive haemodynamic monitoring for closer assessment, and possibly pharmacological intervention. Large amounts of fluid are required despite peripheral oedema or absence of overt fluid loss. All types of shock may lead to adult respiratory distress syndrome (ARDS), disseminated intravascular coagulation (DIC), and ischaemia of liver, gastrointestinal tract, kidneys (acute renal failure) and pancreas.[6]

Assessment of systemic perfusion in children

For specific assessment of systemic perfusion:

- Urine volume should average 0.5 to 2 mL/kg/hour.
- Perfusion of extremities should be warm with pink nailbeds.
- Capillary refill should be brisk (less than 2 seconds).
- Peripheral pulses should be strong and equal.
- Colour should be consistent and mucous membranes pink.
- Arterial pressure and heart rate should be appropriate for age and clinical condition. Tachycardia is an early sign of distress; bradycardia is ominous as young children are dependant on a high heart rate to maintain cardiac output.

Indirect evidence of poor systemic perfusion in infants is temperature instability, hypoglycaemia, hypocalcaemia, fluid imbalances, apnoea, feeding difficulties, abdominal distension and metabolic acidosis. Other indirect evidence of poor systemic perfusion in children is irritability, then disorientation or lethargy.

Assessment of low intravascular volume

- Decreased urine volume with high specific gravity.
- Dry mucous membranes.
- Poor skin turgor, sunken fontanelle in infants.
- Central venous pressure (CVP) or pulmonary artery wedge pressure (PAW) will be low. CVP less than 5 to 10 mmHg is usually inadequate if decreased myocardial function is present.
- Calculate child's circulating blood volume (75 to 85 mL/kg); consider all blood lost as a percentage of blood volume.

GOALS FOR TREATMENT OF SHOCK

- Optimise circulating volume by replacement with type of fluid lost.
- Improve cardiac output by increasing blood volume and, if unresponsive, then consider inotropes.
- Relieve respiratory insufficiency by administration of oxygen or intubation and mechanical ventilation.
- Treat underlying disorder, e.g., by administration of antibiotics in septic shock.
- Diagnose and treat organ damage resulting from hypoperfusion (e.g., acute renal failure).

Treatment of hypovolaemic shock in children

Most children with acute circulating insufficiency will respond to volume expansion.[2] Restoration of an adequate intravascular volume is the goal of therapy for all 3 forms of shock. Adequacy of preload is critical to maintain cardiac output. Decreased contractility requires higher than normal level of preload to maintain stroke volume, therefore the aim of fluid therapy is to optimise preload.[6]

Intravenous access for fluid resuscitation is one of the main priorities. The line must be as large as possible to facilitate the infusion of large volumes. Access is usually through a central line. Dual lumen is advantageous as one line is used for infusions, while the other is available for CVP monitoring. If venous access cannot be obtained, then intraosseous placement of needle and infusion is indicated. The tibia is the usual site for intraosseous needle placement.

The goal is to maximise perfusion (usually CVP 8 to 15 mmHg). PAW of less than 8 to 10 mmHg is usually inadequate if myocardial dysfunction is present (PAW more than 18 to 25 mmHg may produce pulmonary oedema). Administer 10 mL/kg of fluid over 15 minutes; this may need to be repeated. The type of fluid to be administered depends on type of losses and fluids available. A further 10 mL/kg may be given if there is no improvement. Improvement is demonstrated by decreased heart rate, increased peripheral perfusion, increased blood pressure, urine output more than 1 mL/hour (an indwelling catheter if required for accurate estimate). Some children may require more than 20 mL/kg to restore adequate circulating blood volume. Ensure an adequate hematocrit level to maintain oxygen content.

Ventilation

Children in severe shock require intubation and ventilation. The lung is sensitive to poor perfusion. Acidosis causes hyperventilation and thus an increase in the work of breathing, which may lead to respiratory muscle fatigue. Ventilation may need to be considered early to reduce oxygen demand, and in order to facilitate placement of central lines.

Other therapies

Treat acid-base and electrolyte imbalances which depress myocardial function. The following parameters should be monitored: arterial blood gases; blood glucose; calcium; electrolytes (corrected for optimal myocardial contractility). Biochemical abnormalities such as severe metabolic acidosis, hypoglycaemia and hypocalcaemia are common.[7,8]

NURSING RESPONSIBILITIES

Nursing diagnosis

Potential for hypoxia due to metabolic disturbance, and poor perfusion.

Nursing intervention

Ensure adequate oxygenation, preferably by mechanical ventilator support. It is advisable to intubate the child before respiratory arrest occurs. If the child is not intubated, ensure adequate airway protection as the child's condition may deteriorate suddenly. Control and minimise oxygen demands by keeping the child normothermic.

Nursing diagnosis

Potential for alteration to cardiac output due to inadequate circulating volume, or vagal stimulation.

Nursing intervention

The child should be attached to an ECG monitor immediately. The heart rate sound may need to be turned up so that the rate is audible during procedures that may affect vagal stimulation (e.g., intubation) or while the health workers are concentrating on difficult procedures which may distract their attention (e.g., the insertion of central lines).

- Prepare transducers for CVP monitoring and arterial monitoring.
- Inotropic and chronotropic support/vasodilatation may be required. They should not be used in the presence of hypovolaemia. Verify dose, dilution, and rate at least once per shift.
- Label infusion tubing carefully. Be aware of the desired effects, side and toxic effects.
- Check compatibility of all drugs prescribed.
- Add dilutional fluids to total fluid intake.

Nursing diagnosis

Inadequate circulating volume due to loss of fluid or shift of fluid to 'third space'.

Nursing intervention

Immediate intravenous access is required. Intravenous access needs to be the largest bore cannula that can be inserted. A double lumen central line is preferred as it can be used for the infusion of large amounts of fluid quickly, and administration of inotropes, while the second lumen can be used for monitoring of CVP. If the child is peripherally shut down, a peripheral cutdown may be required, or insertion of an intraosseous needle into the tibia.
Monitor the child's fluid and electrolyte balance accurately.

Nursing diagnosis

Potential for metabolic acidosis due to acid base disturbance.

Nursing intervention

- Early administration of fluid boluses will improve tissue perfusion. Vasodilatation therapy may be required if tissue perfusion does not improve.
- Sodium bicarbonate may be required at half correction (body weight × base deficit × 0.3). Electrolytes, particularly calcium and potassium, require close monitoring. Hypocalcaemia predisposes the child to hypotension, tachycardia, myocardial depression and acidosis. Hyperkalaemia is potentially fatal and may occur as a result of correction of pH. (See acute renal failure.)
- Hyperglycaemia and hypoglycaemia may be due to severe stress. Blood glucose levels should be closely monitored.

Nursing diagnosis

Potential for development of cardiogenic shock.

Nursing intervention

- Monitor child's response to therapy; if child fails to respond to repeated doses of inotropes, consider complicating factors.
- Keep child warm — avoid cold stress.

SEPTIC (DISTRIBUTIVE) SHOCK

Endotoxins cause vasodilatation and thus relative hypovolaemia. The decreased contractility causes leucocyte and platelet aggregation, capillary leak and therefore oedema, hypovolaemia and shocked lung syndrome. Infectious organisms or toxins produce changes in myocardial function, vascular resistance and permeability, and decrease oxygen utilisation, resulting in distributive shock. This form of shock has elements of both hypovolaemic and cardiogenic shock.[2]

Assessment

Early septic shock results in hyperdynamic cardiovascular function. Increased pulmonary vascular resistance (PVR) and decreased systemic vascular resistance (SVR) are only seen with maldistribution of blood flow. Late septic shock presents as cardiogenic shock, which has a high mortality.

Treatment

- Prevention or early recognition of the cause is essential.
- Administration of appropriate antibiotics.
- Ensure optimum heart rate, reduce oxygen demands.
- Volume administration to maximise cardiac output and perfusion.
- Titrate inotropic agents as needed to maximise perfusion.

Once a patient develops low cardiac output, management is similar to cardiogenic shock — increased PAW, intrapulmonary shunting, low cardiac output and acidosis are ominous. Monitor for signs of ARDS.

Monitoring of the Critically Ill Child

The importance of assessment and monitoring cannot be emphasised too strongly. In PICU, all children will have continuous monitoring of several physiological parameters. The most common parameters that are continuously monitored on all children are electrocardiograph and heart rate, respiration and oxygen saturation. Children who are haemodynamically unstable or compromised will frequently have continuous arterial blood pressure monitored, or a very frequent non-invasive assessment of blood pressure, and will often have CVP continuously monitored.[9] Observations are routinely recorded hourly on the PICU flowchart, though with the advent of improved computerised systems, this may change. Monitoring and recording of observations and plotting of trends may seem unnecessary or repetitive, but the importance of continuous monitoring and observation is a significant factor in the evaluation of efficacy of therapies, and allows appropriate interventions to occur which may prevent or minimise the development of life-threatening events and complications.

Vital signs

Monitor pulse, blood pressure and respiratory rate every 15 minutes until stable, then hourly. Monitor temperature at least hourly until stable.

ELECTROCARDIOGRAM (ECG)

Definition

The ECG provides a continuous reading of the heart rate and rhythm. The electrical activity of the heart is monitored through electrodes placed on the skin.

Indications

All children requiring admission to the PICU should be attached to a cardiac monitor for continuous assessment of heart rate and rhythm.

Procedure

The negative electrode (white) is placed above the heart on the right upper sternal border; the positive electrode (black) is placed near the apex of the heart, while the ground electrode (green) is placed on the lower right side to avoid electrical interference from the other electrodes. The electrodes are then attached to a cardiac monitor.

Nursing management

Monitor ECG continuously. Observe for dysrhythmias. Observe for atrial and ventricular rate, *PR* interval, *QRS* duration, appearance of *P* waves, *QRS* complex. Keep rate alarms on at all times.

Complications

Artefact from patient movement is often unavoidable when caring for young or distressed children. Accurate lead placement is also important so that correct rhythms can be read on the monitor.

TEMPERATURE

Definition

The child's temperature should be approximately 37°C if taken rectally and 36°C to 36.5°C if taken per axilla.

Indications

Infants and children, especially those who are shocked, requiring long or multiple procedures, or requiring close observation, are usually exposed to changes in ambient temperature. Because of the large surface-area-to-mass ratio and the inability of infants to maintain body temperature, the risk of hypothermia is ever present. Temperature monitoring is important to avoid cold stress, which increases metabolism and cardiorespiratory demands. There are several methods of measuring temperature, depending on the condition of the child. In stable children, per axilla or tympanic membrane monitoring is sufficient. However, in children who are shocked or shut down, the peripheral temperature may be lower than the core temperature. In such cases, rectal monitoring is required to give an accurate temperature. In unstable children, or those with head lesions that may interfere with thermal regulation, continuous monitoring is necessary. Core-toe ambient temperature gradients supply an accurate indication of cardiac output. The gradient increases with low cardiac output or vasoconstriction. It is especially beneficial in determining the effect of vasodilator treatment.

Nursing management

Provide a warm ambient temperature by the use of overhead heaters if the child is hypothermic and requires exposure for procedures or observation. Warming blankets can also be used to provide warmth from under the child. Care should be taken to ensure that the warming devices are not hotter than desired skin temperature. Warm blankets and rugs can also be used to provide warmth. The aim should be to increase the child's temperature by no more than 1°C per hour. Care should also be taken not to overheat the child. The use of hot water bottles is contraindicated.

Complications

Inaccurate estimation of temperature may be made if the child is severely vasoconstricted and shut down. The peripheries feel cool or cold to the touch, while the core temperature is likely to be extremely high. This is especially so in children with late septic shock.

INTRA-ARTERIAL LINE

Definition

Peripheral arterial cannulation provides continuous display of arterial blood pressure and provides easy access for repeated blood gas analysis without disturbing the infant or child. Repeated stabbing of an artery may give inaccurate readings if the child is distressed.[10]

Indications

All critically ill children requiring continuous blood pressure monitoring or frequent blood gas analysis.

Procedure

The artery (radial, dorsalis pedis, posterior tibial, brachial or femoral) is cannulated and attached to a pressure transducer by a heparin flush line.

Nursing management

Monitor arterial pressure continuously in patients with arterial lines. Keep pressure alarms on at all times. Keep all connections in constant view at all times as patients can exsanguinate in minutes if disconnection occurs. Balance and calibrate transducer according to policy at least, every 8 hours. Use a constant closed heparinised flush solution to maintain patency. Observe for characteristic wave form. Investigate dampening or abnormal appearance. Compare with sphygmomanometer reading every 8 hours.

Check pulse, skin temperature and colour distal to insertion site hourly.

Complications

Bleeding due to accidental disconnection; infection; trauma to artery; haematoma; accidental injection of medication; and fluid overload.[11]

CENTRAL VENOUS PRESSURE (CVP)

Definition

Measurement of right atrial pressure, which reflects circulating blood volume and is thus an indirect measure of hydration status. Normal values are 3 to 15 cmH$_2$O. High values are due in the main to volume overload, pulmonary hypertension and ventricular failure. Low values are due to hypovolaemia, septicaemia and peripheral vasodilation.

Indications

The catheter can also be used for the administration of large amounts of fluid during resuscitation, for venous blood sampling, for the administration of hypertonic solutions or vasoactive drugs.[2]

Nursing management

Before measuring CVP, check zero level of catheter (4th intercostal space in midaxillary line). Before measuring CVP, confirm catheter patency by observation of the wave form and fluctuations with respirations. Measure CVP hourly and as required.

Complications

Readings are artificially increased by positive pressure ventilation. Pressure should be read with transducer at the level of the right atrium. Pressure tubing which will not expand should be used for monitoring. The transducer should be calibrated frequently — at least once per nursing shift. Waveform should be checked for characteristic pattern to ensure that catheter tip is in the correct place. Other complications are as for arterial pressure monitoring.

PULSE OXYMETRY (SaO$_2$)[12]

Definition

Pulse oxymeters are a non-invasive method of monitoring the oxygen saturation of arterial haemoglobin by measuring the absorption of 2 wave-lengths of light passed through an arteriolar bed. By comparing the absorption change at each wave-length during a pulse, both oxygen saturation and pulse rate are determined.[13]

Indications

Children who are at risk of becoming hypoxic.

Procedure

The sensor (ensure it is of appropriate size), containing 2 light sources, is placed across a pulsating arteriolar bed such as a finger, toe, ear lobe or the nose. The sensor should be placed so that it is in direct alignment with the photodetector. The child's skin should be clean and dry. When light is transmitted from the source to the photodetector across the arteriolar vessel, light absorption will vary in relation to changes with the blood volume. The changes in ratio of red to infrared determines the SaO$_2$ value.

Nursing management

Regularly rotate placement of sensor to reduce the risk of heat and pressure injury to the skin.

Complications

Inaccurate readings may be made should the light source and the photoreceptor not be in direct alignment, or should the source not be placed over an arteriolar bed. Other clinical factors which may influence the readings are changes in the oxyhaemoglobin curve. These include changes in body temperature, blood pH, level of 2,3-DPG, abnormal $PaCO_2$ or large quantities of foetal haemoglobin.[12]

CAPNOGRAPHY (END TIDAL CO_2)

Definition

The measurement and graphic display of the CO_2 level appearing at the airway by non-invasive, continuous monitoring of ventilation.

Indications

Any patient who is intubated and who requires continuous monitoring of the CO_2 level where raised CO_2 may be detrimental (e.g., in children at risk of raised ICP).

Procedure

The adaptor is attached to the end of the patient's airway near the end of the endotracheal tube. The characteristic waveform denotes a zero baseline, a rapid, sharp uprise, an alveolar plateau and a rapid, sharp downstroke. This waveform corresponds to the exhalation of CO_2 and the inhalation of CO_2-free gas.[13]

Nursing management

Continuous observation of the waveform. Correct calibration of the adaptor.

Complications

Water and mucus may obstruct flow of gas. If the flow rate is too high and the tidal volume small, some inhaled gas will be aspirated along with the exhaled gas and may give an incorrectly low CO_2 level.

PULMONARY ARTERY PRESSURE

Definition

Determine haemodynamic parameters through direct intracardiac and pulmonary artery pressure monitoring and cardiac output determination. In critically ill children the measurement of intracardiac pressures and cardiac output can aid clinical evaluation in identifying specific cardiopulmonary disorders, allowing for appropriate selection and titration of medical therapy to optimise cardiovascular performance.[14,15] However, pulmonary artery catheters are rarely used in children.

Indications[16]

To ascertain pulmonary capillary wedge pressure and pulmonary artery pressures to aid in the diagnosis and treatment of conditions such as: left ventricular failure; ARDS; cardiogenic shock; septic shock; and after liver transplantation.

Contraindications

Relative contraindications include children with recurrent sepsis or hypercoagulable status, where the catheter could serve as a focus for septic or thrombus formation.

Equipment required

Pulmonary artery catheter; ECG monitor; pressure transducer with sterile flush system; and IV cutdown equipment.

Procedure

The catheter is introduced by percutaneous insertion or cutdown procedure. Under continuous pressure monitoring, the catheter is gently advanced into the right atrium, showing the characteristic pressure waveform of the heart and pulmonary circulation. When removing the catheter, ensure the balloon is fully deflated. During removal of the catheter, the child should have continuous ECG monitoring in case of precipitation of ventricular tachycardia.

Nursing management

Place the transducer at the level of the right atrium for accurate reading. Continuous display of the waveform is recommended. Migration of the catheter into a smaller artery and wedging can be observed by changes in the pressure wave. The pressure monitoring lumen should be kept patent by continuous, slow infusion with heparinised saline. Check IV lines, pressure lines and transducer domes hourly to keep them free of air. Ensure stopcocks and connecting lines remain tightly fitted. Balloon inflation for wedge pressure measurement should be kept to a minimum to prevent perforation of the pulmonary artery. The number of inflations should be recorded. After deflation, the syringe is kept attached to the catheter.[17]

Complications

If the catheter tip migrates to the right ventricle this may cause ventricular arrhythmias. The situation should be reported immediately so that the catheter may be advanced to the pulmonary artery, providing sterility can be maintained. If sterility cannot be maintained, the catheter should be withdrawn to the right atrium. Potentially life-threatening complications include pulmonary artery perforation and pulmonary infarction. Therefore, these catheters should only be used for a short time.[16]

INTRACRANIAL PRESSURE (ICP) MONITORING

Definition

Intracranial pressure monitoring provides the most reliable method of confirming cerebral perfusion pressure (CPP), excluding intracranial hypertension, and assessing response to therapy, especially in the paralysed (muscle relaxed) ventilated child.[18] Continuous intracranial pressure monitoring allows for the immediate recognition of raised pressure, while monitoring via an external ventricular drain allows for the removal of cerebrospinal fluid (CSF) to relieve pressure or for sampling of CSF.[19]

Indications

Increasing intracranial pressure following neurological and systemic disorders such as severe head injury, meningitis, and severe hypoxia can lead to secondary brain damage. As intracranial pressure rises, cerebral blood flow is reduced, especially in damaged areas where autoregulation may be impaired.

Relative contraindications

Localised raised intracranial pressure; collapsed ventricles; lesions occupying the posterior fossa space.

Procedure

Three methods which are currently used are:

1. External ventricular catheter (with or without attachment to a drainage bag) inserted into the frontal horn of a lateral ventricle with fluid connection to an externally placed transducer.
2. Subarachnoid screw (Richmond Bolt) threaded through the dura and connected via a fluid-filled system to an external transducer.
3. Fibreoptic probe, which may be inserted into brain tissue or lateral ventricle.[20]

Nursing management[21]

Monitor ICP continuously in patients with ICP catheters. Use a consistent baseline position, usually 30° elevation of the head of the bed. Level the transducer with estimated position of the ventricles. Verify patency of the catheter by observing characteristic pattern of the waveform. Do not measure pressure when patient is moving, coughing or has the head turned. Never aspirate or flush an ICP line unless specifically directed to do so. Monitor cerebral perfusion pressure by subtracting ICP from mean arterial pressure (MAP). Balance and calibrate transducer at least every 8 hours.

Complications

Infection; trauma to brain tissue; leakage of CSF; brain swelling may collapse lateral ventricle so that the catheter cannot be placed or may render pressure measurements invalid and drainage impossible; error in positioning and calibration resulting in false measurement; perforation of cerebral artery; and blockage of the catheter.

Nursing Care Guidelines for the Ventilated Infant/Child

A large proportion of infants and children requiring admission to PICU have respiratory failure, and require airway and respiratory management. There is a strong seasonal pattern as a consequence of the large number of infants and young children who succumb to lower respiratory infections in the winter months. Approximately 50% of admissions to PICUs are for respiratory problems which require intubation and/or mechanical ventilation. For this reason, we have chosen to review in detail the nursing and medical management of infants and children who require endotracheal intubation and mechanical ventilation.

GENERAL PRINCIPLES

Infants and children who require mechanical ventilation rely on skilled and meticulous nursing care. These patients must never be left unattended and the alarms of all monitoring equipment must always be set at realistic limits and left turned on. Good nursing care will maintain the general condition of the infant/child, and early recognition of any change in vital signs or other parameters can avert major complications.

Children may be intubated orally or nasally.[22] The nasal route is preferred because of easier fixation and comfort for the child. The exceptions for nasal intubation include suspected base of skull fracture, and some facial trauma, including burns. Children tend to bite on and thus occlude an orally placed tube. The endotracheal tube (ETT) may be secured in several ways. When intubated, a child is unable to cry or speak audibly. If a cough is present it is usually very quiet. If it is possible to hear a child talk or cry, it must be questioned whether or not the ETT is correctly placed. All intubated children should also have a nasogastric tube inserted to relieve gastric distension and to either drain gastric secretions or to feed the child. While the child is not receiving enteral feeds, the nasogastric tube should be left on free drainage and aspirated regularly. The child should not be given oral feeds while intubated.

Nasopharyngeal tubes are also used occasionally, and also require suctioning, but do not require the instillation of normal saline during the suctioning procedure. Nasopharyngeal tubes are used for upper airways obstruction such as after tonsillectomy or Pierre Robin Syndrome, and do not enter the larynx. The child is therefore able to cry audibly.

Controversy exists about the use of shallow versus deep suctioning, as injury and fibrotic changes in the carina have been reported as a result of deep suctioning.[23] However, each child should be individually assessed as to whether shallow suctioning of the ETT will remove the secretions. A guide to correct ETT size is age of child divided by 4 plus 4.[2]

CARE OF THE ENDOTRACHEAL TUBE

Due to anatomical differences in the paediatric airway, uncuffed endotracheal tubes are used. A cuffed tube may be considered for adolescents. An air leak around the tube must be present on intubation to minimise the risk of subglottic trauma.[24,25]

Taping: This must be secure. If the strapping is loose, ensure that it is strapped as soon as possible. Any mobility of the ETT in or out can cause damage to the airway.

Length: The length of the ETT should be measured at intubation and regularly afterwards to ensure that the tube has not moved. The tube can be marked at the nares and measured from the lateral nares to the end of the tube. The tape should not be marked to indicate the ETT position, as the tube may slip through the tape and give an inaccurate indication of the tube position.

Table 12.1 Guidelines for suction catheter size

ETT size (in millimetres; internal diameter)	Catheter (French gauge)	Length
2.5	FG 5	20 cm
3.0	FG 6	23 cm
3.5	FG 6	25 cm
4.0	FG 6	28 cm
4.5	FG 6–8	30 cm
5.0	FG 8	32 cm
5.5	FG 8	35 cm
6.0	FG 8–10	
6.5	FG 10	
7.0	FG 10	
7.5	FG 12	
8.0	FG 12	

Kinking: Avoid kinking of the ETT by positioning the ventilator tubing downwards.

Traction: The ventilator tubing should be secured by the expiratory hose to prevent traction on the ETT.

Humidification: This is necessary for all intubated patients. Humidification can be provided by means of a ventilator circuit, or for non-ventilated children, by means of a condenser filter.

Arm splints and restraints: These are particularly important to prevent the child from dislodging the ETT. This is particularly relevant if a child is waking after anaesthesia.

Suctioning of the ETT

The need for ETT suction is assessed according to the requirements of the individual patient. Smaller ETTs (those less than 4.0 mm) may require more frequent suction as do those of children with larger amounts of secretions. Children whose condition is unstable or who have raised intracranial pressure should be suctioned less frequently. Children will usually require oxygenation before, during and after the suctioning procedure, with a higher concentration of oxygen with a rebreathing bag to ensure that the oxygen saturation remains at acceptable limits. During the suctioning procedure, it is important to assess continually the patient's colour, heart rate, chest movement and oxygenation level. For children on high ventilator settings, it may be necessary to suction via a 'bullet' attached to the ventilator circuit so that the ventilator does not require disconnection during the procedure, or the connection of a pressure manometer to the rebreathing bag, so that pressures (including PEEP) can be maintained during the procedure.[26]

The suction catheter should be one that is less than half the diameter of the ETT and the following sizes in **Table 12.1** are recommended. If copious secretions are present in the nose, softer catheters with rounded ends may be used. Longer catheters, such as argyle suction catheters, are available for longer ETTs, which are used for children intubated for croup.

MECHANICAL VENTILATION

Continuous positive airway pressure (CPAP) provides a constant distending pressure while the child is able to breathe independently. The gas flow should be approximately twice the minute volume to avoid rebreathing. CPAP is best delivered through an ETT, as CPAP via nasal prongs loses pressure if the child cries or mouth breathes. The benefits of CPAP include an increase in functional residual capacity, reduction in intrapulmonary shunting and decreased inspired oxygen concentration. It is particularly beneficial in splinting lower airways.[27]

Full mechanical ventilation is required for apnoea, hypoventilation, respiratory failure or pulmonary disease. Ventilation reduces the work of breathing, which is beneficial for children who are shocked, exhausted or where reduced oxygen consumption is required. As children are usually intubated with an uncuffed ETT with a small leak around the tube, some form of pressure ventilation is the most usual method of ventilation. Volume cycle mode is usually reserved for lower airway pathology such as asthma, bronchiolitis or ARDS. A combination of volume and pressure regulated ventilation is becoming more common.[28,29]

Observations

Heart rate is recorded hourly and ECG is monitored continuously by cardiac monitor. Observe for tachycardia, bradycardia, arrhythmias or instability, e.g., bradycardia during

---

Box 12.7 Assessment of adequate ventilation.

- Symmetrical and synchronous chest movement.
- Equal air entry — check with stethoscope.
- Patient's colour.
- Monitor oxygen saturation with oxymeter.
- Arterial blood gas results.
- Patient's behaviour, e.g., irritability, restlessness.

Box 12.8 Ventilator assessment.

- Oxygen and air flow: set to at least 10 L/minute.
- Oxygen concentration.
- Pressure: peak airway or inspiratory pressure (PIP), end expiratory pressure (PEEP), mean airways pressure (MAP), or continuous positive airway pressure (CPAP).
- Rate: set by length of expiratory time.
- Mode of ventilation.
- Humidifier and tubing: sterile water is used to keep humidification of the inspiratory circuit. Expiratory circuit may collect water, which requires emptying away from the patient.
- Manifold temperature should be kept between 35 and 37°C. A lower temperature will cause the water to condense while a higher temperature may cause tracheal burns.
- Inspiratory time: measures the length of inspiration, usually 0.7 to 0.8 second.

ETT suctioning. A computer printout may be used rather than a manual recording of the observations. However, this should be used with some caution.

Respirations are recorded hourly and monitored continuously. Check that respirations synchronise with the ventilator.

Temperature should be taken per axilla and recorded hourly until the condition is stable. Children with loss of skin integrity (such as severe burns), those who are shocked and shut down or those children with loss of autoregulation as a consequence of severe neurological dysfunction require continuous monitoring of core temperature via a temperature probe inserted approximately 3 to 5 cm into the rectum. These children may appear peripherally cool, but have a core hyperthermia, which will lead to increased metabolic rate, with subsequent increase in oxygen requirement. Hypothermia may be present in children on muscle relaxants as they are unable to shiver to maintain normothermia. Children are often nursed with few clothes or coverings, so that they are able to be easily observed. Infants and babies are especially at risk of hypothermia after surgery or if shocked.

Blood pressure should be recorded on admission and hourly on most mechanically ventilated children until their condition is assessed as stable. If the condition is unstable an arterial line will be required to monitor blood pressure continuously.

Oxygen saturation should be monitored in all children with an artificial airway, and all children who are at risk of becoming hypoxic.

End tidal CO_2 should be monitored in all ventilated children in whom high $PaCO_2$ is expected or where a lower than usual $PaCO_2$ is beneficial, such as in children with raised intracranial pressure.

Neurological assessment is recorded on admission on all children to determine the child's neurological status; to ascertain signs of hypoxia in children with respiratory conditions; to determine a baseline reading for children admitted with conditions such as head injury, meningitis, coma, diabetes mellitus, ingestion and poisoning, and neuromuscular disease. Children receiving muscle relaxants to facilitate ventilation should have hourly pupil checks, which may indicate signs of raised intracranial pressure.[30]

Urine output is an important indication of adequate circulation; 1 to 2 mL/kg/hour indicates an adequate renal blood flow and cardiac output. Greater than 3 mL/kg/hour may indicate an osmotic diuresis or diabetes insipidus. Less than 0.5 mL/kg/hour may be due to dehydration, circulatory failure, syndrome of inappropriate antidiuretic hormone secretion, renal failure or obstruction to urinary flow. Muscle relaxants and the administration of morphine may cause oliguria and/or urinary retention. If the child does not have a urinary catheter *in situ*, palpate the bladder and express if necessary.

Fluid therapy

Intravenous fluids are usually restricted to two-thirds the normal daily maintenance while the child is being ventilated mechanically, as the humidification of the ventilator circuit does not allow for expiratory loss.

General nursing care

Positioning: Unless contraindicated (e.g., severe hypotension, spinal injury) all patients should be nursed with the head of the bed raised 15° to 30°. This permits better respiratory effort and allows the apex of the lungs to expand more than if lying completely flat. It also promotes safer nasogastric feeding and assists in venous drainage in patients with head injury.

Blood glucose level should be monitored on children on admission; while receiving nothing orally; infants under 6 months of age; and children with abnormally high or low levels. The levels may be raised in children who are stressed or have received steroids.

Stomach distension should be relieved and prevented by the insertion of a nasogastric tube. The tube also allows for the removal of gastric secretions while the patient is nil orally. Aspirate should be tested for occult blood and sucralfate or antacids administered while the child is nil orally. Appropriate management of the gastrointestinal tract is essential in all critically ill children, and is discussed in further detail later in the chapter. Some children who are fed enterally may require the nasogastric tube to be unclamped and elevated to relieve excess gastric gas caused by excessive crying or swallowing of air.

Bodyweight: Whenever possible children should be weighed on admission. Daily weight is important in patients with cardiac and renal conditions. Children lose 1% to 2% of bodyweight per day while receiving only maintenance fluids.

Sedation is required to reduce restlessness and to minimise the work of breathing. A continuous infusion of morphine after a loading dose will hinder alertness and relieve pain. The administration of midazolam may also be required to reduce anxiety in some children. If voluntary respiratory function is to be overridden completely, for hyperventilation or to prevent the child from fighting against the ventilator, muscle relaxants such as pancuronium may be used.[30] In this case, the child is unable to breathe if the ventilator becomes disconnected and so must be continuously observed.

Children should have their position changed every 2 hours if they are unable to move themselves. Children with raised intracranial pressure, suspected or unstabilised spinal injuries or whose condition is labile may not tolerate movement, but will require precautions against the formation of pressure damage. Surgical gloves filled with warm water may be positioned to cushion the joints. The back of the head is susceptible to pressure in children who are nursed for long periods on their back; the use of egg crate foam pillows can reduce pressure. Sheepskins may also be used to minimise pressure on bony prominences. The use of waterbeds or mattresses may also be indicated.

Passive range of motion exercises are required for children unable to move their limbs for long periods due to unconsciousness or muscle relaxants. Hand and foot splints should be used to prevent foot drop or damage to wrists and hands.

Mouth care should be attended to frequently while the child is nil orally. Swabs containing a glycerol solution are useful in keeping the mouth moist. The teeth can be gently cleansed with a soft toothbrush if care is taken to use a suction catheter to avoid aspiration. The lips should be lightly smeared with soft paraffin to prevent cracking and drying.

Eye care using normal saline and artificial tears is particularly important while the child is receiving muscle relaxants and is unable to blink. The eyes should be kept covered with ocular ointment to prevent corneal ulceration.

The skin should be kept clean and dry and washed as required with warm water and soap. Care should be taken to keep the child warm.

Urinalysis should be undertaken on admission, and daily. Specific gravity can be used as a guide to hydration except when osmotic diuretics or dye have been used. If the child has an indwelling catheter, a specimen should be cultured if a urinary tract infection is suspected.

Intubated children should have their nares inspected for pressure from ETT taping. The tube should be kept positioned downwards to prevent added pressure.

Check for the frequency of bowel movement. Stool softeners may be required during periods of inactivity. Check for bowel sounds.

Nosocomial infection, which may seriously compromise the condition of an already ill child, can be minimised by:

- taking care to wash hands before and after handling any patient;
- ensuring equipment is clean;
- maintaining aseptic techniques for dressings and procedures;
- universal precautions when handling body fluids.

Nursing diagnosis

Ineffective ventilation related to respiratory failure.

Nursing intervention

Frequent recording of vital signs; maintain ventilation at prescribed parameters.[31] Observe for signs of hypoxia, partially blocked, blocked or dislodged endotracheal tube: restlessness; poor air entry; increased heart rate; and increased work of breathing. Cyanosis is a late sign.

Nursing diagnosis

Ineffective airway clearance related to ETT or increased secretions.

Nursing intervention

Suction when required, as established by dyspnoea, coughing, secretions in the ETT, rhonchi or increased airway pressures. Suctioning may be required more frequently when the ETT is of a smaller diameter than is usual or when there are copious thick secretions.[32] Ensure oral and nasopharyngeal secretions are removed by suctioning.

Oxygenate before and after with 100% oxygen with a suction catheter less than 50% diameter of ETT. If the child requires PEEP, use a PEEP valve on the rebreathing bag.

Nursing diagnosis

Potential for pulmonary infection.

Nursing intervention

Depending on amount of secretions, either a condensor filter or a ventilator circuit may be required to replace the normal mechanism for moistening inhaled air. Monitor the humidifier's water level and temperature. Observe for signs and symptoms of pulmonary infection such as fever or purulent secretions. Maintain no-touch technique during suction.[23] Change ventilator circuitry as per protocol. Maintain good oral hygiene.

Box 12.9 Features of infants' airways compared with those of adults.

- Narrowest part of airway is the pharynx.
- Short maxilla and mandible.
- Soft palate is proportionately large.
- Infant's tongue is large.
- Narrow posterior nasopharynx.
- Trachea has minimal smooth muscle until age 4 years.
- All lower airways are present at birth, but true alveoli not present until 2 months.
- Principle muscle of respiration is the diaphragm.

Nursing diagnosis

Potential for accidental extubation.

Nursing intervention

Secure strapping is vital to secure the ETT. The tube may be shorter than usual size-for-age and thus easier to dislodge; copious nasopharyngeal secretions may loosen tapes around the nares. Arm restraints may be necessary to prevent self-extubation, especially in young children and immediately after anaesthesia.

The Child Experiencing Upper Airways Obstruction

Upper airways obstruction is common in infants and young children due to a combination of the physiology of the airway and the frequency of respiratory infections (**Box 12.9**).

Croup and epiglottitis are the 2 most common causes of infectious upper airway obstruction in children. It is important to distinguish between the 2 so that appropriate management can be undertaken.[33] Other, less common, causes of upper airway obstruction that may be seen in young children include: bacterial tracheitis, foreign body aspiration, diphtheria, vascular ring, and retropharyngeal abscess.[34]

LARYNGOMALACIA

A common congenital laryngeal anomaly in which the laryngeal cartilage is flaccid and the arepiglottic folds fall into the glottis on inspiration. Stridor is inspiratory and usually high pitched; may be intermittent, may decrease when the patient is placed prone with the neck extended, may increase with agitation, usually present from birth or first weeks of life. The infant's cry is usually normal. Feeding problems may be associated with increased respiratory distress. Laryngoscopy confirms diagnosis. Treatment is supportive, unless respiratory distress interferes with feeding and growth, in which case a tracheostomy may be indicated.

LARYNGEAL WEB

Symptoms are frequently noted at birth with inspiratory stridor. Diagnosis is confirmed by laryngoscopy. Treatment involves lysis in the case of thin webs. A tracheostomy may be required for treatment of a thick web.

TRACHEOMALACIA

This involves malformed tracheal cartilage rings with lack of rigidity and oval shape to the lumen. Wheezing and stridor are noted on expiration, with collapse of tracheal lumen. Diagnosis is confirmed by fluoroscopy and bronchoscopy, which demonstrate tracheal collapse on expiration. Cartilaginous development eventually improves the airway.

VASCULAR RING

The airway may be narrowed by external pressure from congenital malformations of the intrathoracic great vessels. Infants present with stridor at birth or within the first few weeks of life. Other symptoms include wheezing, cough, cyanosis, recurrent broncho-pulmonary infections and dysphagia. Diagnosis may be confirmed by endoscopy, which reveals indentations secondary to extrinsic pressure. The anatomy of the vascular mal-formations is determined by angiography. Treatment is surgical correction of the vascular malformation.

RETROPHARYNGEAL ABSCESS

Suppuration of the lymphoid tissue around the nodes draining the nasopharynx, sinuses and eustachian tubes may cause pus accumulation in the retropharyngeal space. Presenting symptoms include history of upper respiratory tract infection, sore throat, fever, toxic appearance, meningism, stridor, dysphagia and difficulty handling secretions. Diagnosis is usually made on lateral x-ray, with widening of the soft tissue between the trachea and the cervical vertebrae. Treatment involves surgical drainage and antibiotic administration.

LUDWIG'S ANGINA

This involves rapidly spreading inflammation of the sublingual, submandibular and submaxillary spaces. Symptoms are caused by an oedematous tongue causing airway obstruction.

SPASMODIC CROUP

Spasmodic croup usually occurs during the night in children aged 1 to 3 years. It would appear to be an allergic response rather than an acute infection. Spasmodic croup tends to be present or worse during the night and improves during the day.

CROUP (LARYNGOTRACHEOBRONCHITIS)

It is important to distinguish between croup and epiglottitis so that the correct treatment can be undertaken. Diagnosis may be made from history from parents and physical

Table 12.2 Clinical features of croup and epiglottitis[36]

	Croup	Epiglottitis
Aetiology	Viral	Haemophilus
Age	6 months to 3 years	Infancy to adult
Onset	Subacute (days)	Acute (hours)
Fever	+ +	+ + +
Cough	+ + +	—
Drooling	—	+ +
Activity	Upset	Lethargic
Colour	Pale/sick	Toxic
Obstruction	+ + +	+
Stridor	Inspiratory, high pitched	Expiratory snore
Sore throat	Uncommon	Common
Position	Any	Tripod; sitting up
Course	Gradual worsening or improvement	Unpredictable. Fatal if untreated
Season	Autumn–winter[55]	Throughout the year

assessment of the child. Observation of the child should be continuous — pulse rate, respiratory rate, colour, chest retraction, tracheal tug, sternal recession, degree of respiratory distress, agitation, and oxymetry for degree of hypoxia.[35] Children are able to compensate and maintain oxygenation for some time until they become fatigued, when they may become hypoxic and apnoeic. The absence of stridor may mean that the child is exhausted or has decreased air entry, rather than indicating improvement.[36]

Viruses responsible for croup are: parainfluenza virus 1, 2 and 3; respiratory syncytial virus (RSV); influenza virus; rhinovirus and adenovirus.

Definition

Croup is used to describe a set of symptoms which are caused by acute swelling or obstruction around the larynx due to inflammation and oedema of the glottic and subglottic areas.[37] The symptoms are described in **Table 12.2**.

Physical assessment

Diagnosis is made on physical assessment and the history of the illness. Stridor, or noisy breathing caused by rapid, turbulent flow through an obstructed or narrowed portion of the airway is evident, as the obstruction is inspiratory and often quite loud. An absence of stridor may mean little or no air entry and should be treated as an emergency in the child with croup, and not as an indication of improvement. Inspiratory stridor is indicative of a lesion at the supraglottic or glottic area due to negative pressure during inspiration resulting in inward collapse. Expiratory stridor is more evident with lesions below the vocal cords. The cough is characteristic and described as barking or seal-like.

Nursing management

Observation is extremely important. Pulse rate, respiratory rate, colour, assessment of chest retraction, tracheal tug, sternal recession, signs of distress, or agitation. Pulse oxymetry demonstrates the degree of hypoxia.

Box 12.10 Indications for oxygen therapy.

Hypoxaemia:
- increased respiratory rate
- pallor
- increased heart rate cyanosis
- severe: CNS signs

Box 12.11 Recommended use of nebulised adrenaline.

- *Never* used as a definitive management.
- *Temporary* relief of obstruction for children:
  Who require transfer from one hospital to another
  While preparing for intubation
  Sudden, unexpected deterioration
  Other laryngeal abnormalities

Minimal handling is important and the most appropriate place for the child to be may be the parent's lap. Examination of the child may cause distress, which in turn will increase respiratory requirements, oxygen consumption and obstruction.

Hydration is important and in severe or prolonged courses, the child may require intravenous therapy, as oral fluids may not be tolerated.

Steam inhalation is often advocated for children with croup and may be of some benefit to those children with spasmodic croup. However, for the child with acute, severe croup, the treatment provides a cold, damp atmosphere, separation from parents and most importantly, difficulty in observation.

Oxygen therapy was not considered appropriate in the past due to the risk of masking increasing respiratory failure. However, most children with croup have low oxygen saturation levels as shown by the use of oxymeters. Thus, there is an increasing trend to give these children low concentrations of oxygen to maintain the oxygen saturation above 90%. Decreasing saturation levels are usually a sign of the need for intubation.[37]

Nebulised adrenaline is efficacious in the management of croup, but should never be seen as a cure. Children seen in an outpatient setting and administered nebulised adrenaline should be admitted to hospital and not sent home when the symptoms appear to have abated. Rebound oedema often occurs within 50 to 60 minutes of administration and may result in increased swelling.

The effect of nebulised adrenaline is seen within 5 minutes and usually lasts for an hour, but can be shortlived. Although inhalations can be repeated, the benefits lessen with subsequent treatments. Adrenaline does not alter the course of croup.[38] Some adverse side effects include tachycardia, tachyarrhythmias, headaches, nausea and irritability.

Dosage 1:1000 (0.1%) 0.5 mL/kg/dose with a maximum of 5 mL. Recommendations for the use of nebulised adrenaline are described in **Box 12.11**.

Management

If the child becomes exhausted or hypoxic, an *artificial airway* is required. This occurs in about 2% to 3% of children who are admitted to hospital with croup.[39] Making the decision to intubate is often a delicate balance, predicting the need for an artificial airway before a crisis develops and the child collapses. The child should be continuously assessed for signs of hypoxia, such as restlessness, lethargy, increased $PaCO_2$ to a normal level, inability to mobilise secretions, increased heart and respiratory rate, and loss of stridor. An ETT smaller than the usual size is required to intubate a child with croup, due to the excessive swelling and oedema of the airway. A leak around the ETT should be audible at intubation, though it may disappear afterwards. Conscientious suctioning of the ETT is vital, due to the large volume of secretions and the narrow ETT. The child may require oxygen and CPAP to compensate for the narrow tube.

Extubation is usually successful after 5 days. Assessment for extubation may be made on the development of a leak around the tube and thinning of secretions. If signs of respiratory distress are present after extubation, 1 or 2 doses of nebulised adrenaline may be required. If respiratory distress persists, diagnosis of tracheal trauma may be made on laryngoscopy. Reintubation or a tracheostomy may be required for approximately 6 weeks for ulceration, granulation or stenosis.[25,37]

Antibiotics are only useful in cases of associated bronchitis or suspected tracheitis. For intubated children, careful note should be made of their secretions, which may become purulent and require antistaphylococcal therapy.

Controversy has abounded for many years over the efficacy of *steroids* in the management of croup.[40,41] However, it would seem that the use of steroids results in a significant improvement within 12 hours of administration.[38,42-44]

Possible complications

Respiratory failure, respiratory arrest, hypoxic damage, secondary bacterial infection, acute pulmonary oedema, persistence, or recurrence.[45]

Outcome

Children with a history of croup requiring hospitalisation may have associated altered lung function. Significant reduction in functional vital capacity, forced expiratory volume at 1 minute (FEV_1) and $FEF_{25\%-75\%}$ and elevation of residual volume. There has also been evidence of heightened bronchial reactivity.[46]

Persistence or recurrence may be associated with structural airway abnormalities such as tracheal stenosis.

EPIGLOTTITIS

Haemophilus influenzae infection can lead to meningitis, septicaemia, septic arthritis, cellulitis and epiglottitis.[47] The most important aspect in the management of epiglottitis is diagnosis and minimal handling of the child until an airway is in place. This condition requires urgent intubation. All associated treatment, such as insertion of cannula, direct examination of the epiglottis, throat swab or any other attempt that may distress the child should be delayed until an experienced anaesthetist is present. Meanwhile, the child should be not be moved and should be left with the parents in the most comfortable position. Acute obstruction of the airway, followed by cardiac arrest, is a potential hazard.[48]

Definition

The infecting organism is usually *Haemophilus influenza* type b.[49] Septicaemia may be concurrent.

Haemophilus reaches the epiglottis from the nasopharynx or blood, causing the epiglottis to become swollen, red, softened and floppy, tending to fall backwards blocking the airway from above and circumferentially by swollen and inflamed arepiglottic folds surrounding the larynx. This process occurs rapidly over a few hours and the untreated child may become acutely obstructed. With the inclusion of *Haemophilus* B (Hib) vaccination in the immunisation schedule, the incidence of *Haemophilus* disease should decrease.[47]

Physical assessment

The infected child presents as unable to swallow secretions, drooling, refusing to talk or swallow. She maintains an upright position, usually leaning with her head extended, supporting a sitting position with her arms in what is known as the tripod position. Hypoxaemia is almost always present.

Possible complications

Sudden respiratory arrest, followed by cardiac arrest, can occur unpredictably. Cardiac arrest is likely to be asystolic in rhythm due to either vagal stimulation or hypoxia secondary to airway obstruction.

Box 12.12 Management of a child with epiglottitis.

Minimal handling
No examination of pharynx until intubation
No lateral x-rays
Prop up with pillows in sitting position
Arrange for artificial airway stat.
Antibiotics after airway secured

Nursing management

The child should be nursed propped up with pillows while arrangements are made for the insertion of an artificial airway (endotracheal tube). The child should be accompanied prior to tube insertion by the most experienced paediatric anaesthetic physician available for direct examination of the larynx to confirm diagnosis and to perform the intubation under inhalation anaesthesia. Antibiotics can be administered after blood for cultures has been taken.

Outcome

Complete recovery without sequelae is usual if diagnosis and treatment are appropriate and timely.

Box 12.13 Guidelines for extubation after epiglottitis.

- General toxic appearance has improved
- Lethargy and fatigue have settled
- 12 hours since intubation
- Temperature is less than 37.5°C without use of antipyretics

---

Management

Prophylaxis with antibiotic such as rifampicin is required for families and household contacts if there is a child in the household under the age of 5 years.

Children with Lower Airway Disease

ASTHMA

Definition

Asthma is a leading cause of both acute and chronic illness in children. It is defined as an obstructive disease of the airway which results in bronchial and bronchiolar smooth muscle spasm, increased mucous secretion and inflammation. The fundamental abnormality in asthma appears to be hyperactivity of the airways. The aetiology of this hyperactivity is manifested as increased responsiveness of the airways to cold air, tobacco smoke, chemicals, various drugs and atmospheric irritants. Hyperinflation of the lung occurs early in an asthma attack and maintains expiratory airflow during airways obstruction. During inspiration, airways are pulled open and flow depends on muscular effort. Airways narrow and expiratory flow decreases, but inspiratory flow is maintained and causes lung hyperinflation.[50]

Although the underlying pathophysiological mechanisms involved in childhood asthma are the same as in adult asthma, there are anatomical, physiological, immunological and psychological differences. In general, the younger the child the greater the dissimilarities. The most important differences in early life that predispose to wheezing are: a disproportionate narrowing of the peripheral airways; and decreased elastic recoil of the lung. Decreased elastic tissue predisposes to early closure of the airway during expiration, which in combination with narrow airways produces increased resistance to airflow. An additional factor that contributes to airway obstruction is mucous gland hyperplasia in children compared to adults. When these glands are stimulated, such as during a respiratory tract infection, excessive mucous production occurs and contributes to airway obstruction. The adult diaphragm maintains adequate ventilation during airway obstruction; the highly compliant ribcage in children does not provide rigid support for the diaphragm. There are deficiencies in communication between alveoli and bronchioles, and an increased tendency to develop respiratory tract infections. Young children lack prior exposure to viral infections and thus are prone to frequent upper respiratory infections, which often trigger hyperactivity of the airways, leading to an acute attack.[51]

Pathophysiology of acute unresponsive asthma

Airway obstruction leads to a mismatching of ventilation to perfusion, resulting in hypoxaemia. The respiratory system responds with an increase in alveolar ventilation, which is maintained by a reflex overactivity of the inspiratory muscles, the sterno-cleidomastoids, inspiratory intercostals and the diaphragm. This conscription of inspiratory effort leads to an increased lung volume.[50] The airways are held open, effectively compensating for the airway obstruction. While this compensated state is maintained, alveolar ventilation is protected and the $PaCO_2$ remains low. As muscle fatigue develops, lung volume falls, airways close and respiratory failure supervenes.[52]

Diagnostic procedures

Chest x-ray will show hyperinflation of the lungs and a flattened diaphragm. Attention should be paid to the presence of atelectasis, pneumothorax, pneumomediastinum or pneumonia.

Arterial blood gases show a decreased $PaCO_2$, reflecting hyperventilation. In acute asthma a $PaCO_2$ rising to normal level is a late and ominous sign, associated with failure of the inspiratory muscles, and progression to death can be rapid. Hypoxaemia is always present, often despite oxygen therapy, due to atelectasis and subsequent shunting. Acidosis requires close observation.[53]

A full blood count is required to assure sufficient haemoglobin for oxygenation. Electrolyte levels may be raised due to accompanying dehydration.

Management

Oxygen: Hypoxaemia is consistent with acute asthma. Its correction will enhance bronchiolar responsiveness and reduce cardiac irritability. There is no danger of suppressing respiratory drive in children with acute, severe asthma. Humidified oxygen should be delivered to facilitate the removal of secretions and to deliver oxygen to the lungs.

Beta mimetic bronchodilators: Continuous nebulisation of salbutamol is required in exceptional circumstances. Otherwise, a loading dose of 0.03 mL/kg (0.15 mg/kg) followed by 20-minute doses of 0.01 mL/kg (0.05 mg/kg). However, the more obstructed the patient, the less effective the delivery of the nebulised solution. Continuous intravenous infusion of salbutamol has been shown to reduce the need for mechanical ventilation for children with a rising $PaCO_2$. The infusion is usually commenced with a loading dose and is then titrated according to the response of the $PaCO_2$ level.[54]

Ipratropium bromide: The addition of nebulised ipratropium bromide together with beta mimetic bronchodilators after the first hour and repeated hourly has been shown to improve ventilation.[54]

Corticosteroids help to improve bronchodilator therapy within 4 to 6 hours.[55] Steroids are administered as oral prednisolone or intravenous hydrocortisone (loading dose followed by infusion).

Intravenous therapy is indicated in children who have been vomiting, who are dehydrated or who have severe obstruction. Children with acute, severe asthma are dehydrated from increased insensible loss and incapacity to take oral fluids. Transudation of fluid to the alveolar space due to pressure gradients may precipitate pulmonary oedema if fluid replacement is excessive.

Aminophylline: The addition of aminophylline is indicated in the treatment of children who are not responding to beta mimetic bronchodilators. Routine estimation of serum levels is required as the metabolism of aminophylline is unreliable and a potential for toxicity exists.

Clinical monitoring may be deceptive and thus objective assessment by lung function tests, pulse oxymetry and serial blood gas measurement is expedient.[53]

Mechanical ventilation: A child with progressive respiratory failure as indicated by a rise in $PaCO_2$, or a decreased level of consciousness despite the above measures, requires mechanical support. Past practice has been intubation and volume ventilation of 15 to 20 mL/kg. PEEP of up to 10 cmH_2O is necessary to hold open the airways and allow more air to exit before airway closure. The expiratory time is generally prolonged and the inspiratory time shortened. However, this management is associated with significant barotrauma and high mortality. Neuromuscular paralysis is required to facilitate ventilation. Morphine or midazolam should be administered concurrently to relieve anxiety in a fully conscious child.[50]

CPAP has been shown to reduce airway resistance in acute asthma by holding the lung at a high volume and increasing the elastic traction of the airways.[56] This also reduces the transpulmonary pressure and thus the risk of pneumothorax. The work of breathing is reduced, as is the $PaCO_2$, while total alveolar ventilation is increased.

The use of a well sealed CPAP face mask can deliver the pressure required in older children, and intubation is avoided. This method can also be used early in the course of the illness to deliver nebulised bronchodilators.

VIRAL BRONCHIOLITIS

Infants, especially those under 6 months of age, may be acutely affected by viral bronchiolitis.[57] Most cases are caused by respiratory syncitial virus (RSV).[58] The presenting symptoms are that of lower airway disease such as cough, fever, tachypnoea and wheeze. Some infants present acutely with apnoea. Like asthma, the chest x-ray shows hyperinflated lungs, although rib retractions are also evident on examination. Some infants develop respiratory failure and require ventilation, which may cause the development of air leaks. If the infant is able to tolerate CPAP by the nasal route or ETT, this is preferred, the raised $PaCO_2$ may return to normal and also reduce respiratory rate. Otherwise the management is minimal handling, supplemental oxygen and intravenous therapy. It appears that routine lower airway management — bronchodilators and steroids — does not provide clinical improvement.[57]

NURSING MANAGEMENT OF LOWER AIRWAY DISEASE

Nursing diagnosis

Impairment of respiration related to airway obstruction secondary to bronchial and bronchiolar smooth muscle spasm, increased mucous secretion and inflammation.

Nursing intervention

- Initiate oxygen therapy.
- Administer bronchodilators and corticosteroids, and commence intravenous therapy.

- Observe and record child's colour and respiratory rate.
- Evaluate air exchange by chest auscultation frequently.
- Assess skin colour for cyanosis.
- Assess respirations for depth, rate, retractions, nasal flaring, effort, lung sounds.
- Collect blood gases.
- Record vital signs frequently, including pulse and blood pressure.
- Observe type and rate of respirations, colour, apprehensiveness.
- Assist with diagnostic procedures.

Nursing diagnosis

Potential for respiratory acidosis related to CO_2 retention and metabolic acidosis secondary to tissue hypoxia.

Nursing intervention

- Administer sodium bicarbonate and oxygen to reduce anaerobic metabolism.
- Monitor arterial blood gases and record.

Nursing diagnosis

Potential for tissue hypoxaemia and shock related to decreased arterial oxygen tension.

Nursing intervention

- Administer oxygen.
- Increase ventilation.
- Position for optimum lung expansion in high Fowler's position.
- Administer positive pressure ventilation if ordered.

Nursing diagnosis

Potential for cardiac arrhythmia related to hypoxaemia and drug therapy.

Nursing intervention

- Place on cardiac monitor.
- Evaluate and report increased pulse rate or irregularity.

Nursing diagnosis

Potential for mediastinal and subcutaneous emphysema related to alveolar rupture.

Nursing intervention

- Palpate skin over sternum and neck for extravasated air.

Nursing diagnosis

Potential for altered fluid volume related to increased insensible loss or decreased fluid intake (dehydration) or excessive administration of intravenous therapy.

Nursing intervention

- Evaluate state of hydration (skin turgor, mucous membranes, bodyweight).
- Record fluid intake and output and specific gravity of urine.

Nursing diagnosis

Potential alteration in cardiac output related to impaired venous return secondary to fluctuations in intrapleural pressure.

Nursing intervention

- Observe for variation in radial pulse.
- Observe for greater than 10 mmHg variation in systolic blood pressure between inspiration and expiration (pulsus paradoxus) when taking blood pressure.

Nursing diagnosis

Potential for central nervous system abnormalities related to CO_2 retention and hypoxaemia.

Nursing intervention

Evaluate child's orientation, evidence of somnolence.

Nursing diagnosis

Anxiety related to hypoxaemia, feeling of suffocation, fear of impending death.

Nursing intervention

- Administer oxygen.
- Promote physical comfort.
- Position for comfort.
- Organise care for maximum rest.
- Explain procedures and equipment before use.
- Provide continuous attendance.
- Provide reassurance with calm manner.
- Encourage parents to remain with child.

Nursing diagnosis

Alteration in parental role related to hospitalisation.

Nursing intervention

- Reduce parental anxiety.
- Provide support and reassurance to parents.
- Explain unfamiliar procedures and equipment.
- Facilitate parental visits.

Nursing Management of Children with Acute Neurological Dysfunction

Children who experience acute neurological dysfunction fall into several broad categories. These include head injury, infection of the central nervous system, such as meningitis and encephalitis, metabolic encephalopathy caused by hypoxia, drugs, liver failure and polyneuritis. Apart from polyneuritis, the primary management is aimed at the prevention or control of raised intracranial pressure (ICP) and cerebral oedema.

There is a greater incidence of raised ICP in children than in adults. About 50% of adults with coma resulting from head trauma have raised ICP whereas 75% of children with coma resulting from head trauma have raised ICP. The brain of a child has a higher water content and high cerebral blood flow, which probably accounts for the greater incidence and severity of raised ICP in children.[59]

PATHOPHYSIOLOGY OF SEVERE HEAD INJURY

Traumatic brain damage can be either primary or secondary. The primary injury occurs at the time of the initial insult. This damage can be cortical, subcortical, diencephalic or be a disconnection from rotational shearing forces, often worse on the surface of the brain than at the centre. Secondary injury can be caused by compression (extradural or subdural haemorrhage), ischaemia, hypoxia, hypoglycaemia, epilepsy, hypothermia or meningitis. The secondary causes of injury often overlap. Damage from oedema is due to increased intercapillary distance and thus increased diffusion distance for oxygen, together with the toxic effects of protein secreted. The first response of the brain to raised intracranial pressure is decreased cerebrospinal fluid (CSF) and venous blood flow. Brain shifts may be caused by the volume changes due to further increased pressure. Under conditions of autoregulation the cerebral blood flow is relatively constant over a wide range of cerebral arterial pressure. Cerebral blood volume (total volume of intracranial blood) is influenced by the balance between cerebral blood flow and cerebral venous return.[60] Pressure/volume curve is nearly flat until the critical pressure is reached when there is a steep rise. Increased pressure compromises perfusion. Cerebral perfusion pressure (CPP) is measured by mean arterial pressure minus intracranial pressure.[61]

Normal intracranial pressure is 4 to 16 mmHg. Perfusion autoregulation is at arteriole level and can be lost in areas of damage. A CPP of 50 mmHg is required for minimal, adequate blood flow to the brain. If the CPP is less than 40 mmHg, cerebral blood flow is severely compromised and ischaemia can result. A CPP of less than 30 mmHg is incompatible with life. In children there is no available research for comparable figures, although the normal range is thought to be more than 40 to 50 mmHg.[62]

Secondary injury

Following the primary injury to the brain, secondary injury often takes place while the patient is under the care of health professionals within the acute care setting. This may result in raised intracranial pressure and inadequate cerebral blood flow. Therefore, it is essential that nursing therapies be promptly initiated so that secondary complications are anticipated and possibly avoided.

When the brain is compliant, as cerebral blood flow increases, intracranial pressure will remain within normal limits until compensatory mechanisms are exhausted. At this point a small rise in volume will result in a marked rise in intracranial pressure. The clinical importance of raised intracranial pressure is its detrimental effect on cerebral blood flow and perfusion. Cerebral perfusion pressure (CPP) is closely related to blood flow — mean arterial pressure (MAP).

ASSESSMENT OF A CHILD WITH ALTERED LEVEL OF CONSCIOUSNESS

Pulse

A child with rising ICP typically has a falling pulse rate, although alternating tachycardia and bradycardia may occur.

Blood pressure

Increasing pulse pressure is a late but reliable sign of rising ICP. This occurs when ICP equals diastolic blood pressure. The resulting cerebral ischaemia triggers increased systolic blood pressure, which in turn increases pulse pressure.

Respirations

Fast respirations indicate metabolic acidosis or respiratory alkalosis due to damage to the medulla or to stimulation to the medulla from salicylate poisoning, hepatic encephalopathy or Reye's syndrome.

Irregular or Cheyne-Stokes breathing indicates other medullary damage.

Pupils

Unilateral dilation with decreased reflex is caused by tentorial herniation damage to the 3rd cranial nerve and indicates the need for urgent surgical or medical decompression.

Bilateral fixed, dilated pupils indicate irreversible cerebral damage if present for more than 5 minutes.

Non-reactive pupils may indicate hypothermia, poisoning by atropine or sedatives.

Dilated, non-reactive pupils are caused by mydriatics.

Constricted, non-reactive pupils indicate pontine lesions, opiate administration or a barbiturate coma.

Normal pupils in a comatose child are most likely post ictal or due to metabolic disturbance.

Eye movements

Doll's eye nystagmus: Ice water caloric test. Absence of nystagmus indicates brainstem damage or poisoning; the reflex is retained in metabolic encephalopathy.

Lateral and downward eye movemet indicate 6th nerve palsy — not as ominous as 3rd nerve palsy.

Fundi

Papilloedema occurs 24 to 48 hours after injury. Dilated veins and absence of venous pulsations are an early sign of raised ICP.

Haemorrhages and exudates eye movements occur in association with subdural or subarachnoid bleeds.

Posture

Decorticate: Arms flexed on chest, fisted, legs extended — indicates diffuse cortical damage.

Decerebrate: Rigid extension with pronation of the arms can occur with painful stimuli. It indicates midbrain dysfunction; if unilateral and associated with contralateral 2nd nerve palsy, it indicates tentorial herniation.

Meningitis

CLINICAL MANIFESTATIONS

The symptoms depend primarily on the age of the child; the younger the child the less specific the clinical picture. Fever plus altered state of consciousness is the hallmark of CNS infection.

In the newborn and infants the symptoms are frequently non-specific. They include fever, irritability, cyanosis, lethargy, high-pitched cry, poor feeding, usually no stiff neck, and possibly seizures. The infants who are most at risk of neonatal meningitis are premature infants, and those born after a prolonged labour at full term or after prolonged rupture of membranes.

Most neonatal cases of meningitis are caused by *Escherichia coli* and *Streptococcus* group B.[63] The infection may be contracted from the maternal birth canal, other sick infants, nursery personnel or contaminated equipment.[64] During the first 2 weeks after birth, Gram-negative bacteria, *Streptococcus* group B are the most frequent organisms to cause meningitis. By weeks 3 and 4, the most likely organisms are *Streptococcus* and *Pneumococcus*.

Clinical assessment

The peak age for bacterial meningitis is 6 to 12 months of age. Transmission is by direct contact or droplet from the nasopharynx. The clinical signs of meningitis in infants and children are variable and unpredictable. In infants aged 4 months the most common symptoms include fever, tense fontanelle and neck rigidity. By age 1 to 2 years, the symptoms include, stiff neck, headache, and a positive Kernig's sign. In older children, initially headache, vomiting, mental confusion, lethargy, then seizures, decreased level of consciousness and neck rigidity. While the symptoms may develop over a period, others proceed to deep coma and convulsions within hours of onset. These symptoms are frequently associated with brain swelling rather than herniation. The symptoms include hypotension, abnormal pupil reactions and decreased responsiveness. Older children commonly present with headache and vomiting, mental confusion, lethargy and seizures.[65] Later, decreased level of consciousness and neck rigidity is evident. The causative organism may be any bacteria, but most commonly *Haemophilus influenzae* type b, especially

Table 12.3 Differences between CSF in viral and bacterial meningitis

	Bacterial	Viral
Cells/mm	Increased 30 000–50 000); 95% polymorphs	Increased (less than 2000)
Glucose	Greatly decreased (less than 2.5 mmol)	Normal
Protein	Increased	Normal
Lactic acid	more than 2.5 mM	less than 2.0 mM
Peripheral WCC	Increased	Normal
Gram stain	Usually positive	Negative

if the child is under 5 years of age. *Pneumococcus* infection may follow a middle ear infection. *Meningococcus* may present with an acute onset and is associated with a high mortality rate.

Meningitis is almost always accompanied by septicaemia. This may vary from a mild to severely shocked child requiring full resuscitative measures of volume replacement, ventilation and monitoring.[66]

Viral infections may be diagnosed by a mononuclear response in CSF. The symptoms are similar to bacterial meningitis, but usually milder. However, isolation of the virus in CSF is usually difficult. The diagnosis may be made by culturing virus from stool or acute and convalescent sera. Mumps meningitis may give marked pleocytosis with low CSF glucose level.

Other causes of meningitis include fungal infections. They usually occur in immunocompromised hosts (e.g., patients with leukaemia, HIV infection or children receiving immunosuppressive therapy). They may be diagnosed by antigen in CSF and blood.[66]

Recurrent forms of meningitis may be due to skull fractures, especially after head trauma. CSF rhinorrhoea may be apparent and can be ascertained by an increased glucose level in nasal secretions. If caused by a congenital sinus tract, a check of skin over the entire spine for tract, discolouration, abnormal patch of hair should be made. Other causes may include a parameningeal focus such as mastoids, sinuses or epidural infection.

ASSESSMENT AND MANAGEMENT

A lumbar puncture should be performed as soon as the possibility of meningitis is considered, especially in patients with convulsions and fever, unless papilloedema or other signs of raised ICP are present. The assessment of the child should include the state of consciousness, head circumference, fontanelle tension, circulatory state including blood pressure, hydration, focal neurological signs, dextrostix, white cell count and blood culture.

Electrolytes are particularly important. If serum sodium is less than 130 mmol/L, serum and urinary osmolality should be checked for the possibility of inappropriate antidiuretic hormone (ADH) secretion. Culture swabs should be taken from the nasopharynx and any other focus of infection. *Spinal fluid:* cell count and differential; Gram stain; protein and glucose; bacterial cultures. The differences in pathology results between bacterial and viral meningitis are given in **Table 12.3**.

TREATMENT

Speed is important as irreversible shock may develop in minutes. Broad-spectrum intravenous antibiotics (such as penicillin and cefotaxime) are administered initially until sensitivities are confirmed.[67] Other tests such as skull x-rays, EEG, CT scan, subdural taps are performed as indicated by the clinical course.

NEUROLOGICAL COMPLICATIONS

Seizures: Guard against cerebral hypoxia, vomiting and aspiration. Observe the child for respiratory depression. Nurse in a semi-prone position and ensure an adequate airway. Assess the need for assisted ventilation or cooling. Recurrent, prolonged, focal seizures that are difficult to control indicate a poor prognosis.[68]

Other complications include venous thrombosis, subdural effusion, arterial thrombosis, water intoxication, metabolic complication, excessive hydration. Approximately 80% to 90% of children with bacterial meningitis develop inappropriate ADH secretion (SIADH). Therefore, restrict fluid intake to half or two-thirds maintenance after cautious correction of prior losses.

Cerebral oedema and raised ICP are common. These complications should be anticipated if convulsions are repeated or prolonged, if hypoxia or hyperpyrexia are present, and if therapy is delayed more than 24 hours after the onset of meningitis. Uncontrolled ICP due to cerebral oedema with or without hydrocephalus is the commonest cause of death in children with acute bacterial meningitis.[69]

Dangerous ICP levels may be assessed by tense fontanelle, progressive decreased level of consciousness and signs of herniation such as abnormal pupillary reflexes, decorticate/decerebrate posturing, abnormal fluctuations of heart rate, respiratory rate, or blood pressure. Apnoea is an ominous sign.[70]

Lumbar puncture will still confirm diagnosis 24 to 48 hours after antibiotic treatment, when raised ICP is suspected. In this case, a CT scan is indicated. Despite raised ICP, papilloedema is unusual. If focal complications are present, other pathology such as abscess or subdural effusion should be considered. Sixth cranial nerve palsy may be due to raised ICP. This usually occurs early in the course (within 48 hours) of the infection.

Water intoxication may contribute to raised ICP, especially in the first few days. Therefore, careful monitoring of serum sodium and osmolality and judicious fluid administration are warranted. Subdural effusions are common in infants less than 18 months of age. They should be suspected in the presence of persistent lethargy, fever or seizures. Therefore, infants should have serial head circumference measurements.

Focal neurological signs may be due to arteritis. Thrombus and subsequent infarction may be more symptomatic than hemiparesis. Especially significant is venous thrombus, which presents as intractable seizures with focal signs and blood in the CSF. Brain abscess as a complication of meningitis is rare.

Late complications and sequelae include communicating and non-communicating hydrocephalus, which are most common in infants. Therefore, serial head measurements are important. Usually hydrocephalus will develop within 3 months of the infection. Deafness, which is found in 2% to 3% of children after meningitis, may mimic retardation. Behavioural disorders, recurrent seizures and mental retardation are also common. Visual defects may be secondary to optic nerve or cerebral cortical injury.[67]

Aims of management of raised ICP

The goal of intensive care management is to prevent secondary injury to the already damaged brain. The secondary injury is most commonly caused by hypoxia, hypercapnoea, changes in systemic blood pressure or raised ICP. These all are potential causes of local tissue hypoxia or ischaemia. The initial aim of management is to stabilise homeostasis and to control the ICP[71]:

- Intubation, hyperventilation and neuromuscular paralysis.
- Circulation — maintenance of the arterial blood pressure and cerebral perfusion pressure (MAP minus ICP).
- Control of intracranial pressure by $PaCO_2$ at 25 to 30 mmHg, normalising PaO_2, elevating the head by 30°, fluid restriction to maintain serum osmolality between 300 and 320.
- Early detection and removal of intracranial haematomas.

Pathologic changes associated with raised ICP

Transtentorial herniation: Stupor and coma, Cheyne-Stokes breathing, small, reactive pupils with brisk doll's eyes.

Uncal herniation: Compression of the ipsilateral 3rd nerve and posterior cerebral artery. Both block CSF outflow. Ipsilateral hemiparesis, decortication, decerebration, death.

Foramen magnum: Cerebellar tonsils herniate — rapid death.

Eyes: Optic atrophy if longstanding; bilateral scotoma and bitemporal hemianopia from pressure on chiasma; extraocular movement palsies.

Long tract: Transtentorial herniation, stupor and coma; Cheyne-Stokes breathing; small, reactive pupils with brisk doll's eyes; eventual midbrain and brainstem failure; side with facial involvement.

Treatment of sudden rise in ICP[72]

- Nurse with head elevated, midline.
- Intubate and hyperventilate.
- Hyperventilate by hand bagging.
- Mannitol 1 to 2 g/kg intravenously.
- Correct cause.
- Drain CSF if intraventricular catheter *in situ*.
- Decompress mass lesion if present.

Ventilation of children with raised ICP

Secondary injury to the brain following head injury is the physiological response of the brain to trauma. It manifests as cerebral oedema, raised intracranial pressure and reduced cerebral blood flow. In order to maintain effective cerebral perfusion and prevent secondary insults to the brain, the child should be intubated and ventilated to provide mild hypocarbia (25 to 30 mmHg) with PaO_2 maintained at 80 to 100 mmHg.[73]

A positive inspiratory pressure of 25 cmH$_2$O should provide adequate expansion and ventilation of the lungs. The chest movement should be constantly monitored to ensure adequate ventilation, as well as noting colour, perfusion, pulse rate and arterial blood gases. SaO_2 and $PaCO_2$ should be constantly measured by means of pulse oxymetry and end-tidal CO_2 monitoring.

A positive end expiratory pressure of 3 to 5 cmH$_2$O should be adequate to prevent atelectasis and to minimise intrapulmonary shunting. It is recommended that no higher than 8 to 10 cmH$_2$O be used.[22] A higher level of PEEP may increase intrathoracic pressure, reduce cerebral venous return and cause a rise in ICP. A slightly higher respiratory rate than normal should promote a mild hypocarbia, which should cause cerebral vasoconstriction, lower cerebral blood volume and decreased ICP. Frequent monitoring of arterial blood gases is essential as a level of hypocarbia below 22 mmHg is likely to cause severe vasoconstriction, compromise cerebral blood flow so that cerebral perfusion is endangered.[22,74]

Overall, positive pressure ventilation will result in increased PaO$_2$ and increased oxygen saturation; alteration to PaCO$_2$ and acid-base status; decreased oxygen consumption by decreasing the work of breathing. Cardiac output may be compromised, especially if intravascular volume is depleted through the use of osmotic diuretics, thus again adversely affecting cerebral perfusion. An inspiratory time of 1:2 allows for carbon dioxide to be lowered during the longer expiratory time. If the lungs are otherwise undamaged, an FiO$_2$ of 0.25 should be adequate. These problems associated with ventilation may be overcome by the use of intracranial pressure monitoring.[75]

NURSING MANAGEMENT OF ACUTELY RAISED ICP

Nursing diagnosis

Potential for ineffective respiratory function of a child with a severe head injury.

Nursing intervention

Maintain adequate oxygenation by ensuring a patent airway; administer 6 to 8 L oxygen via face mask. Observe respirations closely and continuously for effort, rate and depth. Auscultate lungs for adequacy of air entry. Insert guedel's airway if breathing becomes obstructed. Prepare for intubation.

Rationale: Increased PaCO$_2$ and decreased PaO$_2$ cause cerebral arterial dilatation, which may compromise cerebral blood flow. Although the brain is 2% of bodyweight, it requires 20% of the total oxygen consumption. Hypoxia below 50 mmHg causes cerebral vasodilatation, increased cerebral blood flow and raised ICP.[75]

Hypoventilation causes raised PaCO$_2$ levels which in turn cause cerebral vasodilatation, increased cerebral blood flow and raised ICP. It has been estimated that an increase in PaCO$_2$ from 40 to 80 mmHg doubles cerebral blood flow.[60] Acidosis, even if mild, will cause vasodilatation, increased ICP and decreased cerebral perfusion pressure.

Nursing diagnosis

Potential for ineffective airway clearance due to decreased level of consciousness.

Nursing intervention

Suction airway if blood, mucus or vomitus are present, checking for the presence of gag and cough reflexes.

Rationale: Although coughing may raise venous pressure and thus cerebral pressure, the airway secretions must be removed to facilitate oxygenation.

Position the unconscious child on his side if possible.

Rationale: Correct positioning allows secretions to drain out of the mouth; the jaw should be supported to prevent obstruction by the tongue and to avoid suffocation. If the child's condition does not allow his airway to be protected, intubation is indicated.

Monitor SaO_2 and blood gases.

Rationale: The PaO_2 should be maintained at 100 mmHg and the $PaCO_2$ should be between 35 and 45 mmHg.

Prepare emergency equipment for intubation.

Rationale: If the child has a poor gag or cough reflex or the Glasgow Coma Scale is less than 7, the child is likely to require intubation to maintain airway patency and to facilitate hyperventilation to alleviate ICP.

Nursing diagnosis

Potential for alteration in level of consciousness due to raised ICP.

Nursing intervention

Continuously assess neurological status; assess for changes in status; prevent secondary cerebral insult; maintain cerebral perfusion pressure. Check apex beat for rate, rhythm, attach to an ECG monitor as soon as possible.

Rationale: Dysrhythmias (bradycardia, junctional escape) are common after head injury.

Check blood pressure and peripheral pulses.

Rationale: Decreased cardiac output further compromises cerebral perfusion; inotropic agents may be required if the child is not hypovolaemic. Hypertension is to be avoided in children who have lost their autoregulatory mechanisms as increases in arterial blood pressure cause an increase in ICP.

Check pupillary size and reaction to light.

Rationale: The 3rd cranial nerve may become stretched as ICP rises, initially causing a dilated, non-reactive pupil. If untreated, bilateral fixed pupils will follow as the pressure increases.

Check the child's response to voice and painful stimuli.

Rationale: Assess the child's level of consciousness and functional state of brain as a baseline, and continue to assess the trend.

Evaluate motor response of all limbs.

Rationale: Determine whether the injury is localised or diffuse.

Monitor core temperature.

Rationale: Hyperthermia increases metabolic demands and cerebral blood flow in an already compromised brain. Increasing temperature raises ICP and reduces intracranial compliance.[2]

Support a restless patient and prevent further injury. Try to settle the child with reassurance, soothing voice, touching, and encourage the parents to talk to and touch their child. Avoid the use of restraints. The child may require sedation.

Rationale: The child may hurt himself or may fall. Agitation further increases intracranial pressure. Restraints will not calm the child. Sedation may be withheld initially as the level of consciousness and pupil reactions may be masked by narcotics.

Check acid-base status. Monitor urine output for volume, colour, specific gravity, glucose.

Rationale: Urine output may be decreased due to fluid restriction, SIADH, or pre-renal failure. Note that specific gravity will be affected by osmotic diuretics, contrast used in CT scan. Glucose may be present in the urine due to stress or administration of steroids.

Palpate bladder for distension; the child may require catheterisation.

Rationale: A full bladder may increase restlessness. An indwelling catheter allows for accurate urinary measure, patient comfort and ease of specimen collection.

Check serum electrolytes, osmolality and urinary osmolality.

Rationale: Electrolyte imbalance may occur due to metabolic disturbances such as diabetes insipidis, SIADH, as a result of the head injury.

Monitor urea and creatinine levels if urine volume decreases.

Rationale: Fluids are restricted to two-thirds maintenance levels (or half maintenance if the child is ventilated) to produce haemoconcentration in order that cerebral blood flow be reduced.

Prepare the child for diagnostic procedures. Observe and monitor the child closely at all times. Emergency and monitoring equipment should accompany the child during investigations.

Rationale: The child is likely to require x-rays and CT scan to evaluate the severity of trauma.

Nursing diagnosis

Potential for deterioration of neurological and/or respiratory status due to secondary injury.

Nursing intervention

Continue baseline assessments of respiratory and neurological status.

Rationale: Continually assess the child and his condition closely for deterioration — a change in status may require immediate management.

Nursing diagnosis

Potential for guilt and anxiety of parents and family.

Nursing intervention

Provide psychological support for the family. Provide explanation and give information to parents and family.

Rationale: In providing explanation and information to parents and family, and involving them in the care of their child, guilt and anxiety will be reduced.

Guillain-Barre Syndrome

DEFINITION

Guillain-Barre syndrome (GBS) is an acute polyneuropathy characterised by symmetrical ascending paralysis that may lead to respiratory failure. GBS is also known as infective polyneuritis, polyradiculoneuritis and Landry's ascending paralysis. It affects all ages, all races and both sexes.[76]

CLINICAL PRESENTATION

The primary presenting symptom is symmetrical, distal peripheral muscle weakness. Although leg weakness is pronounced, arm weakness may also be present. Paraesthesia presenting in a glove and stocking distribution may also be present, as may muscle tenderness.

Diagnosis

Diagnosis is made on patient history, clinical symptoms, progression of symptoms and laboratory results. Diagnosis is based on motor weakness of more than one extremity, varying to total paralysis, with or without ataxia. There must also be loss of deep tendon reflexes (areflexia).

Progression of paralysis reaches peak within 3 to 4 weeks, with relative symmetry of weakness/paralysis. This may be accompanied by mild sensory loss involving cranial nerves, primarily the facial nerve, and variable degree of autonomic dysfunction. Sphincter function is usually not affected, and there is elevation of CSF protein without a rise in cell count or in pressure.[77] Recovery occurs within 2 to 4 weeks after progression stops.

Several variants are now generally recognised.

Cases with subacute onset

These account for the majority of cases, presenting with a rapid onset of weakness in the legs and later in the trunk and arms. The weakness may progress over several days, rarely more than 1 month. There is distal paraesthesia in most children, a few will present with a tingling sensation in the fingers and feet. About half of the children will have a form of facial weakness, about 10% affecting external ocular muscles. Other palsies of cranial nerves are uncommon, and rarely are the sphincter muscles affected. Other signs and symptoms include absence of tendon reflexes and tenderness of muscle and nerve trunks.[78]

About half of those with the classical form of Guillain-Barre syndrome present with a history of infective or viral illness such as coryza, sore throat, fever, myalgia, diarrhoea, measles, mumps, influenza A, infectious mononucleosis, infectious hepatitis or cytomegalovirus infection. Those who present after surgery (about 5% to 10% of cases) have a more severe course than do those with idiopathic infection.

Other cases have been reported following immunisation against rabies, an increased incidence in patients with Hodgkin's and other lymphomas, in patients with autoimmune disease such as hypothyroidism and systemic lupus erythematosus. The overall incidence is 1:100 000/year.

In typical cases improvement is rapid, with satisfactory recovery in 85% of patients within 6 months with some residual disability. Recovery is most rapid in those who have a relatively abrupt onset of weakness.

CSF protein is raised after several days and gradually returns to normal during the recovery stage, although in some children the CSF protein is not conspicuously raised.

A good prognosis is indicated in those who have no evidence of denervation during the period of severe weakness, indicating that the axons remain intact. Nerve conduction velocity measurements may be normal or slow distally or proximally.

Relapsing inflammatory polyradiculoneuropathy

About 3% of patients will experience relapse. Most will occur during the first 6 months after the initial onset. There is usually a history of another antecedent illness before the relapse. The recurrent episode may be of varying severity, but recovery will usually be slower. The clinical features are usually similar to a typical subacute syndrome. The CSF protein rises but may not return to normal. Some clinicians have suggested that initial recovery never really occurs, but rather the illness enters a phase of minimal activity which is provoked into an active relapse by an appropriate antigenic stimulus. Sometimes, several relapses occur and may lead to hypertrophic neuropathy.[79]

Chronic inflammatory polyradiculoneuritis

This is a rare variant of Guillain-Barre syndrome. It usually develops after several relapses, but may also begin as a slowly progressive disorder. Recovery from relapse is incomplete with the disease entering chronic, slowly progressive phases with marked proximal and distal weakness, wasting, areflexis and moderate glove and stocking sensory disturbance. Peripheral nerves are usually enlarged and CSF protein is raised. Investigations reveal no systemic abnormalities. Nerve conduction measurements show a slowing of conduction and EMG studies show features of denervation.[79]

GBS with central manifestations

Autonomic neuropathy may occur in severe cases of subacute GBS leading to sphincter paralysis, postural hypotension, tachycardia (about 5% of all cases), impaired sweating and hyponatraemia. These complications may account for sudden death. Pupillary abnormalities are also common. Hypertension may be attributed to supersensitivity of denervated sympathetic receptors to circulating catecholamines. Abnormalities resolve with recovery of the neuropathy.[77]

Miller-Fisher syndrome

This is a rare acute disorder characterised by external opthalmoplegia, ataxia and areflexia. Gradual recovery usually occurs. It is thought to be a variant of GBS.[78]

CLINICAL MANAGEMENT

While there is no specific treatment, therapy is directed to the management of complications. The major risk is that of respiratory failure; dysphagia caused by bulbar and facial weakness; and circulatory collapse associated with tachycardia and autonomic neuropathy. Respiratory reserve must be carefully monitored during the acute illness and assisted ventilation commenced at the first sign of respiratory distress. Where cases are detected early in the course, plasmapharesis will usually be performed. If there is no response after 3 treatments, it is rarely continued.[79]

AETIOLOGY

Idiopathic, may also be considered an immune reaction in which the primary target is the peripheral nervous system. The immune process may be triggered by exposure to an exogenous agent, a recent infection such as varicella, influenza or mononucleosis;

vaccination against rabies, smallpox, typhoid, mumps/rubella or swine influenza. Other precursors are enteric viruses and tetanus antitoxin injection.

An antigen-antibody reaction occurs causing lymphocytes to become sensitised to the peripheral nerve antigen and to attack the myelin of the peripheral nerve tissue.[80]

PATHOPHYSIOLOGY

Primarily one of segmental demyelinisation of the myelin sheath. Degenerative change affects both cranial and spinal nerve roots in ascending order. There is associated inflammation, oedema and compression of nerve roots. Although the myelin sheath is affected, the structure of the axons is usually spared. Degenerative changes result in slowing or total blocking of nerve conduction, causing total or partial ascending paralysis.[78]

Motor neuron: Situated in the anterior spinal roots, the motor neurons are primarily affected, causing disturbances in movement which are more prominent than sensory disturbances.

Sensory neuron: Situated in the posterior spinal roots, the sensory neurons are also affected, causing sensation disturbance.

Autonomic functioning may be disturbed due to damage of the peripheral nerves, which are joined at the anterior and posterior roots, relaying sensory, motor and autonomic impulses. The most distal axons (the legs) are affected first due to disturbance from the nerve cell which is situated outside the spinal cord. Therefore, the first symptom is leg muscle weakness.

NEUROMUSCULAR EXAMINATION

Muscle strength: Test bilateral, proximal and distal muscle strength.

Bilateral sensory functioning of extremities: Test pain; one and two point discrimination; touch; temperature; and position.

Cranial nerve involvement: Cough and gag reflexes; swallow reflex; speech dysfunction; diaphragmatic movement; ability to manage secretions; facial muscle movement; and eyelid and ocular muscle movement.

Bilateral gross motor movement: Flexion and extension of legs; raising of arms and legs; and grip strength.

Autonomic dysfunction: Absence/presence of diaphoresis; flushing/mottling of skin; pupillary size; fluctuating blood pressure; fluctuating heart rate; and sphincter control.

Altered level of consciousness.

MANAGEMENT

Nursing diagnosis

Alteration in respiratory status due to paralysis of respiratory muscles.

The most frequent complication secondary to phrenic nerve and intercostal muscle paralysis is alveolar hypoventilation. Indications for ventilation are the same as for other children in respiratory failure: vital capacity less than 15 mL/kg; PaO_2 less than 50 mmHg; $PaCO_2$ greater than 50 mmHg; clinical signs of respiratory failure such as diminishing rate and depth of respirations; inability to speak or monosyllabic speech; inability to manage secretions; and altered state of consciousness.

Intervention

Endotracheal intubation and ventilation are instigated. A tracheostomy will be performed within 1 to 2 weeks if there are no signs of recovery. An arterial line is inserted for frequent blood gas analysis or oxymeter monitoring for oxygenation. Chest x-rays are performed intermittently to assess level of diaphragm and integrity of pulmonary beds. Regular physiotherapy accompanied by hyperinflation and suctioning is needed. Evaluate tracheal secretions for signs of infection. Perform modified postural drainage, being careful to avoid extreme position changes which can precipitate hypotension and bradycardia.

Nursing diagnosis

Weaning off ventilator.

Nursing intervention

As the child regains strength, the goal is to avoid fatigue. The ventilator rate is decreased for short periods to allow for spontaneous breathing. Periods of CPAP may be instituted for short intervals to test inspiratory force and vital capacity. Monitoring via blood gases, oxymeter and end-tidal CO_2 may be used to assess the weaning process. The intervals of CPAP can be increased and ventilator rate decreased. Weaning from the ventilator may take several forms. Usually, the rate is decreased for a longer time each day, maintaining full ventilation for the remaining period and overnight.

Before extubation or decannulation protective reflexes (cough and gag) must be present to avoid aspiration; diaphragmatic strength and movement must be adequate to prevent hypoxia and hypoventilation; and the child must be able to manage airway secretions.

Nursing diagnosis

Potential for alteration to fluid and electrolyte status.

Nursing intervention

Perform weekly serum calcium tests. Hypercalcaemia may be the result of calcium mobilisation during prolonged immobility. Monitor serum electrolytes weekly.

Bladder functioning is normally unaffected, but urinary retention may develop. Bladder expression or intermittent catheterisation may be required. Input and output should be strictly recorded for fluid balance.

Nursing diagnosis

Potential for alteration to nutritional status due to bulbar palsy and immobility.

Nursing intervention

Give high caloric feeds to prevent muscle mass loss. Care should be taken to prevent aspiration. Gastric acidity may be increased. Assess bowel sounds regularly to detect an ileus, which may cause abdominal distension and poor absorption of feeds. Stool softeners may be required to prevent constipation, or a change of diet may be required if child develops diarrhoea. Weight should be monitored second weekly.

Nursing diagnosis

Potential for autonomic dysfunction.

Nursing intervention

Treatment should be instigated in the presence of decreased cardiac output. Hypotension is treated with fluid administration and bradycardia with atropine. Hypertension is treated with an antihypertensive agent such as clonidine. Autonomic side effects of GBS are usually transient and do not require aggressive therapy.

The child may become poikiothermic because of the loss of the ability to sweat. Persistent fever above 38.5°C should be investigated by blood and urine cultures to exclude sepsis, urinary tract infection, pneumonia or atelectasis.

Nursing diagnosis

Potential for complications related to immobility.

Nursing intervention

Observe for cardiac arrhythmia if the child is hypercalcaemic. Meticulous skin care is required to avoid pressure area and skin breakdown.

Child's position should be changed every 2 hours. Passive range of motion exercises should be instituted early in the course of the illness to prevent contracture of joints. Splints should be fitted to wrists and feet to maintain alignment of joints.

Eye care is essential if the child's ocular muscles are involved. Instillation of artificial tears is required to prevent exposure keratitis.

Nursing diagnosis

Alteration in the ability to communicate due to motor weakness and bulbar palsy.

Nursing intervention

Recognition of the child's fears and feelings is important. The parents also feel helpless and may be fearful. Communication may be possible by eye signals, head nodding and silent speech if the child has facial control. The use of picture boards and language charts may also be helpful. The nurse should always explain procedures, talk about topics from home and encourage the parents to read stories or to record tapes to be played in their absence. The parents can also assist in the child's daily care. Establishing daily routines is helpful and allows the child to gain some control if realistic choices are given when possible.

Near Drowning in Children

There are over 400 reported drownings each year in Australia. Drowning is the second most common cause of accidental death in Australian children, despite intensive lobbying and changes to local government by-laws. Even though there is increased community awareness and local council initiatives, 50% of these potentially preventable accidents occur in private swimming pools.

The term 'near drowning' is used to describe a survival of at least 24 hours after asphyxia due to submersion. The management of these children is complex, in that children with minimal aspiration may have fatal central nervous system damage.

The major factor which has been shown to increase the incidence of accidental submersion in children is the lack of adult supervision of young children and toddlers. This may be due to distraction of the caregiver, inappropriate delegation to a young child, especially in the case of a preschooler being told to watch a baby in the bath; inadequate pool safety barriers that either allow a child to climb over the fence by using a nearby chair, propping open of the gate 'just for a minute'; inadequate adult education in water safety; insufficient public supervised swimming areas; insufficient water safety and swimming programs in schools. Children with epilepsy have a fourfold increased risk of drowning for their age. Parents/caregivers should be reminded that young children drown silently — they do not usually splash or call out.[81]

Children under the age of 4 years represent 20% of all drowning casualties. Toddlers who are left unattended represent 60% of all children who drown, the majority being in backyard swimming pools.

Other causative factors are domestic instability and parties where the adults present consume alcohol, which diminish the usual vigilance of the parents/caregivers.[82]

PHYSIOLOGY OF DROWNING

Infants and young children may be protected from the detrimental effects of submersion by the 'diving seal reflex'. The effects of cold water and fear may stimulate the trigeminal and laryngeal nerves to produce a combination of bradycardia and shunting of blood to the brain and heart muscle while maintaining blood pressure. Therefore, these children often have a much better outcome than would have been expected from the history of the incident.[83]

Once a child is submerged, the accompanying breath holding is frequently followed by laryngospasm of variable duration until the child becomes unconscious. The resulting asphyxia causes the glottis to relax and permits the lungs to fill with water in most, but not all, who drown. About 10% to 20% of drownings will maintain a tight laryngospasm until death and do not aspirate at all. These are often referred to as 'dry drownings'. The exceptions to minimal aspiration are children who have either been held or caught under the water and who have vigorously struggled to escape. These children are likely to have inhaled water during their struggle. These children, especially if submerged in dirty or stagnant water, are likely to have serious pulmonary damage, caused by inhalation of debris as well as water.

The cerebral insult is usually one of hypoxaemia rather than ischaemia. However, as a result of these insults, the brain cells increase glucose uptake, increase glycolysis and therefore increase lactate production.[83]

In ischaemic episodes, the absence of blood flow means that there will be an accumulation of byproducts of cellular metabolism which leads to cerebral oedema. Five minutes of global cerebral ischaemia leads to irreversible brain damage, whereas, a hypoxaemic insult with PaO_2 of more than 30 mmHg, can be tolerated by a healthy brain for a prolonged period of time, provided cerebral perfusion is maintained.

Following an hypoxic insult, however, the ability of the brain to autoregulate its blood flow is lost and cerebral blood flow is entirely dependant on arterial blood pressure. A low blood pressure and poor circulation may lead to a secondary ischaemic insult to an already compromised brain, further increasing the formation of cerebral oedema.

INITIAL ASSESSMENT AND EMERGENCY MANAGEMENT

The presence and adequacy of respiratory effort must be assessed immediately. If the child is conscious, breathing and coughing, it is likely that hypoxic damage is slight and little water has been aspirated. If respiration is absent or inadequate, such as poor respiratory effort or cyanosis, time should not be wasted. The pharynx should be cleared and expired air resuscitation should be commenced. Central pulses should then be checked, and if absent, external cardiac massage should be commenced.[84]

Those children who have required cardiopulmonary resuscitation should have positive pressure ventilation and oxygen substituted for expired air resuscitation as soon as possible. An intravenous catheter should be inserted and a stat dose of bicarbonate 1.2 mmol/kg given, and repeated with further doses in 5 to 10 minutes. If there is no palpable central pulse, adrenalin 0.25 mg/kg should be given intravenously or via the endotracheal tube (ETT) if one is *in situ*.[85]

Metabolic acidosis is usual after submersion due to tissue hypoxia. It should be treated immediately because of its negative inotropic effect on the heart muscle, its effect on pulmonary hypertension and the aggravation of hypoxaemia.

If circulation is impaired or blood pressure is low, the infusion of colloid and/or inotropic drugs may be required to prevent secondary ischaemic damage to the brain.

Emergency management is that for hypoxia and cardiopulmonary arrest. Essentially the management is airway, breathing and circulation. Reflex swallowing of water causes gastric dilatation and may also cause aspiration pneumonitis. The stomach requires venting to prevent aspiration, especially during cardiac massage and intubation. Once intubated, the child should be hyperventilated to reduce intracranial pressure.

The greater the amount of water aspirated, the more profound the injury and the longer it will take to restore parameters to normal levels. Surfactant can be destroyed so that alveoli collapse. This leads to ventilation–perfusion mismatch in the lung, pulmonary oedema, decreased lung compliance, and increased airways resistance. After fresh water aspiration, it is unlikely that any water will be aspirated from the lungs. The hypertonicity of salt water aspiration may draw water into the alveoli and can often be aspirated from the airways. Metabolic and respiratory acidosis usually persists, although the carbon dioxide level usually returns to normal with adequate ventilation.[82]

Electrolyte imbalance is usually transient and does not require specific therapy. Blood volume changes are also usually transient, although colloid may be lost in salt water aspiration. Haemoglobin and haematocrit are also usually unchanged. Coagulopathy can occur from hypoxia. Very cold water submersion (if body temperature falls to less than 28°C) may cause ventricular fibrillation.[86]

Delayed pathophysiological changes

The delayed changes are mainly those of hypoxia. This includes cerebral oedema, pulmonary oedema, multifactorial hypotension, decreased cardiac output, shock lung, infection, pneumothorax and pneumomediastinum. These delayed changes may predispose to the development of ARDS.[87]

After an hypoxic injury such as occurs in near drowning, cerebral perfusion is largely determined by arterial blood pressure. Thus the prevention of raised ICP is imperative. However, once raised ICP has developed as the result of hypoxia, the neurological outcome is unlikely to be improved with treatment of the raised pressure as cerebral damage has already occurred.[82]

Adult respiratory distress syndrome

Adult respiratory distress syndrome (ARDS) is a complex syndrome of diffuse damage to the alveolar-capillary membrane. Also known as non-cardiogenic pulmonary oedema and shock lung, ARDS is characterised by interstitial and alveolar pulmonary oedema. Other pathology includes massive pulmonary shunt, decreased lung compliance and increased alveolar dead space. The syndrome usually develops 2 to 3 days after the incident. The symptoms of dyspnoea, tachypnoea, and widespread changes on both lung fields may be gradual. Arterial blood gases reveal severe hypoxia.[87,88]

Secondary drowning

Often after submersion, the child's condition may deteriorate after an apparently successful rescue. The conscious child may become unconscious, breathing and the heart may stop. Therefore, careful observation is important. Delayed lung complications are common, even in those who have initially appeared well. In those children who have a history of more than 1 minute of submersion or cyanosis or apnoea, an observation period of 24 hours is required. During this admission, the child should have a chest x-ray and arterial blood gases analysed. These children will often require the prompt administration of oxygen by face mask until normal levels of oxygenation are reached, usually at 24 to 48 hours after submersion. They usually do not require more than 40% oxygen.[89]

If the level of consciousness is depressed, if the child is unable to protect the airway or if an increasing oxygen concentration is required to maintain normal PaO_2, the child may require intubation. If breathing is spontaneous, CPAP may be all that is required. A PEEP of 5 to 15 cmH$_2$O will usually be required to decrease the formation of atelectasis. By improving the ventilation:perfusion ratio, intrapulmonary shunting is minimised. A minimum inspired oxygen concentration that maintains an adequate arterial oxygen level will lessen the risk of non-cardiogenic pulmonary oedema.

There has been a dramatic reduction in the neurological deficits in children after near-drowning over the past decade, mainly due to the prevention of secondary insults.[90]

Additional assessment of the child includes: history of incident; estimated time of submersion; temperature and contamination of fluid; need for, duration and quality of CPR; response of the child to these efforts; past history of the child (e.g., asthma); and other physical injuries (e.g., cervical spine injury).

SPECIFIC NURSING RESPONSIBILITIES

Nursing diagnosis

Alteration in oxygenation related to pulmonary shunting and interstitial oedema, and loss of alveolar surfactant.

Nursing intervention

If the child is not ventilated, monitor carefully for increasing tachypnoea, air hunger, restlessness or confusion. If the child presents after a cardiac arrest, maintain cardiac output by assisting with resuscitation.

Administer bicarbonate; inotropes; muscle relaxants; sedation; and fluids as ordered. Record baseline observations: heart rate; blood pressure; temperature; and neurological observations.

Assist with other procedures — intubation, insertion of nasogastric tube, arterial line, CVP monitoring, indwelling catheter as required.

Continue monitoring by serial chest x-rays, arterial blood gases, oxygen saturation, end-tidal CO_2. Monitor for increased unilateral breath sounds, decreased chest expansion, decreased resistance to hand ventilation, desaturation and deterioration. Monitor for signs of respiratory distress such as stridor, tachycardia, retractions, chest retractions, cyanosis, grunting, decreased lung aeration, nasal flaring, and restlessness. Assess breath sounds frequently and auscultate the chest for rhonchi, wheezing, and rales. Monitor peak inspiratory pressure, especially if volume cycle. Monitor ventilator settings as described in nursing management of the ventilated child.

Check chest x-ray for the placement of ETT, nasogastric tube, formation of pulmonary oedema, chemical pneumonitis and the presence of air leaks.

Effect stomach decompression by inserting a nasogastric tube — water swallowed may cause emesis, aspiration. ETT suction as required by assessment.

Nursing diagnosis

Potential for secondary injury as a result of hypoxic injury to other organs.

Nursing intervention

Monitor for changes in blood volume, haemolysis, arrhythmia, poor cardiac output. Monitor colour, CVP, pulses, arterial blood gases. Administer inotropes as ordered. Assess cardiac output by monitoring systemic perfusion, tachycardia, peripheral pulses, extremities, intensity of peripheral pulses, urine output, concentrated urine, capillary filling time, hepatomegaly and periorbital oedema. Monitor continuously for arrhythmia, particularly if electrolyte imbalance is present. Monitor urine output (0.5 to 1 mL/kg/hour is normal) and specific gravity.

Nursing diagnosis

Potential for infection due to monitoring and infusion lines, and ETT.

Nursing intervention

Check all sites and assess for signs of infection. Check colour, odour and thickness of ETT secretions; culture as required. Check for leucocytosis and fever. Obtain urine sample weekly for culture and sensitivity. Ensure aseptic technique for all procedures.

Nursing diagnosis

Alteration in body temperature due to prolonged submersion and loss of cerebral autoregulation.

Nursing intervention

Monitor central temperature. Warm slowly with convection heating — no faster than 1°C per hour.[91]

Nursing diagnosis

Potential for alteration to nutritional status due to prolonged intubation, stress, bedrest, fluid restriction, hypoxia and respiratory distress.

Nursing intervention

Keep the nasogastric tube on free drainage until feeds commence; check its position on chest x-ray. Test gastric aspirate for occult blood and Ph level. Administer sucralfate to prevent gastric ulceration. Auscultate the abdomen for bowel sounds. Commence nasogastric feeds as soon as possible; grade slowly to full caloric and fluid requirement.

Nursing diagnosis

Potential for skin breakdown due to immobility.

Nursing intervention

Keep the skin clean and dry. Use sheepskins and an egg crate foam pillow for occiput. Turn regularly and perform range of movement exercises for limbs when condition stable. Consult a physiotherapist. Monitor colour and appearance of all limbs.

Nursing diagnosis

Potential ineffective coping of parents related to life-threatening event.

Nursing intervention

Assign a primary nurse to provide continuity. Be non-judgmental with family and friends. Allow for expressions of anger, guilt and sorrow. Allow questions and answer honestly. Explain all procedures, and equipment which may be unfamiliar to the family. Explore support system within the family. Refer to social worker, and chaplains if appropriate.

Acute Renal Failure in Childhood

DEFINITION

Acute renal failure describes a sudden loss of kidney function resulting in a build-up of waste products such as urea and creatinine; a loss of regulation of electrolyte and water concentration; acid-base imbalance; decreased urine output and hyperkalaemia. Acute renal failure may occur as a primary renal disease or secondary to other body system disease. The causes are usually referred to as prerenal, renal or postrenal. In essence, the kidneys can no longer maintain fluid and electrolyte balance and cannot filter metabolic waste products. Acute renal failure disrupts all body systems and may cause problems with cardiac, respiratory, gastrointestinal, neurologic, musculoskeletal, integumentary, genitourinary and endocrine–metabolic functions. Mortality may be high.

Neonates develop acute renal failure as the result of hypoxia, shock or sepsis. It may also occur as a result of umbilical artery or vein catheterisation with the subsequent thrombosis of the aorta, renal artery or vein.

Children may develop acute renal failure (ARF) as the result of major surgery, drug toxicity, toxic ingestion and hypovolaemic shock. Children and infants undergoing cardiac surgery may be at risk of developing acute renal failure postoperatively due to a low cardiac output, or prolonged cross-clamping of the aorta.

CLASSIFICATION

Functional

Causes which usually recover are:

- Haemolytic–uraemic syndrome.
- Acute tubular necrosis due to shock/dehydration.
- Interstitial nephritis.
- Occlusion of ureters or urethra.
- Rapidly progressive glomerulonephritis — treated *early.*
- Acute-on-chronic renal failure.

Causes which do not usually recover are:

- Infarcted kidneys.
- Acute tubular necrosis due to failing heart.
- Rapidly progressive glomerulonephritis — treated *too late.*

Traditional

Prerenal

Prerenal are the most common causes of acute renal failure. Prerenal failure occurs following events which reduce renal perfusion. Typical events include shock, low circulating blood volume or poor cardiac output. Any process that causes a reduction in renal blood flow or perfusion will lead to a reduction in the glomerular filtration rate and thus may potentiate acute renal failure. Theoretically, once intravascular volume is restored and the glomerular filtration rate is restored to normal, then renal function should also return to normal. Clinically, however, this is not always the case. Ischaemic damage may already have occurred as the result of decreased blood flow.

Renal

Kidney failure as a consequence of renal parenchymal damage or disease is referred to as renal failure. This may be a consequence of either prerenal or postrenal failure; a disease process such as haemolytic uraemic syndrome, acute glomerulonephritis, or obstructive causes such as blocked arteries, arteritis, thrombus, embolism, blocked veins, renal vein thrombosis, damaged filter, damaged tubules, acute tubular necrosis, interstitial nephritis, toxins and poisons, crystals blocking tubules such as urate in acute lymphoblastic leukaemia induction. The damage caused is usually referred to as acute tubular necrosis.

Postrenal

This is caused by any disorder that obstructs urine flow from both kidneys. This may be due to obstructed ureters, Wilm's tumour or neuroblastoma, fibrosis, obstructed urethra, or posterior insertion of urethral valves.

CLINICAL SIGNS AND SYMPTOMS

Oliguria or anuria

Occasionally children are seen with non-oliguric or polyuric renal failure. Anuria is usually indicative of obstruction to urine flow. Once acute renal failure develops, the ability of the kidney to regulate fluid volume, and glucose, potassium, sodium and calcium concentrations is seriously impaired.

Acid-base disturbance

A metabolic acidosis usually develops due to the kidney's inability to excrete hydrogen.

Fluid overload

This develops because the kidneys are unable to excrete water. However, in some circumstances, such as burns, ascites or sepsis, a low intravascular volume may be due to fluid shifts to the interstitial or 'third' space.

Blood tests

These will show raised urea, creatinine, potassium and phosphate levels, and decreased sodium, calcium and glucose levels. Microscopy of the urine may show casts or renal tubular cells.

INITIAL MANAGEMENT

Early detection of acute renal failure with prompt intervention is essential. Whenever any critically ill child becomes oliguric, acute renal failure should be suspected. A fluid challenge of 10 to 20 mL/kg, together with a diuretic such as mannitol or frusemide, should be administered. A full blood count, urine specific gravity, osmolality and electrolyte levels should be undertaken.

The ECG, CVP, arterial blood pressure, respiratory rate, blood gases, weight, heart rate, peripheral pulses and perfusion should all be monitored.

Treatment is usually conservative, relying on fluid restriction 300 mL/m^2/day + urine output. Diuretics may be administered. A renal dose of Dopamine 2 to 5 μg/kg/min may be commenced to help perfusion of the kidneys. Metabolic abnormalities require treatment. Nutritional support includes both increased calories and protein.

Drug doses should be carefully monitored as excretion of many drugs relies on the kidneys. If conservative treatment does not restore renal function, dialysis (usually peritoneal) may be required.

There are two phases of acute renal failure: the diuretic phase during which management involves the replacement of losses and the monitoring of potassium levels; and the recovery phase with a return to normal fluid requirements for age and weight. Dialysis may be required if the condition of the infant or child continues to deteriorate despite aggressive therapy.

NURSING DIAGNOSIS

Potential for electrolyte imbalance related to decreased electrolyte excretion, excessive intake or metabolic acidosis.

RATIONALE

Prevent complications of electrolyte imbalance. The kidneys' inability to regulate electrolyte excretion and reabsorption may cause high potassium and phosphate levels, low calcium and either high or low magnesium levels. These electrolyte changes may be rapid and result in cardiac conduction complications such as dysrhythmias. Glucose and insulin may transport potassium into cells temporarily, thus lowering the level. Calcium competes with potassium for entry into heart cells, thus decreasing the effects of hyperkalaemia. Cation exchange resins remove potassium by exchanging it with sodium in the bowel. Acute renal failure causes metabolic acidosis, which in turn increases the release of potassium from the cells in exchange for hydrogen ions. The kidneys cannot excrete phosphate released from cellular metabolism. Aluminium hydroxide binds with phosphate in the bowel and prevents absorption into the bloodstream.

NURSING INTERVENTION

Monitor and document potassium, phosphate, calcium and magnesium levels. Continuously monitor ECG. Note and report peaked, high *T* waves, prolonged *PR* interval or widened *QRS*. If hyperkalaemia is present:

- Give IV glucose and insulin solution.
- Give IV calcium chloride or calcium gluconate.
- Give cation-exchange resins, orally or rectally.
- Give IV sodium bicarbonate solution.
- Limit dietary and drug intake of potassium.
- Give aluminium hydroxide antacid with meals.
- Give calcium and vitamin supplements as ordered.

Limit intake of magnesium and give sodium chloride as ordered.

NURSING DIAGNOSIS

Alteration in fluid volume related to sodium and water retention.

RATIONALE

Maintain adequate hydration but prevent fluid overload. Inability to maintain normal fluid homeostasis results in fluid overload during the oliguric stage and potential dehydration during the diuretic stage. Regular assessment detects signs of imbalances. A careful comparison of input and output is required to prevent fluid overload or dehydration. Fluids should be restricted as the kidneys are unable to eliminate excess fluid. Daily weight may help guide fluid replacement. Fluid restriction causes discomfort of a dry mouth, which may be relieved by frequent mouth care. Diuretics may be given initially in prerenal conditions to increase fluid volume through the kidneys in an attempt to prevent ARF. Vasodilators increase renal perfusion.

NURSING INTERVENTION

Assess for signs of fluid overload and document.

Assess vital signs (blood pressure, pulse and respirations), CVP, mean arterial pressure (MAP), adventitious lung sounds (crackles or rhonchi), peripheral oedema. Assess weight daily.

Report high blood pressure, rapid pulse, rapid respirations, high CVP or MAP, crackles or rhonchi, increasing daily weight.

Report signs of low fluid volume — low haemodynamic parameters, rapid pulse, low blood pressure, dry skin and mucous membranes, poor skin turgor or decreased weight.

Measure intake and output frequently. Restrict fluid intake to measured losses plus basal requirement unless fluid or weight losses are excessive. Provide ice chips and mouth care as needed. Administer diuretics as ordered. Document results. Administer low-dose vasodilators (dopamine) as ordered.

PERITONEAL DIALYSIS

Definition

The removal of the end-products of metabolism and excess water across a semi-permeable membrane (the peritoneum) by the processes of diffusion and osmosis. The dialysing solution is introduced through a catheter into the peritoneal cavity as a continuous or intermittent process.[92]

The peritoneal fluid is normally in chemical and osmotic equilibrium with plasma. Water and molecules move freely across the peritoneal membrane, which is less permeable to large molecules and substances bound to plasma proteins. It is freely permeable to sodium, potassium, chloride, calcium, magnesium, sulphate, urea, creatinine and uric acid. The fluid present within the peritoneal space is an ultrafiltrate of plasma. When the osmolality of the peritoneal fluid is increased, water will move freely from the extracellular fluid and, along with electrolytes, toxins and catabolites into the peritoneal cavity. Thus, these products can be removed when the expanded peritoneal fluid is drained.[93]

Goals of dialysis

- Remove waste products from the blood.
- Maintain a safe concentration of electrolytes.
- Correct acidosis by the addition of bicarbonate to dialysis fluid.
- Remove excess fluid by the addition of glucose to dialysis fluid.
- Control infection by the addition of antibiotics.
- Remove drugs in acute poisoning.

Waste product removal

Apart from urea, creatinine, potassium and phosphate, the body produces other toxins which, not being present in the dialysis fluid, diffuse out of the blood into the dialysis fluid.

Urea is the principal waste product of protein metabolism. It readily diffuses across the membrane. The level in the blood varies according to the diet.

Creatinine is a byproduct of muscle metabolism and is produced each day in direct proportion to muscle mass. It is an indicator of normal renal function and the efficiency of dialysis. It diffuses readily across the membrane.[92]

Electrolyte control

Potassium is normally excreted by the kidneys. If the child is hyperkalaemic, no potassium is added to the dialysis fluid. The levels should be monitored every four hours.

Sodium excess is not excreted in renal failure. Hypernatraemia may occur from the use of hyperosmolar solutions or the addition of bicarbonate to control acidosis.

Calcium and phosphate help to control bone composition. In renal failure, calcium is not properly absorbed from the gut. Phosphate is slow to move across the membrane therefore the levels are high. A phosphate binder such as aluminium hydroxide may be required.[93]

Peritoneal dialysis versus haemodialysis

In the care of children, peritoneal dialysis, although less efficient, is considered to have several benefits over haemodialysis. Peritoneal dialysis:

* is simpler to perform;
* can be instituted very quickly;
* the catheter is relatively easy to insert as opposed to vascular access;
* is more efficient in children than in adults because of the relative larger size of the peritoneal surface area.

Indications for peritoneal dialysis

* Acute renal failure.
* Acute exogenous poisoning.
* Salt intoxication.
* Congenital lactic acidosis.
* Inborn errors of metabolism.
* High ammonia levels in Reye's syndrome and other hepatic syndromes.
* Hydrops fetalis.
* Hyperuricaemia, such as in leukaemia or lymphoma, when uric acid levels rise above 20 mg/100 mL.

The dialysis fluid contains dextrose, either as an isotonic solution (0.5% to 1.5%) or if fluid is to be removed, as a hypertonic solution (2.5% to 4.5%). Electrolytes are also contained in the solution at about normal body fluid composition. They include sodium, chloride, calcium, magnesium and lactate. Although dextrose can cross the peritoneum, a hypertonic solution will nevertheless remove excess fluid, as water and the other electrolytes cross the membrane faster than do the larger glucose molecules. Potassium may also be added to the dialysis fluid if the child has either normal or low levels of potassium. Heparin is added to prevent fibrin formation around the catheter tip. Antibiotics may also be added if peritoneal infection is present. All dialysis fluid is sterile and must be delivered at body temperature. Warming the fluid will dilate vessels within the peritoneum and facilitate the exchange.

Phases of dialysis exchange

Inflow phase is the time required to infuse the required volume. Its is determined by catheter placement, the size of tubing, and the volume to be infused (usually 40 mL/kg).

The diffusion time or dwell time usually varies from 10 to 25 minutes. If the dwell time is greater than 25 minutes, glucose will also diffuse across the membrane. However, if antibiotics have been added to treat peritonitis, the dwell time is usually increased to enhance absorption.

Outflow time is the time required to return dialysis fluid plus any other fluid absorbed from the peritoneal space. As children usually need to lose fluid, the outflow volume should be greater than the inflow volume.

Constant observation of the patient is required throughout the procedure. The recording of vital signs is usually done at the end of the cycle, before the next phase begins. Observations include temperature, heart rate, blood pressure, respiratory rate, pain, leakage, outflow liquid.

Complication of the procedure

There is a risk of peritoneal infection. Therefore strict aseptic technique is required throughout the procedure. Cultures of the returned fluid should be taken frequently, or if the fluid is noted to be cloudy.

Catheter insertion may result in perforation of the bowel or the rupture of blood vessels.

Leakage of dialysis fluid around the wound or into the pleural cavity may result in an inaccurate fluid balance and/or infection.

Inadequate outflow of the dialysis fluid may be caused by: the collection bag being higher than the abdomen; kinked or occluded tubing; pooled fluid in the peritoneal space; fibrin plugs around the catheter tip; or omentum being sucked into the catheter tip.

Abdominal pain may be caused by fluid being too hot or too cold, malposition of the catheter or peritonitis.

Hypoproteinaemia may be caused by loss of protein across the peritoneum, resulting in dizziness and low blood pressure.

Hypertension or hypotension may be caused by removal of too little or too much fluid.

Hypokalaemia may result to the loss of too much potassium.

Hyperglycaemia may result to dextrose diffusing across the membrane.

HAEMOFILTRATION

Continuous arteriovenous haemofiltration (CAVH) is used in fluid overload, and in acute renal failure to control or reduce sodium, potassium, urea or creatinine levels. It may also be used to administer total parenteral nutrition in the presence of acute severe fluid overload, to remove toxins in septic shock, to remove excess fluid or water after extracorporeal membrane oxygenation (ECMO) or cardiac bypass. The system receives blood from an arterial catheter and returns blood to the body via a venous catheter.

In continuous venovenous haemofiltration blood is received and returned via venous catheters. This system is the preferred option when the child's haemodynamic state is unstable and CAVH may compromise the status further.

Definition

Continuous filtration is a process whereby water and solutes can be removed from the blood via a semipermeable membrane or filter. It allows continuous removal of fluid in small quantities, thereby avoiding rapid fluid level changes.

Indications

Haemofiltration is used for acute renal failure, fluid overload, particularly where a patient is haemodynamically unstable or has a coagulopathy or where peritoneal dialysis is contraindicated, for example, after abdominal surgery. Plasmapheresis and haemoperfusion are similar processes, which use filters and different-sized membrane pores. Plasmapheresis removes all the plasma and returns the blood cells. It is used in the treatment of conditions such as Guillain Barre, overdoses of drugs which become protein-bound (e.g., theophylline, digoxin), septic shock and acute lymphoblastic leukaemia if there is an excessively high white cell count. Haemoperfusion uses a charcoal filter to remove toxins and drugs which are protein-bound or lipid-soluble. It is sometimes used in hepatic encephalopathy.

Major complications

- Haemorrhage.
- Fluid and electrolyte imbalance.
- Infection.
- Thromboembolism.
- Air emboli to brain.
- Vascular injury.
- Mechanical failure.

Management of the Gastrointestinal Tract in Critically Ill Children

Infants, children and adolescents with disease or disorders of the gastrointestinal tract may require admission to the intensive care unit for actual or potentially life-threatening events, e.g., acutely bleeding oesophageal varices, fulminant hepatic failure, or following major surgery such as liver transplantation.

Many critically ill infants and children are also at risk of developing complications involving the gastrointestinal tract (GIT), which incorporates the liver and pancreas. Appropriate nursing and medical management instituted on admission to intensive care may prevent these potentially life-threatening complications developing, and allow prompt detection and intervention should they occur.

Possibly the most frequent serious GIT complication seen in the critical care setting is stress ulceration of the stomach. Other complications include diarrhoea, liver failure, paralytic ileus, bowel pseudo-obstruction and pancreatitis.[94] Liver failure and GIT haemorrhage are discussed in detail elsewhere.

Stress Ulceration of the Gastric Mucosa

All critically ill patients are at risk of developing stress ulceration of the gastric mucosa. Patients with burns, head injuries, major trauma, hepatic disease, Reyes syndrome, sepsis and renal failure are at particular risk.[94,95]

Hypoxia with and without hypotension and stress tend to result in a decreased blood flow to the gastric mucosa. This leads to a decrease in the production of gastric mucus, which acts as a protective barrier to the mucosal lining. In addition, some drugs act to decrease cellular integrity, such as aspirin and anti-inflammatories.[94] Acid hypersecretion is also thought to be a factor for some patients, such as head-injured patients.[95]

CLINICAL MANIFESTATIONS

Nasogastric aspirate may become blood-stained, malaena or occult blood may be present in stools. Abdominal pain is rare. Some patients may develop massive haematemesis with resultant hypovolaemic shock.

MANAGEMENT

Prophylactic drug therapy is the usual management for all patients in paediatric intensive care, particularly when the infant or child is fasting. Drug therapy is aimed at control of gastric pH, which aims to neutralise gastric acids and thus prevent erosion of the gastric mucosa. However, allowing gastric pH to rise too high (>6–7) may lead to an increase in nosocomially acquired pneumonia.[96] Gastric tubes require aspiration every 4 to 6 hours, and may need to be left on free drainage for children who are not receiving enteral feeds. Aspirate should be tested daily for the presence of blood, or if coffee-ground aspirate is obtained or if blood flecks are apparent.

Pharmacological agents include antacids to increase pH and H_2 antagonists such as cimetidine and ranitidine. Dosage and safety of the H_2 antagonists remain issues in paediatric patients. Sucralfate is thought to be an effective, safe and cheap alternative to both antacids and H_2 antagonists. The mode of action of sucralfate is to protect the gastric mucosa against gastric acid, bind with bile acids, stimulate epidermal growth and secretion of mucus and bicarbonate, and to increase blood flow.[94]

Early institution of enteral feeds has also been shown to reduce the incidence of gastrointestinal bleeding due to stress ulceration. This may also prevent or minimise the malnutrition which can occur in critically ill children.

Acute Gastrointestinal Haemorrhage

DEFINITION

Acute gastrointestinal haemorrhage is a life-threatening event, which may occur as a consequence of stress ulceration of the gastrointestinal mucosa in critically ill infants and children. Bleeding can be from either the upper or lower GIT. Causes are usually age-dependent. Older children are likely to experience upper GIT bleeding as a result of bleeding oesophageal varices and stress ulceration, while lower GIT bleeding is as a consequence of polyps and anal fissures. Infants will experience upper GIT bleeding associated with stress ulcers and gastritis, while lower GIT bleeding is associated with intussusception and anal fissures.[97] Age-related causes are listed in **Box 12.14**. Acute upper GIT haemorrhage is more commonly seen in intensive care patients, and is often the event requiring admission to intensive care. Bleeding from the lower GIT tends to be less dramatic and serious. Management of acute life-threatening upper GIT haemorrhage is presented here.

CLINICAL MANIFESTATIONS

Upper gastrointestinal haemorrhage usually presents as sudden haematemesis — coffee-ground vomitus is usually indicative of slower bleeding. Malaena may be present. Patients may experience tachycardia, nausea, a sensation of abdominal fullness. Although pain is not usually a feature, these children and their families are usually terrified at the sight of such a lot of blood, and fear they may die. Hypovolaemic shock may develop rapidly where blood loss is large, therefore the child must be assessed for signs of shock immediately. Adequacy of peripheral perfusion is assessed by taking peripheral pulse, looking specifically for tachycardia, quality of pulse (whether it is feels strong, faint or thready), temperature of peripheries (does the child feel cool?), and adequacy of urine output. Hypotension is a late sign of shock in children — therefore **do not** assume hypertension or normal blood pressure rules out hypovolaemic shock.

PRIORITIES OF CARE

Acute upper GIT haemorrhage is a medical emergency! Emergency management of an infant or child consists of: 1) fluid resuscitation and stabilisation; 2) determination of specific underlying cause; and 3) specific treatment of the underlying cause.

Assess the degree of blood loss and assess for signs of shock. If the child is shocked, management of hypovolaemic shock must be instituted immediately. (See Management of Hypovolaemic Shock earlier in this chapter).

Cannulation of a large central vein is a priority, so that intravenous fluid therapy may be instituted, CVP monitored and blood can be taken for urgent crossmatch. Consider use of a large-bore dual lumen central venous line (CVL) to allow concurrent rapid infusion of fluid and continuous CVP monitoring.

An intra-arterial line may also be inserted to allow continuous blood pressure monitoring and provide access for frequent blood tests.

Fluid replacement initially will be with plasma expanders such as 5% normal serum albumen (NSA), stable plasma protein solution (SPPS). Fresh frozen plasma (FFP) may be available. Once blood has been crossmatched, this becomes the fluid of choice. The aim of fluid resuscitation is to restore a normal circulating volume, as demonstrated by return to normal heart rate, urine output of at least 1 mL/kg/hour and good peripheral perfusion.

Ninety-five per cent of upper GIT haemorrhages are due to either bleeding oesophageal varices secondary to portal hypertension or gastric mucosal bleeding.[98]

Box 12.14 Causes of GIT bleeding in infants and children.

Upper GIT

Infants   *Children*

Stress ulcers   Oesophageal varices
Gastritis   Ulcers
Vascular malformations   Gastritis
Oesophagitis   Oesophagitis

Lower GIT

Infants   *Children*

Intussusception   Polyps
Anal fissures   Anal fissures
Colitis   Colitis
Meckel's diverticulum   Intussusception
Inflammatory bowel disease   Inflammatory bowel disease
Bowel duplications   Meckel's diverticulum
                                             Haemorrhoids
                                             Vascular malformations

---

Insertion of a wide-bore nasogastric tube for diagnostic purposes and to commence saline lavage should be attended once intravenous access is ensured. Blood in the stomach is diagnostic of an upper GIT bleed, however the absence of blood in the stomach does not exclude this diagnosis.

Should blood be aspirated from the stomach, saline lavage should commence. Room temperature saline is recommended, as it is just as effective as iced saline to stop bleeding and has the advantage of facilitating removal of gastric debris and clots to enhance endoscopy.

A wide-bore tube must be used, as clotted blood and debris from the stomach may occlude a narrow tube, and will require the child to be subjected to re-insertion. In a cooperative older child, it may be possible to attend to both cannulation and insertion of nasogastric tube simultaneously.

For a child with known hepatic disease and/or known portal hypertension with oesophageal varices, a Sengstaken-Blakemore tube should be inserted instead of a nasogastric tube. The Sengstaken-Blakemore tube has 3 channels and a gastric balloon and oesophageal balloon, which may be inflated to apply pressure on bleeding oesophageal or gastric varices, and thus stop or slow bleeding. The 3rd channel allows aspiration and lavage to the stomach.

For uncontrolled bleeding, regardless of cause, intravenous administration of the vasoconstrictor drug vasopressin may be commenced. A continuous infusion is usually maintained until bleeding has been controlled for 12 hours.[99] To counteract the potentially adverse effects of vasopressin, glyceryl trinitrate (GTN) may be added as an infusion, given sublingually or as a skin patch.[99]

Once bleeding has been controlled and the child's condition has been stabilised, endoscopy can be performed to determine the site of bleeding. Sclerotherapy to oesophageal varices may be performed at this time. Sclerotherapy involves injecting a sclerosing agent into or around the varices. Direct cautery to a bleeding ulcer or erosion may be possible, as may the direct application of clotting agents. For uncontrolled bleeding, surgery may be necessary.

ONGOING MANAGEMENT

Monitoring

Haemodynamic status should be continually monitored to evaluate adequacy of fluid resuscitation and signs of re-bleeding. Nasogastric tube should be left on free drainage and aspirated every 4 to 6 hours to monitor for recommencement of bleeding. Urine output must be maintained at > 1 mL/kg/hour. Children may be at risk of developing acute renal failure as a consequence of hypovolaemia.

Monitor for complications such as coagulopathy, shock, hepatic encephalopathy. All stools should be tested for blood.

Anxiety

Both the child and the parents will be extremely scared and anxious during acute GIT bleeding and for some time afterward. If the child's condition and management allows, parents should be encouraged to stay with their child. Significant mortality is associated with upper GIT haemorrhage, particularly if the child is in end-stage hepatic failure.

Nursing care of Sengstaken-Blakemore tube

Insertion of the tube can be traumatic for the child, as it is a wide-bore tube. Explanation, reassurance and having a parent in attendance may help minimise the trauma associated with insertion. Test the 2 balloons and 3 lumens before insertion. The tube should have lubricant applied to ease insertion. Once in place, the gastric balloon should be inflated to hold the tube in position. A chest x-ray should be taken to confirm correct placement of the tube. The oesophageal balloon can now be inflated to a pressure of 20 to 40 mmHg.[95] Occasionally, traction is applied to the tube to apply further pressure to the varices. Ensure that the tube is securely and comfortably taped.

The balloons must be deflated every 6 to 8 hours to prevent pressure necrosis of the oesophagus and stomach. Prior to deflation, aspirate the gastric port to check for bleeding; if bleeding is occurring, the balloon should not be deflated at that time. Inflation pressures of the balloons should be checked regularly.

The gastric port should be aspirated regularly to check for the presence of bleeding. Patency of this lumen should be maintained by frequent saline irrigation.

Acute Hepatic Failure

Hepatic failure may occur as a consequence of almost all forms of liver disease. The liver is a complex, multifunctional organ, which is essential for life. There are varying severities and forms of liver failure. Patients experiencing fulminant hepatic failure and hepatic encephalopathy, regardless of underlying cause, are critically ill, and will require admission to the PICU. Many PICU patients are also at risk of developing some degree of liver dysfunction, therefore liver function of all critically ill patients requires careful monitoring and management.

A brief review of liver functions is necessary to understand the physiological events which transpire in liver dysfunction and liver failure. Hepatic functions can be divided into 3 broad areas: vascular functions, metabolic functions, and excretory functions.

VASCULAR FUNCTIONS

Approximately 29% of resting cardiac output flows through the liver each minute. The greater portion of that blood flow is via the portal vein, with the remainder entering via the hepatic artery.[100] The liver plays an important role in storage and filtration of blood. The liver has the capacity to expand, so that large quantities of blood can be stored when blood volume exceeds needs, and it can supply blood at times when supply is decreased.

The Kupffer cells of the liver are a vital part of the immune system. Much of the blood entering the liver via the portal circulation has gut bacteria present; the Kupffer macrophage cells lining the hepatic sinuses destroy these by phagocytosis.

METABOLIC FUNCTIONS

The liver performs a large number of metabolic functions, including the metabolism, synthesis and storage of many important substances.

Carbohydrate metabolism

The liver stores glycogen, performs gluconeogenesis and converts galactose and fructose to glucose. As a result of these functions, the liver plays a vital role in the maintenance of normal blood glucose level. An excess of glucose is converted to glycogen and stored in the liver ready to be re-converted to glucose in the event of a low blood glucose level.

Fat metabolism

The liver has specific functions in the metabolism of fats. These include:

- conversion of fatty acids to supply energy for other bodily functions;
- conversion of carbohydrates and proteins to fats;
- formation of most lipoproteins; and
- synthesis of large amounts of phospholipids and cholesterol.

Protein metabolism

The body is able to survive without most of the processes for the metabolism of fat and carbohydrate which occur in the liver. However, the protein metabolic processes which the liver performs are vital for survival, and death would occur within days of their cessation.[100] The most important of these processes are:

- formation of plasma proteins;
- deamination of amino acids;
- formation of urea to allow excretion of ammonia; and

- reformation among amino acids and other compounds which are necessary for many metabolic functions.

All of the plasma proteins, except some of the gammaglobulins, are synthesised by the liver. The ability to synthesise certain amino acids and other chemical substances from amino acids is among the most important of all hepatic functions. The function of urea formation is also essential, as without urea the ammonia levels in the plasma would rise rapidly. This in turn leads to hepatic encephalopathy and death.

Other metabolic functions

The liver synthesises several blood coagulation factors. These include: fibrinogen; prothrombin; accelerator globulin; and clotting factors VII, IX, X. Factors VII, IX and X and prothrombin require vitamin K. In the absence of vitamin K these substances cannot be synthesised, so that coagulopathies develop.

The liver also acts as a reservoir for the fat-soluble vitamins and iron. Vitamins A, B12 and D are stored in large quantities. Iron is stored as ferritin.

Excretory functions

Excretory hepatic functions include detoxification of drugs and hormones.

PATHOPHYSIOLOGY

Acute liver failure affects every body system. The major cause of death in children experiencing acute liver failure is cerebral oedema, frequently associated with coning of the brain stem.[101,102] Haemorrhage, usually of the upper GIT, may also be a cause of mortality in these children. Up to 70% of patients in acute liver failure will experience GIT bleeding as a consequence of either portal hypertension with subsequent varices formation, or stress ulceration. Approximately 30% of patients experiencing acute liver failure will die from GIT haemorrhage.[103] Management of acute GIT haemorrhage and management of the child with raised ICP are covered in greater detail earlier in this chapter. Management of the child with acute hepatic failure represents one of the greatest challenges in intensive care.

Children in end-stage liver failure may present acutely with fulminant hepatic failure, or acute bleeding from varices.

FULMINANT HEPATIC FAILURE

Definition

Fulminant hepatic failure refers to liver failure with encephalopathy which occurs within 8 weeks of illness onset.[102] There is massive hepatocyte necrosis which results in acute failure of synthetic, storage and detoxification functions. In other words hepatic failure results in a lack of substances normally made by the liver and a build-up of substances which the liver removes or breaks down.[95] Mortality from fulminant hepatic failure ranges from 60% to 90%.[94]

Causes

Liver failure is seen most commonly in children with chronic liver disorders.[95] Other causes include viral hepatitis as a result of Hepatitis A, Hepatitis B, Hepatitis C, Herpes

---

Box 12.15 Causes of hepatic failure.

Chronic liver disease	Hepatitis B	Paracetamol poisoning
Drug sensitivity/toxicity	Wilson's disease	Iron poisoning
Viral hepatitis	Reye's syndrome	Vitamin A poisoning

---

simplex, cytomegalovirus (CMV) or Epstein Barr virus; drug-induced hepatitis, hepatitis as a consequence of poisoning (paracetamol overdose, poisonous mushrooms, industrial solvents, pesticides), Wilson's disease, and Reye's syndrome.[94,103]

Clinical features

As previously mentioned, all body systems are affected when the liver fails. As a general rule, the more rapidly hepatic failure develops, the more severe the symptoms will be.

CNS symptoms range from a slight alteration in function to coma. The cause of encephalopathy is unknown, but accumulation of substances from the gut are implicated, and appear to have a damaging effect on the blood–brain barrier.[98,99] The most serious complication is cerebral oedema, causing raised ICP, and is associated with a very high mortality rate.[103]

Bleeding and coagulopathies such as disseminated intravascular coagulopathy (DIC) may occur. Production of clotting factors is impaired, so that bleeding can occur suddenly, and is frequently from the GIT, nasopharynx and respiratory tract. Intracerebral bleeding may also occur. Prothrombin time is used as an indicator of recovery.

Respiratory failure may develop as a result of worsening neurological condition. Hypoxia is a frequent event requiring mechanical ventilation.

Renal failure occurs in approximately half of all patients with hepatic encephalopathy, and indicates a poor prognosis.[103] It is associated with acute tubular necrosis and hepatorenal syndrome. Hepatorenal syndrome is largely unexplained and difficult to treat, but improves as liver function is restored.

Metabolic disturbances include respiratory alkalosis, hypoglycaemia, hypothermia (though patients with hepatitis often develop fever). Electrolyte disturbances include hypokalaemia, hyponatraemia, hypomagnesaemia, hyperammonaemia.

Treatment

Treatment of fulminant hepatic failure is largely supportive. Prevention of bleeding and appropriate management of raised ICP are vital, and if these can be prevented or minimised, children will have a much better prognosis.

Care of the Child Undergoing Liver Transplantation

Liver transplantation, once regarded as experimental, is now regarded as a therapeutic treatment for end-stage liver disease, acute fulminant hepatic failure and certain inborn

---

Box 12.16 Paediatric conditions for which liver transplant is performed.

Extrahepatic biliary atresia after failed Kasai

Alpha-1-antitrypsin deficiency

Tyrosinaemia

Wilson's disease

Hepatitis B

Glycogen storage diseases

Familial hypercholesterolaemia

Crigler-Najjar syndrome

Hepatoblastoma

Alagilles syndrome

Familial cholestatic disorders

Budd-Chiari disease

Oxalosis (also receive kidney)

---

errors of metabolism.[104–109] The first human liver transplant was performed in 1963 in the United States by Dr Thomas Starzl, and in 1987 the first long-term survivor received a transplanted liver. This was a 13-month-old boy with hepatoma.[109,110] With the advent of the immunosuppressive drug Cyclosporin A, survival rates increased dramatically, and liver transplant centres were established. The first successful liver transplant performed in Australia was in 1985 in Brisbane. The recipient was a 2-year-old girl with biliary hypoplasia.[103] The first cut-down liver from an adult donor was transplanted in Sydney in 1986 into a 2-year-old girl with biliary atresia.[106]

Two types of transplant can be performed. Orthotopic liver transplant is where the diseased liver is removed and the donor liver is sited in the correct anatomical position. Orthotopic transplant is most common, and almost exclusively used in paediatric transplant due to anatomical size of the recipient. Heterotopic liver transplant is where the diseased liver remains in place, and the donor liver is placed in an ectopic position.[103]

INDICATIONS FOR TRANSPLANTATION

Children with progressive, irreversible hepatic conditions, either as a consequence of a chronic liver condition or acute, life-threatening hepatic failure, which are unresponsive to conventional medical treatment are considered for transplant. Paediatric conditions amenable to liver transplantation are listed in **Box 12.16**.

Biliary atresia is the most common paediatric condition requiring liver transplant. It is usually only performed after failed hepatoportoenterostomy (Kasai procedure). Absolute contraindications include sepsis outside the biliary tract, infection with the human immunodeficiency virus (HIV), malignancy outside the liver and severe cardiopulmonary disease.

Timing of transplantation is aimed to occur before the development of life-threatening complications, such as uncontrolled varicele bleeding, severe coagulopathy and encephalopathy unresponsive to management. The aim is also to have the child in good nutritional status.

THE OPERATION

The 3 phases of the operation are: (i) donor hepatectomy; (ii) recipient hepatectomy the child will be put onto venovenous bypass while anhepatic to improve cardiovascular stability, decrease blood loss and better chance of survival[105]; and (iii) implantation of donor liver (or prepared segment of donor liver if an adult donor used in small child) followed by anastomosis of hepatic vessels and reconstruction of the biliary tract.

POSTOPERATIVE NURSING CARE

All children are nursed in intensive care following liver transplantation.[111] On admission, the child will be intubated, ventilated and muscle relaxed. The management of the child immediately on return requires a team approach as there are many important procedures that are required almost simultaneously. An ECG monitor should be attached immediately.

The child will have been intubated for several hours during the procedure and will require suctioning of the ETT.

The ventilator requires attachment, with assessment of airway and respiratory status. Breathing may be compromised by the large abdominal mass (the new liver which will be oedematous initially) pressing against the diaphragm and lungs.

Assessment of haemodynamic status can be attended to once airway and ventilation are satisfactory. Blood transfusion is frequently in progress, and there are many vascular lines *in situ*. Frequently there are 2 arterial lines, one of which can be removed and the other connected to a transducer to monitor arterial blood pressure. Other catheters such as CVP lines or pulmonary artery catheters should also be connected to transducers to enable readings of central venous pressure and pulmonary artery pressure.

Two to 4 large abdominal drains will be *in situ* to drain fluid from the operative bed. The drains may or may not have irrigation attached. They will require attachment to continuous suction as soon as respiratory and haemodynamic factors are satisfactory.

The child will usually be nursed flat for the first 24 hours without being turned side to side to prevent haemodynamic instability, hypertension, which may compromise vascular grafts, and movement of large drains. For infants and very small children who have received a cut-down adult liver, the abdomen may be left open, and covered with a synthetic skin membrane. The child will return to the operating theatre in 2 to 3 days for closure of the abdomen once swelling and oedema have subsided. Intravenous flucloxicillin may be administered until the abdomen is closed. Very careful pressure care may still be performed. The child should be nursed on sheepskins and a foam mattress.

Monitoring

Continuous ECG, arterial blood pressure, CVP monitoring are standard. Vital signs and urine output are recorded hourly. Temperature is monitored rectally. The child may be cool from the long period in theatres and may require gentle warming with an overhead heater. Accurate fluid balance recording is essential.

Fluid administration

Blood transfusion is required to replace intraoperative losses initially. This can be considerable — many times the child's circulating blood volume. The child will then receive reduced maintenance fluids while ventilated. Electrolytes will be added as required; common additives include potassium chloride, potassium phosphate and magnesium sulphate. Additional dextrose is not usually required unless the patient is an infant. Total parenteral nutrition usually commences 24 to 48 hours postoperatively. If coagulopathy develops, FFP and/or platelets should be considered.

Drug management

Adequate analgesia and sedation is required. Morphine usually commences at 40 µg/kg/h and is adjusted as required to provide adequate pain relief. Midazolam may be considered while the child is muscle relaxed and ventilated.

Antibiotic therapy is often given as prophylaxis for 48 hours. Mycostatin 100 000 U/mL is given orally every 6 hours.

Immunosuppressive therapy consists of methylprednisolone and cyclosporin. Sucralfate should be given every 6 hours while the child is nil by mouth.

Investigations

Blood tests include urea and electrolytes, blood glucose, haemoglobin, haematocrit, bilirubin, liver function tests performed twice daily for the first few days and more frequently if there are derangements. Full blood count, white cell count, cyclosporin levels, magnesium, calcium, protein and amylase levels are monitored daily. Arterial blood gases are taken as required. Blood for bacterial, viral and fungal cultures is taken daily.

Chest x-ray should be attended to as soon as practicable on return from theatre to determine the position of ETT and ventilation. It is not uncommon for these children to develop a right pleural effusion.

Specific liver investigations such as nuclear medicine scans (DISIDA scan) and liver biopsy will be attended to as per transplant protocol.

POTENTIAL PROBLEMS

Serious complications may include sudden intra-abdominal haemorrhage as a consequence of hepatic artery rupture. Sudden hypotension, tachycardia and frank blood draining from abdominal drains may indicate this. Urgent laparotomy is required.

Primary graft non-function rarely occurs and is due to prolonged ischaemia intra-operatively. This is detected by development of coagulopathy, hypoglycaemia, raised serum bilirubin and ammonia in the first 48 hours. Should this occur, immediate retransplantation is indicated.

Postoperative fluid overload may occur followed by fluid shift over the next 24 hours. Therefore, close haemodynamic monitoring is required.

The child is at great risk of developing infections as a consequence of immunosuppression and is thus nursed in protective isolation.[112,113]

Hepatic artery thrombosis is the most serious technical complication and accounts for up to 40% of children requiring retransplantation.

Other complications that may arise include hypertension associated with fluid overload, pain and immunosuppressive therapy. This may require intravenous administration of diuretics and sodium nitroprusside while receiving nil orally, or oral antihypertensives when able to take fluids.

DISCHARGE

The child may be discharged to the general ward as early as 3 days postoperatively. However, some children experience complications which require a longer stay in the intensive care unit.

REFERENCES

1. Blumer JL. The critically ill child and the pediatric intensive care unit. *In:* Blumer JL, ed. *A practical guide to pediatric intensive care.* 3rd ed. St Louis: Mosby, 1990.
2. Hazinski MF. Cardiovascular disorders. *In:* Hazinski MF, ed. *Nursing care of the critically ill child.* 2nd ed. St Louis: Mosby, 1992.
3. McCrory JH, Downs CE. Cardiopulmonary resuscitation in infants and children. *In:* Blumer JL, ed. *A practical guide to pediatric intensive care.* 3rd ed. St Louis: Mosby 1990.
4. Sayer JW, Brzoska MR. Oxygen administration. *In:* Blumer JL, ed. *A practical guide to pediatric intensive care.* 3rd ed. St Louis: Mosby 1990.
5. Perkin RM, Levin DL. Shock in the pediatric patient. Part I. *J Pediatr* 1982; 101: 163–169.
6. Perkin RM, Levin DL. Shock in the pediatric patient. Part II. *J Pediatr* 1982; 101: 319–332.
7. Rice V. Acid-base derangement in the patient with cardiac arrest. *Focus Crit Care* 1987; 14 (6): 53–61.
8. Jeffers LA. The effect of acidosis on cardiovascular function. *J Assoc Nurse Anesthetists* 1986; 54 (2): 148–150.
9. Sanders MB. Venous catheters. *In:* Blumer JL, ed. *A practical guide to pediatric intensive care.* 3rd ed. St Louis: Mosby, 1990.
10. Jordan W. Arterial catheters. *In:* Blumer JL, ed. *A practical guide to pediatric intensive care.* 3rd ed. St Louis: Mosby, 1990.
11. AACN Thunder Project Task Force. Arterial catheter complications and management problems. *Crit Care Nursing Clin North Am* 1993; 5: 557–561.
12. Carroll P. Clinical application of pulse oximetry. *Pediatr Nursing* 1993; 2: 150–151.
13. Sayer JW. Noninvasive blood gas monitoring. *In:* Blumer JL, ed. *A practical guide to pediatric intensive care.* 3rd ed. St Louis: Mosby, 1990.
14. American Edwards Laboratory. Hemodynamic measurements made with swan ganz catheter.
15. Wetzel RC, Tabata BK, Rogers MC. Hemodynamic monitoring considerations in pediatric critical care. *In:* Rogers MC, ed. *Textbook of pediatric intensive care.* 2nd ed. Baltimore: Williams and Wilkins, 1992.
16. Pope J. Pulmonary artery catheters. *In:* Blumer JL, ed. *A practical guide to pediatric intensive care.* 3rd ed. St Louis: Mosby, 1990.
17. American Edwards Laboratory. Procedure for insertion & maintenance of swan ganz catheters.
18. Horner A, Mechsner WK. Bedside insertion of ICP monitoring devices. *Crit Care Nurse* 1985; 5 (4): 21–27.
19. Smith SL. Continuous intracranial pressure monitoring. Implications and applications for critical care. *Crit Care Nurse* 1983; 4: 42–51.
20. Ostrup RC, Luerssen TG, Marshall LF, Zornow MH. Continuous monitoring of intracranial pressure with a miniaturised fiberoptic device. *J Neurosurg* 1987; 67: 206–209.
21. Hazinski MF. Neurologic disorders. *In:* Hazinski MF, ed. *Nursing care of the critically ill child.* 2nd ed. St Louis: Mosby, 1992.
22. Arnold J, Castro C. Endotracheal intubation. *In:* Blumer JL, ed. *A practical guide to pediatric intensive care.* 3rd ed. St Louis: Mosby, 1990.
23. Runton N. Suctioning artificial airways in children: appropriate technique. *Pediatr Nursing* 1992; 18 (2): 115–118.
24. Arnold J. Extubation. *In:* Blumer JL, ed. *A practical guide to pediatric intensive care.* 3rd ed. St Louis: Mosby, 1990.
25. Arnold J. Postintubation syndrome. *In:* Blumer JL, ed. *A practical guide to pediatric intensive care.* 3rd ed. St Louis: Mosby, 1990.
26. Kerr M, Menzel L, Rudy E. Suctioning in the paediatric intensive care unit. *Heart Lung: J Crit Care* 1991; 20(3): 30.
27. Gillis J, Gratten-Smith T, Kilham H. Artificial ventilation in severe pertussis. *Arch Dis Childh* 1988; 63: 364–367.

28. Witte MK. Acute respiratory failure. *In:* Blumer JL, ed. *A practical guide to pediatric intensive care.* 3rd ed. St Louis: Mosby, 1990.

29. Chatburn RL. Assisted ventilation. *In:* Blumer JL, ed. *A practical guide to pediatric intensive care.* 3rd ed. St Louis: Mosby, 1990.

30. Gronert BJ, Brandon BW. Neuromuscular blocking drugs in infants and children. *Pediatr Clin North Am* 1994; 41: 73–89.

31. Benjamin PK, Thompson JE, O'Rourke PP. Complications of mechanical ventilation in a children's hospital multidisciplinary intensive care unit. *Respiratory Care* 1990; 35: 873–878.

32. Arnold J. Airway obstruction. *In:* Blumer JL, ed. *A practical guide to pediatric intensive care.* 3rd ed. St Louis: Mosby, 1990.

33. Mauro RD, Poole SR, Lockhart CH. Differentiation of epiglottitis from laryngotracheitis in the child with stridor. *Am J Dis Childh* 1988; 142: 679–682.

34. Wiatrak BJ, Cotton RT. Diagnosis and treatment of lesions of the upper airway, Part II: the child. *Sem Resp Med* 1990; 11: 235–247.

35. Dawson K, Cooper D, Cooper P, Francis P, Henry R, Isles A, et al. The management of acute laryngotracheobronchitis (croup): a consensus view. *J Paediatr Child Health* 1992; 28: 223–224.

36. Skolnik NS. Treatment of croup. *Am J Dis Childh* 1989; 143: 1045–1049.

37. Eigen H, Westkirchner DF. Laryngotracheitis (croup). *In:* Blumer JL, ed. *A practical guide to pediatric intensive care.* 3rd ed. St Louis: Mosby 1990.

38. Eden AN. Twenty-two years and the same questions about croup treatment. [Letter; comment] *Pediatrics* 1989; 84: 941.

39. McEniery J, Gillis J, Kilham H, Benjamin B. Review of intubation in severe laryngotracheobronchitis. *Pediatrics* 1991; 87: 847–853.

40. Myer CM 3rd, Holmes DK. Management of croup. [Letter; comment] *Am J Dis Childh* 1990; 144: 267.

41. Tibballs J, Shann FA, Landau LI. Placebo-controlled trial of prednisolone in children intubated for croup. *Lancet* 1992; 340: 745–748.

42. Freezer N, Butt W, Phelan P. Steroids in croup: do they increase the incidence of successful extubation? *Anaesthesia Intensive Care* 1990; 18 (2): 24–28.

43. Kairys SW, Olmstead EM, O'Connor GT. Steroid treatment of laryngotracheitis: a meta analysis of the evidence from randomised trials. *Pediatrics* 1989; 83: 683–693.

44. Smith DS. Corticosteroids in croup: a chink in the ivory tower? [Editorial] *J Pediatr* 1989; 115: 256–257.

45. Fanconi S, Burger R, Maurer H, Uehlinger J, Ghelfi D, Muhlemann C. Transcutaneous carbon dioxide pressure for monitoring patients with severe croup. *J Pediatr* 1990; 117: 701–705.

46. Quan L. Diagnosis and treatment of croup. *Am Fam Physician* 1992; 46: 747–755.

47. Harris A, Hendrie D, Bower C, Payne J, de Klerk N, Stanley F. The burden of *Haemophilus influenzae* type b disease in Australia and an economic appraisal of the vaccine. *Med J Aust* 1994; 160: 483–488.

48. Eigen H. Epiglottitis. *In:* Blumer JL, ed. *A practical guide to pediatric intensive care.* 3rd ed. St Louis: Mosby, 1990.

49. Gorelick MH, Baker MD. Epiglottitis in children, 1979 through 1992. Effects of *Haemophilus influenzae* type b immunisation. *Arch Pediatr Adolescent Med* 1994; 148 (1): 47–50.

50. Hill JH. Acute severe asthma. *In:* Blumer JL, ed. *A practical guide to pediatric intensive care.* 3rd ed. St Louis: Mosby, 1990.

51. Knott AM, Long CE, Hall CB. Parainfluenza viral infections in paediatric outpatients: seasonal pattern and clinical characteristics. *Paediatr Infect Dis J* 1994; 13 (4) 269–73.

52. Royall JA. Adult respiratory distress syndrome in children. *Sem Resp Med* 1990; 11: 223–234.

53. Dawson KP. The asthma clinical score and oxygen saturation. *Aust Clin Rev* 1991; 11: 20–21.

54. Levin RH. Advances in pediatric drug therapy of asthma. *Nursing Clin North Am* 1991; 26: 263–271.

55. Uchida DA, Brugman S, Larsen GL. New insights into the mechanisms and treatment of childhood asthma. *Sem Resp Med* 1990; 11: 211–219.

56. Sayer JW, Brzoska MR. Oxygen administration. *In:* Blumer JL, ed. *A practical guide to pediatric intensive care.* 3rd ed. St Louis: Mosby, 1990.

57. Morgan WJ. Viral respiratory infection in infancy: provocation or propagation? *Sem Resp Med* 1990; 11: 306–313.

58. Rashotte J. The seasonal invader. *Can Nurse* 1989; 11: 28–32.

59. Kraus JF, Rock A, Hemyari P. Brain injuries among infants, children, adolescents and young adults. *Am J Dis Childh* 1990; 144: 684–691.

60. Robinet K. Increased intracranial pressure: management with an intraventricular catheter. *J Neurosurg Nursing* 1985; 17: 95–104.

61. Jones CC, Cayward CH. Care of ICP monitoring devices: a nursing responsibility. *J Neurosurg Nursing* 1982; 14: 255–261.

62. Montague D. Intracranial pressure measurements. *In:* Blumer JL, ed. *A practical guide to pediatric intensive care.* 3rd ed. St Louis: Mosby, 1990.

63. Ackerman AD. Meningitis, infectious encephalopathies and other central nervous system infections. *In:* Rogers MC, ed. *Textbook of pediatric intensive care.* 2nd ed. Baltimore: Williams and Wilkins, 1992.

64. Whitley R, Arvin A, Prober C, et al. Predictors of morbidity and mortality in neonates with herpes simplex virus infections. *N Engl J Med* 1991; 324: 450–454.

65. Bonadio WA, Mannenbach M, Krippendorf R. Bacterial meningitis in older children. *Am J Dis Childh* 1990; 144: 463–465.

66. Goldfarb J. Infections of the central nervous system. *In:* Blumer JL, ed. *A practical guide to pediatric intensive care.* 3rd ed. St Louis: Mosby, 1990.

67. Shelton MM, Marks WA. Bacterial meningitis: an update. *Neurol Clin* 1990; 8: 605–617.

68. Tait VF, Dean JM, Hanley DF. Evaluation of the comatose child. *In:* Rogers MC, ed. *Textbook of pediatric intensive care.* 2nd ed. Baltimore: Williams and Wilkins, 1992.

69. Dean JM. Altered states of consciousness. *In:* Blumer JL, ed. *A practical guide to pediatric intensive care.* 3rd ed. St Louis: Mosby, 1990.

70. Rashotte J, Patry L. Acute bacterial meningitis. The pathophysical sequence of events. *Can Crit Care Nursing J* 1990; 5: 6–14.

71. Davis RJ, Dean JM, Goldberg AL, Carson BS, Rosenbaum AE, Rogers MC. Head and spinal cord injury. *In:* Rogers MC, ed. *Textbook of pediatric intensive care.* 2nd ed. Baltimore: Williams and Wilkins, 1992.

72. Walleck C. Intracranial hypertension: interventions and outcomes. *Crit Care Nursing Q* 1987; 10 (1): 45–57.

73. Sherman CB, Dacey RG, Peirson DJ, Winn HR. The use of hyperventilation in head injury. *Respiratory Care* 1986; 3: 1121–1127.

74. Staller AG. Systemic effects of severe head trauma. *Crit Care Nursing Q* 1987; 10 (1): 58–68.

75. Rekate HL. Increased intracranial pressure. *In:* Blumer JL, ed. *A practical guide to pediatric intensive care.* 3rd ed. St Louis: Mosby, 1990.

76. Covert CR, Brodie SB, Zimmerman JE. Weaning failure due to acute neuromuscular disease. *Crit Care Med* 1986; 14: 307–308.

77. Swash M. Clinical aspects of Guillain-Barre syndrome: a review. *J Roy Soc Med* 1979; 72: 670–673.

78. Sumner AJ. The physiological basis for symptoms in Guillain-Barre syndrome. *Ann Neurol* 1980; 9: 28–30.

79. Hughes RAC, Kadubowski M, Hutschmidt A. Treatment of inflammatory polyneuropathy. *Ann Neurol* 1981; 9: 125–133.

80. Tarby T. Guillain-Barre syndrome. *In:* Blumer JL, ed. *A practical guide to pediatric intensive care.* 3rd ed. St Louis: Mosby, 1990.

81. Cass DT, Ross FI, Gratten-Smith T. Child drownings: a changing pattern. *Med J Aust* 1991; 154: 163–165.
82. Christensen DW, Dean JM, Setzer NA. Near drowning. *In:* Rogers MC, ed. *Textbook of pediatric intensive care.* 2nd ed. Baltimore: Williams and Wilkins, 1992.
83. Beyda DH. Pathophysiology of near drowning and treatment of the child with a submersion incident. *Crit Care Nursing Clin North Am* 1991; 3 (2): 273–279.
84. Beyda DH. Prehospital care of the child with a submersion incident. *Crit Care Nursing Clin North Am* 1991 3 (2): 281–285.
85. Biggart MJ, Bohn DJ. Effect of hypothermia and cardiac arrest on outcome of near drowning accidents in children. *J Pediatr* 1990; 117: 179–183.
86. Elixson EM. Hypothermia-cold water drowning. *Crit Care Nursing Clin North Am* 1991; 3: 287–292.
87. Eigen H. Adult respiratory distress syndrome. *In:* Blumer JL, ed. *A practical guide to pediatric intensive care.* 3rd ed. St Louis: Mosby, 1990.
88. Leach SC. Continuing care for the near-drowning child. *Crit Care Nursing Clin North Am* 1991; 3: 307–317.
89. Witte MK. Near-drowning. *In:* Blumer JL, ed. *A practical guide to pediatric intensive care.* 3rd ed. St Louis: Mosby, 1990.
90. Luttrell PP. Care of the pediatric near-drowning victim: a nursing challenge. *Crit Care Nursing Clin North Am* 1991; 3: 293–306.
91. Orlowski JP. Drowning, near drowning and ice-water submersions. *Pediatr Clin North Am* 1987; 34: 75–92.
92. Lowrie L, Stork JE. Peritoneal dialysis. *In:* Blumer JL, ed. *A practical guide to pediatric intensive care.* 3rd ed. St Louis: Mosby, 1990.
93. Stork JE. Acute renal failure. *In:* Blumer JL, ed. *A practical guide to pediatric intensive care.* 3rd ed. St Louis: Mosby, 1990.
94. Rogers EL, Perman JA. Gastrointestinal and hepatic failure in the pediatric intensive care unit. *In:* Rogers MC, ed. *Textbook of pediatric intensive care.* 2nd ed. Baltimore: Williams and Wilkins, 1992.
95. Barnard JA, Hazinski MF. Pediatric gastrointestinal disorders. *In* Hazinski, MF. *Nursing care of the critically ill child.* 2nd ed. Baltimore: Mosby, 1992.
96. Tryba M. Sucralfate vs antacids or H2 antagonists for stress ulcer prophyllaxis: a meta-analysis on efficacy and pneumonia rate. *Crit Care Med* 1991; 19: 942–949.
97. Tuggle DW. Advances in pediatric surgical critical care. *Surg Clin North Am* 1991; 71: 877–886.
98. Laurence BH. Acute gastrointestinal bleeding. *In:* Oh TE, ed. *Intensive care manual.* 3rd ed. Sydney: Butterworths, 1990.
99. Bosch J, Navasa M, Garcia-Pagan JC, DeLacy AM, Rodes J. Portal hypertension. *Med Clin North Am* 1989; 73: 931–953.
100. Guyton AC. *Textbook of medical physiology.* 8th ed. Philadelphia: Saunders, 1991.
101. Katelaris PH, Jones DB. Fulminant hepatic failure. *Med Clin North Am* 1989; 73: 955–970.
102. Rogers EL. Hepatic encephalopathy in the ICU. The 16th Australian and New Zealand Scientific Meeting on Intensive Care, Canberra 1991.
103. Hawker F. Liver transplantation. *In:* Oh TE, ed. *Intensive care manual.* Sydney: Butterworths, 1990.
104. Coleman J, Mendoza MC, Bindon-Perler PA. Liver diseases that lead to transplantation. *Crit Care Nursing Q* 1991; 13 (4): 41–50.
105. Munoz SJ, Friedman LS. Liver transplantation. *Med Clin North Am* 1989; 73: 1011–1039.
106. Kendrick T. A two year review of paediatric liver transplantation. Paper presented to The 14th ANZ Scientific Meeting on Intensive Care, Gold Coast, 1989.
107. Sheets L. Liver transplantation. *Nursing Clin North Am* 1989; 24: 881–889.
108. Treem WR, Etienne NL, Hyams JS. Pediatric liver transplanation: part I. Choosing and caring for the transplant candidate. *Soc Gastroenterol Nurses* 1990; 1: 261–269.

109. Whitington PF. Advances in pediatric liver transplantation. *Advanced Pediatr* 1990; 37: 357–89.

110. Shepherd RW. Liver transplantation in children. *Med J Aust* 1990; 153: 509–510.

111. McHugh MJ. Intensive care aspects of organ transplantation in children. *Pediatr Clin North Am* 1987; 34: 187–199.

112. Shaefer M, Williams L. Nursing implications of immunosuppression in transplantation. *Nursing Clin North Am* 1991; 26: 291–311.

113. Vargo RL, Rudy EB. Infection as a complication of liver transplant. *Crit Care Nurse* 1989; 9 (4): 52–62.

Chapter 13

Care of the Infant, Child and Adolescent with Burns

Lynne Brodie

Burn injuries are a major cause of morbidity in children, not only in Australia but throughout the world. Data collected by the Victorian Injury Surveillance System over a 3-year period from 1989–1991 showed that burns were the 4th highest cause for presentation to hospital in the 0 to 14 age group.[1] Figures provided by the New South Wales Department of Health reveal that in this state alone during 1992 over 800 children required hospital admission for burns.[2] A substantial number of others would have received treatment by a local general practitioner or an outpatient facility.

This chapter aims to discuss a wide range of treatment issues and provide a practical guide for nurses caring for paediatric burn patients, irrespective of where the child is managed. There are many different methods of treating burns. Each burns unit develops specific protocols based on experiences and resources. The approach will therefore focus on common underlying principles rather than specific treatments.

Burns management is very much a team effort and many aspects such as surgery and scar management are discussed only in relevance to the nurse's role. Physiology relating to burn injuries is briefly discussed. There are many excellent texts and papers on the topic. It is hoped that the references will allow the reader to explore areas of specific interest.

Burn Prevention

Although accurate figures are difficult to confirm, estimates suggest that every year thousands of young children are admitted to Australian hospitals with burns. The majority are toddlers scalded from hot liquids, and most sustain their injuries at home.[3] The cost in monetary terms is enormous, but the human cost lies in the pain, treatment and long-term consequences of burns.

According to Achauer,[4] prevention is the most effective and least expensive form of burn treatment. Preventive programs need to target both educational and environmental change. The first involves changing human behaviour and the second usually necessitates legislation and the development of new technology.

Scald caused by a child pulling a jug of boiling water from a bench top.

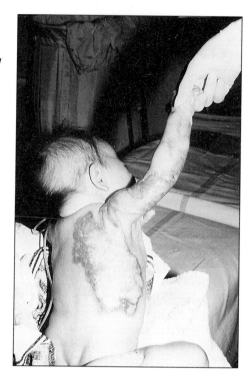

However, it has been noted that passive measures 'that protect the public through product modification, environmental redesign or control, and legislation are generally more effective in preventing injuries than active measures that depend on persistent, long-term behavioural or lifestyle change'.[5]

For over 30 years burn prevention programs have been developed by child safety centres located at the major paediatric hospitals throughout Australia. The Child Accident Prevention Foundation of Australia has been very concerned about the high incidence of burn injuries that occurs in the paediatric population. The Foundation has developed a broad range of educational aids for use in the media, schools, health centres and other relevant places. Other organisations, such as state fire services, the specialist burns units and the Australian and New Zealand Burns Association are committed to prevention. Despite such measures, burn injuries remain one of the most common childhood accidents. Like other childhood accidents such as drownings, the majority could have been prevented with better understanding of the dangers, and attention to simple safety measures.

A prospective study conducted at the Adelaide Children's Hospital in the early 1970s revealed the causative factors involved in burn injuries.[6] More recent research supports these earlier findings.[7,8] Approximately 60% of scald accidents surveyed happened in the kitchen and most involved hot liquids being pulled or tipped from the table or stove, while 20% occurred in the bathroom, where frequently children were unsupervised. Almost 70% of scalds occurred in children aged between 1 and 3 years. The severity of such injuries was highlighted in a recent campaign, 'Hot Water Burns Like Fire', conducted by the NSW Department of Health.[9]

In contrast, the majority of flame burns occur outside and involved older children. Main ignition agents were matches, flammable liquids and domestic heaters or fires. The extent of injury was more severe than for scalds. Ignition of clothing was the main determining factor affecting severity.

Behavioural measures which significantly reduce the risk of burn accidents in the home include simple steps such as turning the handles of pots away from the front of the stove, choosing appliances without dangling cords, not using table cloths that overhang the table when there are young children present, storing chemicals in childproof containers out of reach, keeping matches and lighters out of a child's reach, maintaining and using electrical appliances correctly, and choosing clothing that is flame resistant.[10,11]

As mentioned, most paediatric scald injuries happen through hot liquids being accidentally pulled or splashed onto the child. Precautions such as ensuring children are not in the immediate area when hot liquids are being prepared, taking care when drinking hot tea and coffee, and the use of safety products such as jugs with retractable cords would significantly reduce these accidents. Similarly, supervising young children during bathtime, running the cold water first, and placing appliances such as hair driers and shavers away from the bath or sink are practical measures that will reduce the incidence of bath burns. Improved technology such as safety taps and temperature controls on hot water systems has a significant role to play, as do simple design measures such as positioning taps out of the reach of young children. However, none of these steps can surpass that of continuity of supervision.

It is known that a high proportion of burn injuries occur when an adult is distracted or leaves the child, even for a very short period. In reality there are few parents who can be attentive 100% of the time in their care of children. Burns can and do happen in the most organised of households. It is true, however, that burns tend to happen more in families where, for whatever reason, simple safety measures are ignored.

Prevention of burn injuries therefore remains a challenging one. There is little evidence to show that education alone is effective and it is impossible to legislate for the majority of situations in which children sustain burns, although establishment and enforcement of standards has been shown to be of great benefit in reducing morbidity and mortality associated with burns.[12]

It has been demonstrated that careful and accurate data collection is a vital component in the planning of any prevention campaign.[13] This is one area still poorly coordinated throughout Australia. More thorough research is required into the specific circumstances surrounding burn accidents so that high-risk groups and contributing behaviours can be targeted.

First Aid

An article published in 1979 stated that 'methods of first-aid treatment of burns are varied, imprecise and sometimes harmful'.[14] Despite concerted efforts by many individuals and organisations to clarify and disseminate information on first aid, this statement still applies today. Far too often, members of the burns team see patients presenting for treatment who have received inappropriate first aid measures. In many cases no first aid has been attempted.

GENERAL PRINCIPLES

There are several first aid principles that apply to any burn, irrespective of how the injury occurred. The first is to remove the patient from the source of heat. The second is to prevent ongoing damage by cooling the wound with water. Pegg recommends that, except for minor burns, medical advice should be sought once first aid has been initiated.[15] Home remedies and creams should not be applied as they will hinder accurate assessment of the wound and may cause further damage. The need for resuscitation needs to be assessed. Patients who have sustained electrical burns, smoke inhalation or asphyxia may need immediate resuscitation and the ABC of first aid should be instituted.

SCALDS

The child should be removed from the immediate area and cold water applied for approximately 30 minutes.[16] Any clothing that is retaining heat should be removed. Woollen garments can be deceptive, as they may not appear to be moist. Jewellery should be removed. The burn should then be covered with a clean, dry sheet or dressing and medical attention sought.

It is particularly important *not* to continue cooling to the point where the child becomes cold, as this may cause further problems such as hypothermia. Use of ice is not recommended, as time is often wasted in collecting it and direct application of ice to a burn can cause further tissue damage.

FLAME BURNS

The first principle with flame burns is to prevent the child from running and fanning the flames.[17] The motto: STOP DROP ROLL is widely taught to school children. Flames can be smothered by any means available. Methods include rolling the child on the ground, covering the area with a blanket or other heavy material, or using cold water to extinguish the flames. Again, the area should be cooled for 30 minutes.

Clothing that retains heat should be removed. To avoid burning the face or hair, garments should not be pulled over the head. Any clothing adherent to the wound should be cooled and left intact. Remove any jewellery that may retain heat or cause constriction. Cover the burn with a clean, dry sheet or dressing and seek medical help.

CHEMICAL BURNS

Chemical burns to the skin are uncommon in children.[16]

People administering first aid should first protect themselves by avoiding direct contact with the chemical. A pair of rubber gloves is adequate. The chemical should be diluted by flushing the area with copious amounts of water, and clothing should be removed. If the chemical has splashed into the eyes, hold the lids open and flush the eyes with gently running water. Further medical information can be obtained by phoning the poisons centre attached to major paediatric hospitals. If the child has ingested chemicals, expert advice should be sought.[18]

ELECTRICAL BURNS

The severity of an electrical injury is determined by resistance of the skin and internal body structures, type of current (AC is more dangerous than DC) and the frequency, intensity and duration of the current.[19]

Domestic supply

If the child has been burned by current from domestic power supply (240 V), remove the source of current by either turning the switch off, or disconnecting the plug. The rescuer needs to take care not to become the next victim. If the wires are live, push the child away from the current, using an insulated material such as dry wood or a wad of newspaper. The area should then be cooled with water.

High voltage

No attempt should be made to remove the child from a high voltage source unless one is specifically trained to do so. Await expert help, then resuscitate and cool the area. Electrical burns are often more extensive than they initially appear.[20]

CONTACT BURNS

Contact burns account for a large percentage of minor burns in children and are generally managed on an outpatient basis. However, they often involve priority areas such as the hands and feet and expert medical opinion should be sought. First aid involves application of cold water as for scald injuries.

Referral of Children to Specialised Units

In 1981, a working party was established by the Australian Health Ministers through their Standing Committee, to consider issues relating to super-speciality services, which included the management of burns.[21] Recommendations were made regarding the types of services, transfer of patients, data collection, first aid and burns prevention. Recommendations also included the criteria for admission to burn units, and the coordination of services to improve transport of severely injured patients.

CRITERIA FOR ADMISSION TO A BURNS UNIT

The national guidelines include the following recommendations for referral of patients to specialised burn units:

- Adults with 10% or more of body surface involvement.
- Children with 5% or more of body surface involvement.
- Burns to the hands, feet, perineum and inner joint surfaces.
- Special burns (electrical and chemical) or other selected cases involving loss and/or destruction of skin, requiring the special facilities of a burns unit.

The guidelines stress that consultation should take place on all patients meeting this criteria before a decision is made to transfer. The document also states that, in some cases, patients with smaller burns may require admission because of other factors such as social problems or medical complications.

As a result of the working party's report, each state and territory developed protocols for the transfer and management of burn patients. In New South Wales a circular was published in 1983, and revised in 1988.[22] The document reiterates the importance of consultation and referral and sets out the organisation and clinical protocol for the triage and management of major burns in New South Wales. Recommendations relating specifically to paediatric burn management are detailed below.

IMMEDIATE TREATMENT FOR BURNS — CHILDREN[23]

- Apply cold water packs to relieve pain (*Note*: hypothermia is a potential complication and must be avoided).
- Administer morphine, preferably intravenously. The initial dose is 100 µg/kg and this dose may be repeated after half an hour. Further morphine may be given in a dosage of 50 µg/kg/hour.
- Cover burn area with a clean sheet.
- Secure intravenous access by percutaneous cannulation. If cut-down becomes necessary, it is desirable that it be done through non-burned skin.
- Insert urinary catheter if burn more than 20%.
- Give booster dose of tetanus toxoid.
- Fluid replacement.
    Replacement formula is:
    Weight in kg $\times$ 2 $\times$ % burn = volume in mL in 1st 8 hours given as colloid.
    Time is calculated from the time of burn. Maximum burn figure for calculation = 50%.
    Maintenance:
    One-third of normal daily requirements is given as 3.75% dextrose and 0.225% sodium chloride (N/4) over each 8-hour period.
- Airway management.
    Evidence of hoarseness, mild stridor, restlessness, redness in hypopharynx or respiratory distress should initially be managed with humidified oxygen. For patients burned in an enclosed space or who are unconscious, careful observation is essential. Intubation and controlled ventilation should be instituted if deterioration occurs.

Classification of Burn Injury

MINOR BURNS

A burn can be considered minor in children if:

- the surface area is less than 5%;
- there is no full-thickness skin loss;
- priority areas are not involved (hands, feet, face, perineum inner joint surfaces);

An extensive full thickness flame burn.

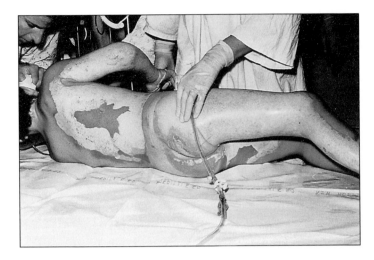

- there is no respiratory involvement;
- the burn is not an electrical or chemical burn;
- there are no complicating factors such as other injuries or pre-existing illness.[24]

MAJOR BURNS

Burn injuries that fall outside the description of a minor burn are classified as major. There is usually no confusion between the 2 when factors such as burn surface area, depth and respiratory involvement are considered. However, some burns are 'borderline' or there are other complicating factors such as exacerbation of pre-existing illness or suspected abuse. It is recommended that the child be admitted if any doubt exists about the suitability for home or outpatient management.[24]

INITIAL ASSESSMENT AT HOSPITAL

Initial assessment should determine the cause of burn, extent of body surface involved and any associated injuries.

Assessment of the burn surface area

This task is routinely performed by the medical officer, but it is important that nurses understand the procedure as situations may arise, particularly in country regions, where a skilled medical assessment may be initially unavailable. The 'rule of nines' commonly used to assess adults is unreliable in children because of the changes that occur in surface area with age. An example of these differences is provided by comparing the surface area of the head of a newborn baby (19%) with that of an adult (10%).[25]

Assessment of body surface area is therefore best determined by use of a chart that accounts for these age-related differences (**Figure 13.1**). If the burn has occurred in patches, assessment of area can be very difficult and it is useful in such cases to try to estimate the number of times the child's palm covers the area. The palm of the hand is approximately 1% of body surface area.[26]

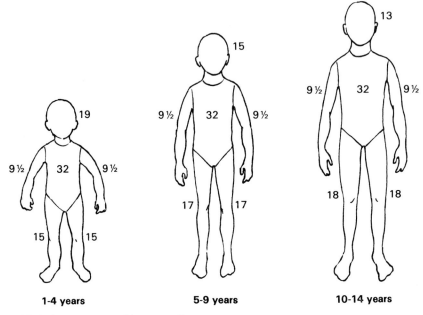

Figure 13.1 Assessment of burn surface area.

Table 13.1 Characteristics of burns of varying depths

	Superficial partial	Deep partial	Full thickness
Appearance	Red, blanches with pressure	Red to mottled pink and white slow to blanch with pressure	Brown, black, white or red, leathery texture
Sensation	Painful to touch temperature change and exposure to air	Increased	Decreased
Blisters	Large, thick walled, increase in size	Easily broken weeping	Thin and do not increase

Adapted from Dyer.[38]

Assessment of depth

This task is often extremely difficult in children, particularly in scald injuries. In Australia the terms 1st, 2nd and 3rd degree are rarely used. It is usual to describe the depth as partial or full thickness. Partial-thickness burns are further divided into superficial or deep.[16] The major characteristics used to assess depth are listed in **Table 13.1**.

Management of minor burns

Any burn, regardless of extent, causes a great deal of distress for both the child and parents. The child is likely to be frightened and in pain, which often makes assessment difficult. A first priority is to provide adequate pain relief. Narcotics are safe and effective when used appropriately. As intravenous access is generally not required for fluid replacement in minor burns, oral or intramuscular pain relief is usually given.[24] Keeping the burn covered with a sterile handtowel or saline pad helps relieve the pain until analgesia takes effect.

A clear history of how the burn occurred is essential. Facts such as whether the accident happened indoors or out, the intensity of heat and presence of smoke may alert the medical officer to possible respiratory involvement or other complications not immediately obvious.[27] First aid measures should be documented and, in cases where inappropriate measures have been taken, it may be necessary to attend to the burn wound as a priority, to remove clothes or heat-retaining jewellery and apply cold water.

Unfortunately, a great many substances are used as first aid measures other than the recommended cold water. These include common remedies such as fat, butter and antiseptic ointments, but may include a wide array of more exotic preparations. In such cases it is advisable to remove the substance by gentle washing so that no further tissue damage occurs.

Management of the burn should be based on the same principles that apply to treatment of any wound.

- Aseptic technique should be used to minimise the risk of contamination.
- Care must be taken to prevent further tissue damage.
- Pain should be minimised.

It is usual practice in burns units to wash the burn using a dilute antibacterial agent. In many outpatient centres other agents, such as saline or soap flakes dissolved in water, are still used and there have been no studies which contradict this practice. The burn surface should be gently washed and any loose skin removed with a sterile cloth. Intact blisters are usually left.[24] The area is then carefully dried.

The choice of dressing is unit specific, but the following are widely used throughout Australian hospitals.

1. A topical antibiotic cream such as Silvazine (Smith and Nephew) is applied to sterile handtowels, gauze or non-adherent dressing, and then covered with a layer of wool roll such as Webril (Kendall) or surgical pad. A crepe bandage or netting secures the dressing. The wound is assessed daily or as stipulated by the doctor until healed.
2. Transparent occlusive dressings such as Opsite (Smith and Nephew) or Tegaderm (3M) are applied to the cleaned wound and allow for easy visualisation of the burn. It is important to leave a wide enough margin around the perimeter of the burn and application of Tinc Benz Co at approximately 5 cm from the wound edge aids adherence of the dressing.[28] The dressing is then left intact until the area heals and is checked at regular intervals. The child can be bathed normally while the dressing is intact. Collection of excessive exudate can be aspirated and the puncture site patched with a smaller occlusive dressing.
3. Omiderm (Dermatech Laboratories) is the dressing of choice for minor partial-thickness burns at Royal Alexandra Hospital for Children. After cleansing, the burn area is moistened with water or saline and the dressing applied. Lyofoam (Seton Healthcare Group) is then placed over the Omiderm to absorb excessive exudate and the area bandaged.[29]
4. Excellent results with dressings such as Fixomull (Beiersdorf) and Duoderm (Convatec) have also been reported.[30,31]

A healing scald injury, managed on an outpatient basis with omiderm.

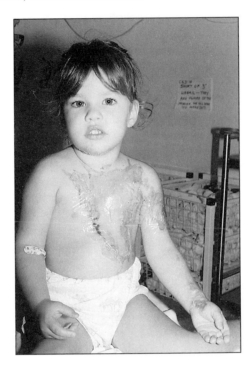

As mentioned, minor burns are generally managed on an outpatient basis or by the local doctor, but require expert assessment both on initial presentation and during the management phase to provide optimal treatment. If distance or family circumstances preclude regular follow-up, it may be necessary to manage the burn on an inpatient basis until the extent of injury is clear. Minor burns generally heal quickly with minimal scarring. Nevertheless, like any wound they can become infected or may be deeper than they initially appeared.

Parents require advice on pain relief and assessment of the progress of the wound. They need to be able to monitor the child's temperature and note any offensive discharge or excessive pain which might indicate infection. Parents should be advised that once the burn heals, the skin is particularly vulnerable to sunburn and use of sunscreens and protective clothing is recommended.

ASSESSMENT AND MANAGEMENT OF MAJOR BURNS IN THE ACUTE PERIOD

The acute period refers to the first 48 to 72 hours after burn injury, when the focus is on treatment of any respiratory problems and prevention of hypovolaemic shock. The priorities in assessment are the same as those for any major trauma. The primary assessment includes airway, breathing and circulation. Secondary assessment involves a head-to-toe examination of the child to detect associated injuries.[32] In specialised units, many aspects of resuscitation occur almost simultaneously with medical officers and nurses working together to initiate well established protocols.

Respiratory burns are associated with increased mortality and extended length of hospitalisation.[33] Situations where the child has been burnt in an enclosed space, such as a house fire or car, pose a high risk of respiratory complications such as carbon monoxide poisoning, and in such circumstances 100% oxygen should be administered immediately.[16]

Priorities of care

Assessment of airway adequacy

History should focus on the circumstances surrounding the burn. Was the child burned in an enclosed space? Were smoke or potentially dangerous chemicals involved? Check for evidence of soot in the nostrils and mouth, singed nasal hairs, stridor, mouth burns, hoarseness, agitation and irritability.

Burns to the face, neck and chest may cause problems due to pressure from oedema and constricting eschar. Note any pre-existing respiratory problems, e.g., asthma, upper respiratory tract infection.

A baseline chest x-ray and blood gases should be obtained. Closely monitor respiratory rate and effort. Airway problems may not be immediately apparent — if present they are likely to worsen.

Maintaining adequate ventilation

Administer humidified oxygen 100% by face mask if ordered. Assist with intubation if necessary. Monitor and record vital signs closely.

Relief of pain and anxiety

Administer analgesia as ordered. A small dose of morphine diluted and given slowly intravenously is recommended. Intramuscular analgesia is poorly absorbed and should not be used in the acute period.[34] Narcotic infusions are often used. Most children are alert enough to be extremely anxious and where possible parents should be encouraged to stay with their child to provide reassurance. Parents will need to have procedures explained and are likely to be very distressed. The presence of the social worker can be very beneficial at this time.

Prevention of hypovolemic shock and electrolyte imbalance

A large-bore intravenous cannula should be inserted as large volumes of fluid need to be given quickly. Most formulae for fluid are based on the child's weight and burn surface area and colloids are often used.[24,35] Monitor input hourly. Blood is taken for baseline electrolyte, urea and creatinine levels.

Monitoring urine output

A urinary catheter is inserted and output recorded hourly. Assess colour, specific gravity and the presence of protein or blood. An adequate output is 0.5 to 2 mL/kg/hour.[35]

Assessment of circulation

Check the child's colour and peripheral circulation. Circumferential burns may cause constriction of blood flow which in turn may lead to ischemia and tissue necrosis if circulation is not restored. Escharotomy may be indicated. The nurse needs to report any symptoms such as decreased peripheral pulses, numbness, pain or colour change.[25]

Decompression of gastrointestinal tract

The smaller stomach capacity of children and delayed emptying may lead to rapid gastric distension and ileus.[36] A nasogastric tube should be inserted for burns greater than 15% and left on free drainage. Check pH and give antacids as ordered. It is policy to delay oral fluids in major burns until resuscitation is well established.

Assessment of eyes

Formation of oedema is rapid following facial burns. The eyes should be examined as soon as possible, before swelling of the lids causes the eyes to close tightly. Debris can be removed by gentle irrigation with saline. Antibiotic ointment may be used prophylactically.

Other

Once the above measures have been taken, other aspects such as checking tetanus immunisation status, bathing and dressing the wound, management of fever and correct positioning can be attended to. Close monitoring of the child's response to fluid resuscitation is vital so that adjustments can be made and complications avoided. These include fluid overload, acute renal failure, electrolyte imbalances, respiratory distress and gastrointestinal problems such as duodenal erosion.[37] Progress is assessed by means of vital signs, general physical appearance and laboratory data.

DRESSING BURN WOUNDS

At the 7th International Congress on Burn Injuries held in Melbourne in 1986, Pinnegar detailed the progress in burn care over the centuries.[39] Since the discovery of fire, a vast number of differing plant, animal, mineral and chemical remedies have been used to treat burns. Tea leaves were popular in ancient Chinese society while the ancient Egyptians used a mixture of goat milk and expressed breast milk. A vast array of poultices made from such ingredients as vinegar, honey, alcohol, egg, scraped potatoes and various oils have been widely used along with ointments of zinc, calomine, carbolic acid, alum and hydrogen peroxide to name a few. It is of interest to note that treatments such as aloe vera and potato skins have received renewed attention in recent years in developing countries.[40] Other remedies have withstood the test of time despite new techniques and technology. The first documented use of nitrate of silver was by Samuel Cooper in 1821 and silver nitrate dressings are still used in some centres, although less frequently than Silvazine (Smith and Nephew) which was introduced in the late 1960s. The other widely used topical antibacterial cream developed in the 1960s, mafenide acetate (Sulfamylon, Winthrop Laboratories) is rarely used in paediatrics because of the pain caused on application, and is no longer available in Australia.

Over the past 10 years, a wide range of synthetic and biological dressings have been developed. An overview of current burn wound dressings is provided by Queen et al.[40]

Management of the Burn Wound

There are 2 main ways in which burns are managed. These are commonly referred to as the open (exposed) and closed methods. The advantages and disadvantages of each are outlined below.[41,42]

OPEN METHOD

This method is suitable for burns that are not full thickness. The child is nursed on clean sheets and the burn is left open to the air to dry. An overhead heat lamp may be used to facilitate this process. An eschar forms in approximately 48 hours. The child is usually bathed several times per day. The eschar will eventually separate to reveal either a healed area or a surface that requires some grafting. The advantages are that the burn surface is easily visible and the time involved in caring for the burn is minimised. The cost of dressings is avoided.

The disadvantages are that movement is restricted and restraint may be necessary until the eschar forms. The child can then move around the unit, but cannot play outside and direct contact with parents and staff is minimised. A warm environment is necessary, which may make working conditions unpleasant for nursing staff.

CLOSED METHOD

Although the actual techniques used vary from unit to unit, the principle is that the child is bathed at least daily and dressings applied to the burn surface. This method is the one of choice in most Australian paediatric units. It is generally felt that this method provides for optimal care of the child's physical and emotional needs. The healing process can still be monitored during bathing. Between dressing changes the child can play more freely and when appropriate, enjoy walks outside the unit. Parents and staff can hold and comfort the child. Risk of injury to the healing surface is reduced.

Disadvantages are that dressings are expensive both in time and cost and are often distressing for all involved. The healing wound may easily be damaged during dressing changes.

Another form of closed dressing involves use of occlusive dressings which remain intact for varying periods following application. Until recently this type of management has been mainly restricted to treatment of outpatient burns, but with the availability of new and improved dressings the technique may play a major role in future burns care.[43,44]

Principles of Bathing and Dressing Burns

AIM

The aim is to remove soiled burn dressings and replace them with clean dressings, using a technique that does not damage the healing burn wound and is as least traumatic as possible to all concerned. This is best achieved in a unit specifically designed for burns management, staffed by skilled, experienced nurses. The following overview is based on the procedures used at the Royal Alexandra Hospital for Children (RAHC), Sydney.[45]

PREPARATION FOR BATHING/SPONGING

Provision of adequate analgesia

Analgesia is given prior to the bath, allowing sufficient time for it to work. Oral morphine, codeine, vallergan and midazolam are often used at RAHC. A combination of these drugs is individually prescribed for each child. If a narcotic infusion is in progress, the rate is increased before starting the procedure. Nitrous oxide may be used, following strict protocols for administration.

Explanation for child and parents

Most children are extremely anxious and fearful of the bath and these feelings often intensify throughout their hospitalisation. Adequate explanation will be necessary both for the child and parents, and factors such as the age of the child, degree of injury and stage of treatment need to be considered.

Environmental considerations

Ideally, the bathroom and dressing area should be adjacent but separate for infection control purposes. A special stainless steel burns bath that can be height adjusted is desirable. Free-standing dressing tables facilitate the dressing procedure and overhead heating helps reduce heat loss. Easy access to sterile stock and facilities for disposal of soiled dressings are required. Use of distraction techniques such as music and overhead murals are becoming more common in paediatric burns units.

Removal and discarding of soiled dressings

This procedure can be performed wherever practical. The nurse and parents wash their hands. Minimum requirements for all involved are sterile gloves and a clean gown. Outer bandages may be removed prior to the bath. Adherent dressings should be soaked off in the bath or sponged off beforehand. Soiled dressings are discarded into a pedal bin in a manner that does not contaminate surrounding areas.

BATHING PROCEDURE

The child is placed into a warm bath to which a dilute solution of hibitane gluconate 20% has been added. If inhaled nitrous oxide is being used, time is allowed for it to take effect. Adherent dressings are soaked off and the wound gently washed with a sterile handtowel to remove cream and slough. Scissors and forceps may be used to trim loose tissue but extensive debridement of eschar is only performed in the operating theatre. The therapist may be present to perform passive exercises and encourage active movement. The surgeon may also wish to review the child. Parents and children often ask questions about the appearance of the burn and the opportunity should be taken for education about the healing process.

Table 13.2 The bathing procedure

Principles and rationale	Points of emphasis
The procedure should be done as quickly and efficiently as possible to decrease pain, anxiety and complications such as heat loss.	Experienced staff should attend to the bath whenever possible. Heat lamps are used when applicable.
Adequate analgesia is essential.	Nitrous oxide is being increasingly used along with other analgesics.
Bathing aims to decrease the number of contaminating organisms	The bath is filled to a suitable depth to immerse the wound. A solution such as Hibitane 1:2000 is added to the bath.
Soaking adherent dressings reduces risk of trauma to the healing wound.	Once dressings have soaked off, the burnt areas are washed with a sterile handtowel, using enough pressure to remove all old cream, slough and loose skin. Scissors and forceps are not routinely used except for minor trimming. Debriding is performed in the operating theatre.
Provision of diversional therapy helps decrease pain and anxiety.	Tapes, music, overhead pictures and presence of parents and/or therapist are useful diversional techniques.
Bathtime provides an opportunity for active and passive exercises as the warm water helps relax the child.	The physiotherapist is often present to perform passive exercises and promote movement of stiff joints.
Bathtime provides an opportunity to monitor wound healing and educate the parents and child.	The surgeon may wish to be present to review the burn and the parents and child should be given explanations about the appearance of the burn and evidence of healing.

CLEANING PROCEDURE FOR BATH

At the completion of each bath the bath and surrounding areas are cleaned thoroughly using hypochlorite solution to prevent cross-contamination. It is important that staff wear protective gloves to avoid the irritant effects of the cleaning agents. As a safety measure, all cleaning solutions should be kept in an area inaccessible to children.

BURNS DRESSING PROCEDURE

Minimum requirements for routine dressing are as follows:

- Clean gown.
- Drawsheet for dressing table.
- Sterile dressing sheet.
- Sterile dressing.
- Sterile gloves.
- Topical antibacterial cream.
- Sterile scissors and spatula.
- Bandages and tape.

Ideally, the dressing should be prepared before bathing to minimise the time the child spends with the burnt area exposed. This helps to decrease anxiety and pain. The dressings are prepared using an aseptic technique.

Following the bath the child is weighed, then placed on the dressing table and covered with clean towels. Overhead heaters are turned on if needed. The nurse and parents discard their dirty gowns and gloves and the nurse dons a clean gown and sterile gloves. Swabs are taken routinely on admission and thereafter weekly, following grafting or more frequently if the burn appears infected.

It is difficult to outline the steps involved in performing a complex procedure such as a burns dressing. Ultimately each unit develops its own protocols and there is a multitude of techniques, dressings and creams that are effective. Children with extensive burns may not be able to be bathed in the acute phase as they may be intubated and physiologically unstable. Commercially made dressings such as Exu-Dry (Frastec) have been useful in decreasing the time taken to perform large dressings in these very sick children. The following section provides a guideline for dressing specialised areas.[45]

DRESSING SPECIFIC BODY AREAS

Arms

Omiderm may be used for small, partial-thickness burns.

Antibacterial cream applied to sterile handtowels such as Daylees is a useful dressing for large areas. Elevating the arm and bandaging from the fingers upwards will help reduce oedema. If the axilla is burnt it will be necessary to incorporate the trunk. The correct bandaging technique is to bandage from the inner surface of the upper arm to the outer over the shoulder, to help maintain correct posture. Bandages are secured with tape as clips are easily removed and may be dangerous to young children.

Hands and fingers

In the acute period, the hands and fingers may be very swollen and preservation of circulation is the priority. Elevation of the limb will help decrease oedema and escharotomies may be needed. It is important to separate the web spaces between the fingers and this can be easily achieved by applying Bactigras between and around each finger. The hand is then bandaged using Webril and a crepe bandage. The tips of the fingers should be left unbandaged to facilitate circulation checks and can be covered with Bactigras. Splints are often used by therapists to maintain burnt hands in a functional position. Individual finger bandages can be used once oedema has decreased, to allow for increased movement.

Trunk

Omiderm covered by Lyofoam to absorb exudate is a useful dressing when the burn involves only a small area and is not full thickness. A crepe bandage secures the dressing. For larger or deeper areas, antibacterial cream applied to a sterile Daylee towel is preferred.

Legs and feet

It is important to maintain the legs in a functional position and bulky dressings behind the knee should be avoided. Splints may be necessary to keep the legs straight. Again the

Daylee dressing is effective. The legs are bandaged from the feet up (distal to proximal) to help decrease oedema. The trunk is incorporated when the burn involves the upper thigh, to help keep the dressing from slipping. If the feet are burnt, web spaces should be separated and a dressing applied to provide protection during mobilisation.

Head and face

Applying dressings to these areas can be difficult and takes practice and patience. To secure the dressing, it is often necessary to apply a somewhat larger dressing than the area of burn would indicate, which may give the appearance of a much more extensive injury. Fortunately, most children are unconcerned about such detail.

Antibacterial creams such as Sivazine, Neosporin or Bactroban can be used on the face by applying a small amount to a tulle dressing which conforms to the contours of the face. Strips of Webril can then be applied over the top and the area bandaged. This type of dressing is often the one of choice for partial-thickness burns of the face as the open method of management involves frequent cleaning and is likely to be painful on these types of burns. A closed dressing also helps prevent children from scratching and damaging the healing wound.

Bactigras alone is often used and at least 2 layers should be applied to avoid crusting. Bactigras may be used in conjunction with antibacterial creams. Eye, nose and mouth care are attended to at the time of the dressing. Burns involving the scalp require the hair to be trimmed or shaved for accurate assessment before dressing.

Ears

Tullegras can be folded to make an ear plug in the external meatus to avoid accumulation of cream in the ear canal. The rest of the ear can be dressed with Silvazine cream applied to gauze or Bactigras, taking care to separate burnt surfaces such as the head and back of the ear. The cartilage of the ear has a poor blood supply and is easily damaged. Donut sponges can be used to avoid pressure on the ear while the child is in bed.

Neck

A collar can be made using antibacterial cream applied to a sterile Daylee covered by Webril. Once oedema has subsided, Jobst or soft foam collars will help keep the dressing in place.

Perineum

A catheter is indicated for most perineal burns and meticulous catheter care is necessary. Bactigras covered with Silvazine can be wrapped around the penis and scrotum and secured with strips of Webril. The same dressing applies for females. Silvazine applied to a Daylee or non-stick dressing can be used to line nappies.

Nursing Management of the Child Who Requires Grafting

The need for grafting is determined by the surgeon. The timing of the grafting procedure varies from unit to unit. In units where early grafting is the policy, the child is usually

Split skin grafting to a full thickness flame burn.

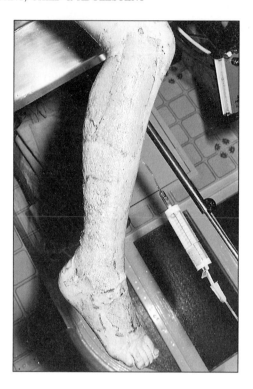

taken to the operating theatre very soon after admission. The burn is assessed under a general anaesthesia and a decision is made about grafting.[46,47] Areas of full-thickness greater than approximately a 20 cent coin do not generally heal without significant scarring. Depth of burn is therefore the primary determinant for grafting. The amount that can be grafted at any one session is dependent on the child's condition and the surgeon's policy. Deep, partial-thickness burns are usually grafted to achieve a better cosmetic and functional result.[25] Some surgeons prefer to wait for a period of approximately 10 to 14 days until the areas that will require grafting are obvious before proceeding with surgery.

Split skin autographs are the most common type of grafts used. Very deep burns may require use of more complex procedures such as flaps.[4,27] In adult units, the graft may be left open, but the closed method of management is usual for children because of difficulties they have in complying with restricted movement in the early postoperative period. Grafts are easily damaged and young children are not noted for their ability to keep still. Split skin grafts are usually sutured or stapled into position and then covered with layers of protective dressing. Splints are often used to further protect the new grafts. More recently, other dressings such as backed gauze (Hypafix) have been used to secure grafts.

Various techniques are used to dress the donor site. One method involves application of an antibacterial cream and a protective dressing. Alternatively, if there is a large enough area around the donor site to allow for correct application, a transparent occlusive dressing may be used.

Dressings are usually left intact for 5 days. Regular pain relief is provided and a morphine infusion may be necessary for the first few days. The child is generally restricted to bed rest for the first 48 hours after surgery and then, depending on the site that has

Table 13.3 Management of paediatric skin grafts

Principles of graft care	Nursing intervention
1. To minimise risk of damage to newly grafted areas.	Movement is minimised through restricting the child's activity, use of splints, adequate pain relief and sedation as needed. The postoperative dressing changes are performed by experienced nurses.
2. To detect and report signs of infection or bleeding that may compromise graft take.	Dressings are checked regularly and excessive exudate is reported. The area is outlined using a felt pen. It may be necessary to reinforce the dressing or the surgeon may order the blood to be aspirated from under the graft. Monitor temperature.
3. To promote healing by providing optimal nutrition.	High protein, high caloric foods are encouraged. Nasogastric feeds may be necessary and in severe burns, TPN is often needed.

been grafted, gentle ambulation such as sitting out of bed or short walks in a stroller may be allowed, at the surgeon's discretion.

POSTOPERATIVE BATH AND DRESSING

Every unit has a protocol for graft care and postoperative dressings. The following protocol is that currently used at the RAHC.[29]

Most postoperative dressings are removed in the unit. In some cases, where further grafting is necessary or the child is particularly fearful and unable to cooperate, the dressings are changed under general anaesthesia.

On the 5th postoperative day, the child is given a premedication. Nitrous oxide is commonly used during the procedure to provide further sedation and pain relief. Outer dressings are removed before bathing. The child is then placed into a bath to which hibitane gluconate 20% has been added. Any staples are removed. The grafts are gently washed and any overlapping areas are trimmed, using sterile scissors. As much of the donor site dressing as possible is removed without causing damage to the healing process. Omiderm used over donor sites is easily removed by soaking.

If Hypafix has been used to secure the grafts, preparation is necessary approximately 4 hours before the dressing change. Liberal amounts of vitamin A cream are applied to the dressing which is then covered with plastic film and bandaged so that the cream soaks into the dressing. The dressing is then easily removed during the bath.

The dressing procedure follows that for a routine burns dressing except that Bactrigras or Hypafix are the dressings of choice.

GRAFT FAILURE

Technical errors during the grafting procedure may result in graft failure.[48] On rare occasions, grafts may mistakenly be applied upside down. Grafts that are too thin may

Table 13.4 Causes of graft failure

Cause	Nursing intervention
1. Inadequate graft bed due to compromised blood supply, movement of graft, systemic disease or infection.	Note the appearance of the graft. Pallor or blackness may indicate graft failure. Report any concerns. Administer antibiotics if ordered. Use aseptic technique.
2. Haematoma	Aspirate, deroof or roll blood under graft to the edges as ordered.
3. Movement	Restrict activities as indicated by position of graft. Immobilise the area, using splints.

fail to take. Grafts must be firmly secured using sutures or staples, to prevent the grafts slipping or rolling.

In order to try and prevent unrealistic expectations, it is important that the parents and child understand what the new grafts will look like. A graft that has taken well is an occasion for celebration by the professionals involved. However, to the parents and child, the graft may appear ugly, disfiguring and frightening. Their idea of plastic surgery is likely to be far removed from that of the medical and nursing team and, despite seemingly adequate explanation, it is not unusual for the response to be one of shock and disappointment. Educational material such as photos of grafts may be useful preparation. Observation of other children in the unit who have had grafting performed and discussion with other parents may also be useful.

Scar Management

The burn that occurs in seconds may cause lifelong disfigurement and disability which affect the child both physically and emotionally. In Australian burns units, scar management is largely the domain of physiotherapists and occupational therapists, but the nurse as 24-hour caregiver plays a central role in ensuring that the programs and strategies developed by the therapists are carried out. A detailed discussion of scar formation and management is beyond the scope of this section and references are therefore provided for the interested reader.

THE HEALING PROCESS

Because of the complexity of wound healing and the insidious nature of burn scar formation, it is extremely difficult to predict what the burn will look like once the healing process is complete.[49,50] It is known that the deeper the burn the more intense will be the scarring. The length of time the burn takes to heal and the presence of infection are other important factors. Children are reported to form hypertrophic scars more than adults.[51,52] Some individuals are prone to a type of scar formation known as keloid. Keloid scars are often confused with hypertrophic scars and the differences are listed in **Table 13.5.**

Table 13.5 Differences between keloid and hypertrophic scars

Keloid scars	Hypertrophic scars
Tumour-like appearance which invades surrounding normal skin.	Scar stays within the boundaries of the wound and often forms at the junction of unburned skin and grafts.
Increased warmth, tenderness and itchiness usually present.	Usually only itchiness is a feature.
Remain florid, raised and do not improve over time.	Initial hard, red, whorl like appearance; gradually flattens and becomes pale and softer.

Adapted from Linares.[53]

Contracture formation is a problem that can cause severe disability if untreated. All scars and free grafts tend to shrink. This process is associated with scar maturation and is often not evident at the time of discharge.[54]

STRATEGIES FOR SCAR MANAGEMENT

It is essential that a program aimed at preventing and minimising contracture and scar formation be initiated within the first few days following a major burn injury. Prophylactic measures include correct positioning, early splinting and exercise programs which aim to maximise function and counteract the effects of immobility and the tension applied to joints and muscles by the healing tissue. During the first week or so, oedema formation and resuscitation priorities may restrict exercises and correct positioning, but if the child is allowed to remain immobile and assume the position which he finds most comfortable, the task of initiating prophylactic measures becomes very difficult. Young children usually cannot understand the rationales behind these measures and it is also sometimes difficult for parents to accept their necessity. By providing education and encouraging parents to become involved in their child's care, the support so necessary for compliance with treatment is usually forthcoming.[55]

Passive and active exercises are best performed during and following the bath. As the child's condition improves, normal activities can be resumed. Early mobilisation is encouraged in most units and the provision of both structured and unstructured play is an excellent way of ensuring that the child maintains as much function as possible. Medical play is increasingly being used by specially trained therapists to help children cope with frightening and unpleasant experiences.[56]

The importance of discharge programs and follow-up care is well accepted by all involved in burn management and some units have nurses who work in a liaison role between the hospital and community. Regular assessment by the surgeon, nurse and therapist may be necessary for several years following major burn injury.[57]

Adjuncts to scar management

There is a wide range of products that are used throughout Australia to help prevent and to treat scar formation.[58,59] The most commonly used are pressure garments which are individually tailored to the child's needs. These garments are worn continually for as long as necessary, which may be several years in some cases. They are removed daily for bathing and skin care. The aim of the garment is to provide pressure over the maturing scar to help prevent hypertrophic scarring. Water-based emollient creams are applied to the skin under the garments. Oil-based creams damage the fibres of the commercially made garments. Some units make their own elasticised garments.

Specially designed clear plastic face masks are also commercially available. They are used in conjunction with moulds to apply pressure to facial scars. Other products include silicon gel, adhesive stretch gauze bandages, a wide variety of moisturising creams, elastomer moulds and splints. Burns physiotherapists and occupational therapists have become experts in scar management and often develop their own techniques for problem scars and difficult cosmetic problems. They also check for complications such as re-gressed skeletal growth that may result from prolonged application of compression garments.[60]

Long-term problems such as hair loss and keloid and hypertrophic scars require specialist management. Some children with hair loss opt for wigs, but in most cases young children find them hot and irritating and prefer to stay as they are or wear a cap. Surgical intervention may be appropriate for severe scarring but may not be required until the onset of adolescence where, for example, breast development is being impeded by scar tissue. Clever use of make-up may also be helpful in some cases, but experience has shown children and parents rarely request such products.

Itching can be a major problem for many children and is often very difficult to con-trol. Strategies include antihistamines, moisturising creams, cool compresses and non-irritant clothing.[61]

Pain Management

THE NATURE OF BURNS PAIN

It is well accepted that the pain of a burn injury is intense. It is also well documented that, in general, the deeper the burn, the less intense the pain, because nerve receptors have been damaged or destroyed.[62,63] However, there are many factors other than depth that can significantly influence the degree of pain experienced by the patient. Individual differences in pain thresholds and responses to analgesia have been observed and the importance of cultural factors and emotional aspects such as temperament are also in-creasingly being recognised.[64]

Due to the protracted nature of burn injuries, pain is often prolonged and variable. Pain may be well controlled during the acute resuscitation phase and early management period, but may become more difficult to control as treatment continues over weeks or months, particularly if multiple grafting sessions are needed.

Although burns units develop their own specific protocols for pain relief, several points can be generalised. In the acute period following a major burn, physiological processes occur that make the intravenous route the preferred method of analgesic administration. Hypovolaemia and peripheral vasoconstriction mean that drugs admin-istered intramuscularly are likely to be poorly absorbed. Once hypovolaemia has been corrected, overdose can occur through rapid absorbtion of the medication.[65]

The second point relates to findings of a patient's pain ratings when compared with staff ratings of the patient's pain. Nursing and medical personnel who work with burns patients have consistently underestimated the severity of patients' pain.[66] Concerns by professionals about possible overdose or addiction may also interfere with the provision of adequate analgesia. There are many myths surrounding pain and pain management which, in turn, become barriers to the effective provision of pain relief. There appears, however, to be a growing recognition of the complexity of pain, its assessment and management.

Patient-controlled analgesia administered intravenously, and inhaled nitrous oxide are increasingly being used for both children and adults.[67,68] Hypnosis, relaxation and visualisation techniques have also been used successfully in paediatric burns units.[69] Many centres now have access to pain specialists for consultation by unit staff. Such specialists can advise staff on aspects of pain management as well as raise the consciousness of professionals in this area.

EFFECT OF CHILDREN'S PAIN ON NURSES

Pain management is a routine part of the nursing role. However, when the patient experiences pain on a daily basis during the course of routine nursing procedures, the nurse is likely to have a great deal of difficulty performing the tasks required.[70,71] In a survey of perceived stressors among burns unit nurses, issues relating to pain and children were rated as major stressors. Perry and Heidrich asked 180 nurses working in 93 burn units throughout the United States to respond to the question 'how does the patient's pain affect you?'. Feelings commonly expressed included frustration, guilt and emotional exhaustion. Comments concerning the responses of children (such as 'I hate you' or 'the other nurses never hurts me') were commonly reported. Concerns about becoming hardened to the pain experienced by their patients were also expressed.[72] A recent Australian study supports these findings.[73]

Sandroff provides 10 coping strategies used by burn nurses. These include becoming an expert in pain assessment, avoiding stereotyping patients, focusing on the task and learning to express one's feelings.[74] The unusual dynamics that may arise from the situation of having to inflict pain regularly in the course of treatment may lead to hostility from the child and parents. Adler points out that this hostility is largely an expression of the child's and parents' own anxiety, anger and guilt, but cautions that staff need to examine their interactions with the patient critically to avoid assuming all criticism is displaced anger.[75]

Nutritional Support

The past 20 years have seen enormous advances in all aspects of nutritional support for burns patients. Research has led to a better understanding of the physiological processes involved and new techniques for measuring energy requirements such as indirect calorimetry have been developed.[76] Use of continuous feeding pumps to deliver high-protein, high-calorie formulas, increased use of parenteral nutrition and the availability of a vast array of nutritional supplements have meant that in developed countries, patients with severe burns no longer suffer from the effects of uncontrolled severe weight loss that can lead to death.

The metabolic response to major burn injury is both dramatic and profound. The pattern has been extensively studied. It has been shown that the hypermetabolism and severe catabolism that characterise this metabolic response are proportional to the size of the burn injury and exceed that of any other injury.[77] Burned children are at particular risk from a nutritional standpoint because of their high metabolic requirements, decreased caloric reserves and increased surface area in relation to weight.[78] A detailed account of the physiological changes that occur is provided by Souba et al.[79]

There are a number of other aspects that impact on nutrition. Burned children are often anorexic. Pain, lack of activity, depression and general malaise decrease appetite. In extensive burns, frequent grafting sessions also interrupt feeding regimens. So does the need to fast before administration of nitrous oxide used for dressing changes. Children may have had poor diets prior to the burn injury. Other considerations include food allergies, food preferences, religious restrictions and complications such as paralytic ileus or sepsis. Diarrhoea is often a major problem and can be caused by factors such as hyperosmolar feeds, lactose intolerance, hypoalbinaemia and administration of drugs such as antibiotics.[80]

The dietitian needs to take all these factors into account when calculating the child's nutritional requirements and develop a plan which is workable for all concerned. The dietary plan requires cooperation from nursing staff in the daily monitoring of parameters such as weight and intake and output. Laboratory tests may be ordered to further monitor progress.[81] Nurses can play a key role in encouraging and rewarding children for eating. They should also be involved in reinforcing the need for supplementary feeds, explaining the use of equipment such as enteral feeding pumps, and educating parents about suitable food choices for their child.

The actual regimens for feeding burned children vary from unit to unit. Some units have aggressive approaches to feeding that include the instigation of enteral feeding immediately following admission and the continuation of feeds during surgery over multiple grafting sessions. Others take a more conservative approach and wait several days before introducing enteral feeds. There are many controversial issues still to be resolved. Does early feeding increase the risk of paralytic ileus?[82] Can enteral feeding be safely continued during surgery? What is the most accurate formula for calculating the energy requirements of burned children?[83] Regardless of the protocols adopted by various units, there is general acceptance that the complexity of nutrition in the burn-injured child requires the skills of specialist dietitians as part of the burn team.

Psychological Aspects

Most people can identify with feelings of self-consciousness and will have worried at some stage about bodily imperfections which have caused varying degrees of distress. It is also highly likely that most nurses will have had some experience with people who have physical scars or disabilities and will have wondered how they cope and how we would cope if it happened to us. Such musings, however, could not possibly prepare us for the significant emotional hurdles to be overcome in the event of ourselves or our loved ones suffering burns.

Acceptance of changed appearance is one of the most difficult emotional hurdles faced by the burned child and his family. More immediate problems include disruption to family routine, uncertainty regarding the prognosis, confusion, fear and anxiety about treatment, pain, guilt, and feelings of loss of control.[84] This section focuses on some of these issues from the perspective of the child, parents and siblings.

RESPONSES OF THE CHILD

In the early post-burn period children are often unaware of what is happening. They have been transported to a strange, frightening place full of unfamiliar people, sights and sounds that they cannot fully comprehend. They may be in shock, and pain, medication and medical procedures serve to heighten their distortion of events.[85]

How children react following this initial period of disorientation is determined by a multitude of factors, including the severity of the burn, age and level of cognitive, social and emotional development, premorbid personality, and parental responses. Children's responses may vary over time and the process of adaptation is a long-term one for children with major burns. Despite these different influences, the problems reported in the literature are remarkably consistent.[75,86,87] They include:

- ongoing anxiety and fear
- lack of trust in the parent and caregivers
- interpreting the burn as punishment
- feelings of inadequacy arising from forced dependence on others
- hostility towards caregivers because of the painful procedures
- insecurity about school and future plans
- fantasies of abandonment and mutilation
- depression
- nightmares.

If the nature of burns and the associated treatments are considered, it is not difficult to see how some of these problems arise. One of the first tasks of infancy, according to Erikson, is the development of trust. This primarily arises from basic needs being met by the parents. The child learns that the parent will protect and comfort him. The treatment required following a major burn injury involves many situations where the parents cannot prevent pain or protect their young child. If the child is very young, development of trust may be jeopardised.

Depending on their level of cognitive reasoning ability, young children may perceive the pain, and the parents' failure to stop it, as a consequence of being bad. Pleas such as 'tell them to stop mummy' and 'I'll be good if they stop hurting me' are commonly heard on paediatric burns units.[88]

It is also common for children to perceive the caregivers as 'torturers'. After all, it makes no sense to a child to be told his treatment will make him better, when a considerable amount of care provides evidence to the contrary. It is beyond the cognitive capacity of young children to comprehend the long-term benefits of short-term pain and discomfort. Children frequently believe that if they hurt themselves, a bandaid and a kiss from the parent are often all that is needed. The injured part is rested and the bandaid left intact. The looks of disbelief as the nurse removes the dressings and then proceeds to wash the burn, sometimes causing bleeding, strongly suggest that young children fail to understand the rationales for their treatments. Since children are usually taught that nurses are kind, the child may interpret what is happening in terms of his own badness and view the treatment as punishment.[89] Children aged between 3 and 6 years tend to be

Play is an invaluable form of therapy to help young children cope with their burn injuries.

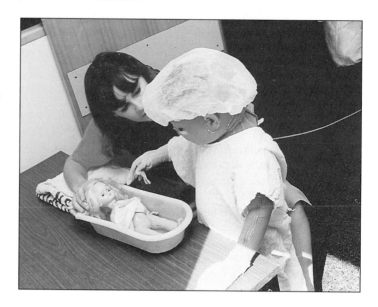

particularly vulnerable to fantasy and may distort the circumstances of the accident and their role in it, as well as the treatments involved.[85]

There are many ways of helping children cope with hospitalisation following a burn injury. Encouraging parents to be involved in as much of their child's care as possible provides security and normality. Play, as well as providing a valuable outlet for release of frustrations and anger, is also an excellent way of gaining cooperation with therapy programs such as exercise routines, and provides necessary diversion from the more painful aspects of burn management. Seeing a child enjoying play is very reassuring for parents who have fears about their child's recovery and adjustment. Medical play carried out by trained therapists can be particularly valuable in helping children to work through their fears and understand aspects of treatment.[56]

It is important to structure children's days so that they know what to expect and can look forward to free time. In units where closed dressings are used, the child may be allowed to go for walks and be involved in play programs with other children. As treatment progresses, family outings can be arranged so that the child spends time away from the unit. Schoolwork is encouraged for older children and is an important part of returning the child to normal life and routines. Some children may spend months away from school, and their eventual return to school will be made easier if they have managed to keep up with their peers. Liaison between the hospital teacher and the child's school is of great benefit. Many units also have a school visiting program where a member of the team visits the school and talks to the other children and teachers about aspects of treatment such as the need for special pressure garments and the special needs of the burned child. This may be limited to the child's class, or in some cases is carried out within the context of a broader educational program involving all teachers and children at the school.[90]

Children also need to feel that they have some control over what is happening to them. Seemingly simple steps such as encouraging them to help with their dressings and taking responsibility for their exercises, splints and other treatments can help give them this sense of control.

One of the major hurdles for the older child is learning how to deal with teasing and comments from others. While it is impossible to prepare children fully for the range of reactions that they may have to face, it is important that the issue is not ignored. Role play has been very useful in preparing children for such situations. Bernstein identifies some typical responses of burned children to teasing, including avoidance and aggression.[91] He points out that the problem with both of these solutions is that the child will increasingly become an outsider and miss out on forming friendships with children who are not concerned with the scars. Although many children work out for themselves the best way of dealing with teasing, it is important that the parent is ready to listen and support the child in meeting these challenges. Self-help groups for children and their families such as the BEES group (Burns Educational and Emotional Support) initiated in Melbourne, play a vital part in helping some families cope. Some units also hold an annual camp for children. Such camps provide an opportunity for the child to share experiences with others, learn new ways of dealing with problems, have fun, renew old friendships and make new friends.

DEVELOPMENTAL ASPECTS

For the child who is burned at an early age, it may be some years before he becomes aware that he is different.[92] Very young children remember little of the actual accident or subsequent hospitalisation, even though there may be significant physical and psychological trauma. Between the 2nd and 3rd years children begin to realise how they differ from others, but these differences may not greatly concern the child until he reaches school age and becomes generally more competitive. By this time many factors will determine how he copes: his own personality and temperament; the response of his teachers and peer group; and of course the attitude of his parents and significant others with whom he has been interacting up to this point.[93]

For the older child the reality of what has happened is more acute. The memory of the accident is likely to be vivid, as well as the time spent in hospital. Children can imagine what others will think, interpret their responses and compare their changed appearance with their previously incorporated body image. It is common, however, for older children not fully to realise fully the impact of what has happened until they leave the unit and return home and to school. It may be months or even years before the psychological effects of their burn injuries become apparent.

FACTORS THAT INFLUENCE LONG-TERM ADAPTATION

It is important to realise that the way in which the child copes emotionally will be an individualised response influenced by a multitude of factors. While this may appear to be a very obvious statement, there is a common tendency to predict and make assumptions about how the child can be expected to behave. The assumption is often made that the worse the injury, the worse the psychological problems. This is not necessarily true.[94] Some children with major burns involving extensive, lengthy treatments and hospitalisation cope extremely well, while others with a relatively minor injury have a great deal of difficulty.[95] Extent of scarring does not appear to be a major predictor of psychological adaptation following burn injuries.[96] The way in which the child's parents cope appears to be much more important. If parents have difficulty coming to terms with the child's changed appearance, it is highly likely that the child will also experience problems.[97]

Ideally there should be recognition and acceptance of the child's appearance from the outset. Questions should be answered as honestly as possible and the child should be helped to deal with other people's questions in the same way. Normal activities should be encouraged, and children should be allowed to pursue interests and hobbies at their own pace. Obviously, parents and children will need a great deal of help to achieve this ideal situation. No matter how insignificant scarring may appear to those familiar with burnt children, it can never be regarded as insignificant by the child and the parents.

PARENTAL RESPONSES

In the first few days following the accident, parents are in a state of confusion and distress. They have to adjust to what has happened, absorb information about treatment, and handle their emotions of anger, fear and guilt. At the same time they have to comfort and support their child. One of the biggest hurdles parents face is their feelings of guilt.[98] Irrespective of whether or not they were present when the accident happened, many parents feel they should have been able to prevent the burn injury. Fears, insecurities and guilt about being a good and capable parent are common. Guilt is perpetuated by the pain that the child experiences. Parents often feel a sense of helplessness and despair at being unable to protect their child from the daily pain of the treatments. Pre-existing problems between parents or other family members are often exacerbated, and may interfere with much-needed support from loved ones. Moreover, guilt may persist for a long period as the scars and long-term follow-up treatment are constant reminders of the accident.[99]

A typical response on the part of parents is to spend all their time with their sick child. Children may become aware that they are being treated differently and may become demanding and difficult to handle. Other siblings often become jealous and angry about the attention shown to the sick child and this may create additional problems. Guilt and anxiety may also become diffused, and many parents find that they are more easily upset and worried about issues that may have nothing to do with the accident. Sometimes there are pre-existing problems such as breakdown of the marriage or financial difficulties, which have already placed a strain on the parents' emotional resources. Parents need to be kept fully informed of their child's progress and encouraged to discuss their feelings in an atmosphere of acceptance and warmth. They need to be reassured that what they are feeling is normal and will gradually fade. Nurses need to be empathic and listen to the issues causing concern. Expert help from the team social worker, psychologist or psychiatrist may be necessary in some cases.

The long periods spent supporting their child in hospital can place enormous stresses on even the most organised family. Parents need to feel that it is all right to have time away from the ward, and may in some cases have to be strongly encouraged to take breaks and get adequate rest, particularly once the acute stage has passed. Provision of facilities for parents at ward level, regular parent meetings and practical help from members of the burns team contribute to easing stress and distress.

RESPONSES OF SIBLINGS

Most of the studies in this area have focused on the effects on siblings of the chronic illness or death of a child. According to McKeever, many of the existing research findings are undermined by shortcomings in design which makes interpretation of results confusing and hazardous.[100] It seems, however, that despite these weaknesses, patterns emerge which may be of help to professionals in understanding the effects of trauma such as burns on siblings. Findings suggest that a chronic illness or disability in a child is likely to be a major stressor for the sibling. Lobato et al argue that sibling relationships are intense, complex and extend beyond the traditional notions of jealousy and rivalry.[101] They state that even from a very young age, the relationship is an extremely rich one and that by 1 year of age, children spend as much time interacting with their siblings as they do with their mothers. Given the richness of this relationship, it is highly probable that one child's illness will affect healthy siblings. The needs of siblings should be not be overlooked.

Another consistent finding is that siblings are often poorly informed about their sibling's illness. It has been reported that siblings often fantasise about what has happened and hold fears that the same may happen to them. Children too young to understand what has happened are particularly vulnerable when a parent and sibling suddenly disappear.

Despite the paucity of research in this area, it is apparent that health professionals have a role to play in helping siblings deal with the crisis of a burn injury. In consultation with the parent, age-appropriate information should be provided about the treatment and information updated regularly. Parents need advice about involving siblings. There should be provision for siblings to visit frequently, not only for their own sake, but for the positive contribution they in turn can make to the sick child's recovery.[102]

Special Needs of the Adolescent Who has been Burnt

Adolescence has been described as a transitional phase, a time of learning to become an adult and relinquishing the behaviour of childhood. Traditionally this stage of development has also been considered a particularly turbulent one. More recent thinking suggests that this 'storm and stress' aspect of adolescence is largely a myth. This is not to deny the enormous physical and emotional changes that accompany the onset and progression of puberty. It has been pointed out that stresses that affect adolescents are usually spread over many years and do not reflect a state of constant turmoil as depicted in the media.

For the teenager who sustains a burn injury, however, the sequelae can indeed bring about a period of great turmoil. Burn treatment involves weeks and sometimes months of painful procedures, with loss of independence and disruption to the normal process of growth and development. There may be permanent damage that will significantly impact on the adolescent's concept of self. He will have to develop a revised body image and come to terms with the response of others to his changed appearance. The adolescent is often demanding, regressive, defiant and, above all, angry in response to his changed situation. Where he may have been responsible for the accident and/or others may have been injured, the process may be even more problematic. Frequently, initial compliance with treatment gives way to intense feelings of guilt and non-compliance. It is essential that health professionals understand these responses within the context of the trauma of burn injuries.

WAYS OF HELPING THE ADOLESCENT

One of the first questions an adolescent asks following a burn injury is 'What do I look like?' It is important that the teenager see for himself the extent of his burns and be given time to clarify what the implications are. It is important to stress from the start that all burns are different and that comparison with others is to be avoided. At a time when a significant amount of time is spent in self-appraisal, appearance may become the major focus and it is essential that questions be addressed as openly as possible. Depending on the teenager's stage of maturation, issues such as the effect of the burn injury on future employment, relationships, sexual performance or childbearing can cause anxiety. Once the extent of the burn is clear, counselling and therapy may be needed to help the adolescent express fears and worries. Involving teenagers who have suffered similar injuries or showing photographs of teenagers with similar burns has proved to be very useful. Although it may seem that adolescents strive to be different, there is a strong wish for conformity and to be part of the group. A program of visiting the school and explaining aspects of the burn to the peer group has helped smooth the way for many teenagers to resume their lifestyle.

Following a severe burn injury, it may be necessary for pressure garments and splints to be worn and these can be a particular point of contention for the adolescent. Some units have experimented with techniques such as allowing the teenager to 'decorate' the pressure garment or modifying the time spent wearing the garment in order to increase compliance.

PROMOTING INDEPENDENCE

One of the most difficult issues for the teenager to come to terms with is the loss of independence at a stage when they are being encouraged to be more responsible for their own actions. Some units may not have separate facilities for adolescents, or it may not be possible to provide these during the acute phase of management due to the specialised nature of burn injuries. It is important that, when possible, the teenager is involved in decisions about aspects of management. This may involve relatively minor aspects such as the timing of the bath and dressing, allowing him to pace the procedure and be involved in formulating regimens such as splinting and exercising. On the other hand, it may involve the teenager being involved in major decisions such as the need for, or timing of, further surgery. Guidelines and limits need to be established, but cooperation is much more likely if the adolescent feels he has some control and input into his management.

RESPECTING PRIVACY

The need for privacy is taken for granted in adult hospitals but in paediatric settings this aspect is often overlooked. Firstly, children generally do not demand privacy in the same way as adults do. Secondly, the unit may not be designed to ensure that privacy needs are easily met. It is imperative that adolescents be given privacy and that their needs in this regard are respected, particularly with bathing and dressing procedures where they may feel extremely self-conscious. It is not uncommon for adolescents to request that they wear swimming costumes or underwear during the bath, and these wishes need to be understood and incorporated into the procedure. Allowing time alone during procedures may be necessary. The provision of mirrors is essential, not only for this age group, but also for younger children who often express the need to look at their burns.

PROVISION OF AGE-APPROPRIATE ACTIVITIES

While this aspect seems self-evident, it is an issue that needs to be emphasised in a paediatric setting. Computers are particularly popular and can be both educational and recreational. The involvement of the school teacher may not be enthusiastically received, but is also very important. The teenager who has been burned may spend months away from school and it is essential that these effects be minimised. Having to repeat a year while friends move on should be avoided if possible.

Allowing for more flexibility with regard to rules such as time for 'lights out' is another area to be considered with adolescents. Some rules need to be adapted so that they are more age appropriate. Encouraging friends to visit and staff being prepared to answer their sometimes confronting questions is an essential part of helping the teenager cope with his injury.

Little research has been carried out into the long-term effects of burn injuries on the adolescent. There are few authenticated cases to substantiate reports of an increased incidence of suicide among adolescents who have been burned. Nor is there evidence that a significant proportion become social isolates. Certainly, from experience, it seems that improved treatment techniques, follow-up care and support, contribute to helping the adolescent cope. However, it is likely that the adolescent's own ego strength, the support of the family and peers and the response of the school and community are the significant predictors of how the teenager deals with the crisis of a burn injury.

Child Abuse and Burn Injuries

While most paediatric burn injuries can be classified as accidental, a percentage of children sustain burns in a manner that indicates either intent or neglect. Estimates of the incidence for this form of child abuse vary greatly within the literature. Estimates of inflicted burns in childhood in a 1979 hospital survey, ranged from 6% to 20% of cases.[103] Hobbs believes that deliberately inflicted burns and scalds account for 10% of physically abused children.[104] A retrospective survey conducted in 1985 at the Royal Alexandra Hospital for Children in Sydney found that over a 5-year period, 7.5% of admissions to the burns unit were notified to the Department of Family and Community Services. [105]

The variation in incidence reported in the literature may arise because of differences in the definition of abuse and procedures for notification. The task of deciding whether a particular case warrants notification is often a difficult one. Every day, children are in situations where the potential for spilling hot water onto themselves or getting too close to a fire exists and all parents go through periods of stress when supervision is not as close as it should be. It is the task of professionals caring for the child to decide whether, on the balance of circumstances, abuse has occurred and intervention is warranted. One of the most important aspects of the admission routine involves the taking of an accurate and detailed report of the circumstances surrounding the burn injury. A review of the previous medical record may also be productive as there have been reports of a high incidence of repeat injury in children who sustain non-accidental injury.[106] Factors which should alert professionals to the possibility of abuse-related burns are well documented.[107,108] Criteria consistently reported include isolated burns to the buttocks, the outline of a radiator, iron or cigarette butts, well demarcated burns to the feet or hands (which suggest that the extremities have been forcibly immersed) and multiple haematomas or scars at various stages of healing. More subtle indicators include prior hospitalisation for accidental trauma, the account of the injury being inconsistent with the age or developmental stage of the child, unexplained delay in presentation for treatment and concurrent evidence of neglect such as malnutrition.[109,110]

Caring for a child who has been abused provides special challenges for the burns team. The child may be particularly fearful and distrusting of adults, withdrawn and depressed. The treatment itself may hold added terrors if, for example, the child was burnt by immersion in a bath. The dysfunctional relationship which exists between abusive parents and their child commonly prevents the helpful or useful participation of parents throughout the child's hospitalisation.[111] If parents of abused children are unable or unwilling to support their child throughout treatment, it is important to involve someone who is close to the child to provide love and support. There are many reasons why parents abuse their children and the topic is a particularly sensitive and emotive one. Nurses as primary caregivers need to be aware of the dynamics underlying child abuse in order to provide what is always an extremely difficult aspect of burns care.

The Stresses and Challenges of Burns Nursing

The first encounter with a child who has sustained a significant burn injury can be one of the most distressing in a nurse's career. The pain the child experiences, the disbelief and confusion of the family, and the urgency that surrounds the situation often leave the nurse feeling overwhelmed and helpless. Interestingly, many nursing students are fascinated by the nature of such injuries and request to visit burns units during clinical experience. Despite this initial interest, burns nursing is not generally perceived as a desirable choice for new graduates. The challenge facing this speciality is the attraction and retention of capable and committed nurses. It has been argued that nursing managers need to respond more to the emotional needs of their staff to prevent high attrition rates.[112]

Bernstein proposed that nurses pass through well defined stages in the process of adaptation and adjustment to working in a burns unit.[91] Initial idealised expectations of themselves as caregivers is soon threatened by the severity of patients' conditions and the pain involved in treatment. In order to reach a stage of acceptance and commitment, they need to develop more realistic objectives and useful coping strategies. Most of the stress reported by nurses at a regional burns unit in Minneapolis, USA, contained an emotional component, with issues relating to pain, abused children, the dying patient, uncooperative patients and interstaff conflicts.[113] The most commonly reported coping methods for dealing with work-related stress were talking with co-workers and maintaining a sense of humour. Sandroff lists strategies such as becoming an expert judge of pain response, focusing on the task and avoiding identification with the patient.[74]

Hinsch found that when nurses have mastered the coping mechanisms required to work on a burns unit, they tend to stay in that area for long periods.[70]

The rewards are certain for those nurses who successfully learn to deal with the stresses involved in nursing the burned child. There is much satisfaction in being involved in the long-term care and rehabilitation of the child. Burns nursing demands a comprehensive knowledge of all aspects of patient care and specialised skills that will prove invaluable throughout a nursing career. Rewarding relationships develop between the nurse, the child and family. Children's progress can be followed as they often return to the unit for visits and retain links with the staff through support groups and camps. Perhaps most important of all is the experience of belonging to a team, and the support that accompanies the team approach to burns care.

REFERENCES

1. The Victorian Injury Surveillance System Draft Paper. *Burns: an overview of child and adult thermal injury patterns in Victoria, 1989–1991.* Melbourne: Health Department, 1992.
2. NSW Health Department. *Health Information Centre Inpatient Statistics 1992/93. Separations and average length of stay by hospital and age group for patients with burns.* Sydney: The Department, 1993.
3. Phillips W, Mahaira E, Hunt D, Pegg SP. The epidemiology of childhood scalds in Brisbane. *Burns* 1986; 12: 343–350.
4. Achauer BM, ed. *Management of the burned patient.* Connecticut: Appleton and Lange, 1987.
5. Linares AZ, Linares HA. Burn prevention: the need for a comprehensive approach. *Burns* 1990; 16: 284.
6. Savage JP, Leitch IOW. Childhood burns. A sociological survey and inquiry into causation. *Med J Aust* 1972; 1: 1337–1342.
7. Gordon PG, Ramsey GC. *A survey of thermal injuries.* Parkville, Vic: CSRIO, 1983.
8. NSW Health Department. *Health Information Centre Inpatient Statistics 1992/93. External cause by age group for patients with burns.* Sydney: The Department, 1993: 27–59.
9. NSW Health. *Scalds Prevention Campaign Bulletin.* Sydney: NSW Health, 1994.
10. Wagner MM, ed. *Care of the burn-injured patient: a multidisciplinary approach.* London: Croom Helm, 1981: 1–4.
11. Maley MP. Children under five and butane cigarette lighters. *J Burn Care Rehab* 1988; 9: 423–424.
12. McLoughlin E. The causes, costs and prevention of childhood burn injuries. *J Dis Child* 1991; 144: 677–683.
13. Bouter LM, van Rijn OJL, Kok G. Importance of planned health education for burn injury prevention. *Burns* 1990; 16: 198–202.
14. Solomon JR, Brooksbank M, Swift W. First aid treatment of burns. *Aust Fam Physician* 1979; 8: 785.
15. Pegg SP. Emergency care. First aid in burn injuries. *Emergency* 1982; 4: 13–15.
16. Martin HCO. First aid treatment of burns in children. *Mod Med Aust* 1992; June: 38–42.
17. Shun A. First aid management for burns. *The Children's Hospital Camperdown Clinical Bulletin* 1993; December.
18. Sykes RA, Mani S, Heibert JM. Chemical burns. *J Burn Care Rehab* 1986; 7: 342–346.
19. Thompson JC, Ashwal S. Electrical injuries in children. *Am J Dis Childh* 1983; 137: 231–235.
20. Bush A. What to look for when the patient suffers an electrical injury. *RN* 1987; 9: 39–43.
21. Australia (1982) Standing Committee of the Health Ministers' Conference. Super Speciality Services Working Party. *Guidelines for burn treatment.* Canberra: AGPS, 1982.
22. NSW Department of Health. *Burn Services in NSW. Organisation and clinical protocol.* Sydney: The Department, 1988. [Circular no. 88/25.]
23. NSW Department of Health. *Burn Services in NSW. Immediate treatment of paediatric burns.* Sydney: The Department, 1988. [Circular no. 88/25 1988.]
24. Kilham H, ed. *The Children's Hospital Handbook.* Section 9. Sydney: Allen Press 1993.
25. Herndon DN, Rutan RL, Alison WE, Cox CS. Management of burn injuries. *In:* Eichelberger MR. *Paediatric trauma prevention, acute care, rehabilitation.* St Louis: Mosby Year Book, 1994: 570–571.

26. Wilson GR, Fowler CA, Housden PL. A new burn area assessment chart. *Burns* 1987; 13: 401–405.

27. Constable JD. The state of burn care: past, present and future. *Burns* 1994; 20: 318.

28. Cockington RA. Ambulatory management of burns in children. *Burns* 1987; 15: 271–273.

29. Royal Alexandra Hospital for Children. *Nursing policy and procedure manual.* Sydney: RAHC, 1994.

30. Wood F, Sperring B. *Patient guidelines caring for your minor burn using Fixomull retention dressings.* Perth: Royal Perth Hospital, 1993.

31. Hermans MHE, Hermans RP. Duoderm, an alternative dressing for smaller burns. *Burns* 1986; 12: 214–219.

32. Advisory Committee, Nebraska Burn Institute. Initial assessment and management. *Advanced burn life support course instructor's manual.* Lincoln: The Institute, 1987: Chapter 1:7.

33. Bayley EW. Care of the burn patient with an inhalation injury. *In:* Trofino RB. *Nursing care of the burn injured patient.* Philadelphia: F.A. Davis, 1991: 325, 348.

34. Solomon JR. Primary care of the acute burn. *Current Therapeutics* 1987; 28 (5): 113.

35. Martin H. Basic burns care: fluid resuscitation. *ANZBA Bulletin* 1994; 14: 9–11.

36. Bernardo LM, Sullivan K. Care of the pediatric patient with burns. *In:* Trofino RB. *Nursing care of the burn injured patient.* Philadelphia: FA Davis, 1991: 255.

37. Carvajal HF. Resuscitation of the burned child. *In:* Carvajal HF, Parks DH. *Burns in children: paediatric burn management.* Chicago: Year Book Medical, 1988: 78–98.

38. Dyer C, Roberts D. Thermal trauma. *Nursing Clin North Am* 1990; 25: 90.

39. Pinnegar MD, Pinnegar FC. History of burn care: a survey of important changes in the topical treatment of thermal injuries. *Burns* 1986; 12: 508–517.

40. Queen D, Evans JH, Gaylor JDS, Courtney JM, Reid WH. Burn wound dressings — a review. *Burns* 1987; 13: 218–228.

41. Martin CJ, Ferguson JC, Rayner C. Environmental conditions for treatment of burned patients by the exposure method. *Burns* 1992; 18: 273–282.

42. Konop DJ. General local treatment. *In:* Trofino RB. *Nursing care of the burn injured patient.* Philadelphia: FA Davis, 1991: 43.

43. Hermans MHE. Treatment of burns with occlusive dressings: some pathophysiological and quality of life aspects. *Burns* 1992; 18 (Suppl 2): S15-S18.

44. Staso MA, Raschbaum M, Slater H, Goldfarb IJ. Experience with Omiderm — a new burn dressing. *J Burn Care Rehab* 1991; 12: 209–210.

45. Royal Alexandra Hospital for Children. Nursing guidelines for routine bath and dressing of a burn wound. *Nursing policy and procedure manual.* Sydney: RAHC, 1994: 04.04.

46. Parks DH, Wainwright DJ. The surgical management of burns in children. *In:* Carvajal HF, Parks DH. *Burns in children: pediatric burn management.* Chicago: Year Book Medical, 1988: 156–172.

47. Heimbach DM. Early excision and grafting. *Surg Clin North Am* 1987; 67: 93.

48. Rudolph R, Fisher J, Ninnerman J. *Skin grafting.* Boston: Little Brown, 1979: 113–114.

49. Lawrence JC. The aetiology of scars. *Burns* 1987; 13: S3-S14.

50. Dziewulski P. Burn wound healing: James Ellsworth Laing Memorial essay for 1991. *Burns* 1992; 18: 466–478.

51. Dobke MK. Burns in children — a continued challenge. *J Burn Care Rehab* 1993; 14: 17–20.

52. Bayley EW. Wound healing in the patient with burns. *Nursing Clin North Am* 1990; 25: 218–221.

53. Linares HA. Hypertrophic healing: controversies and etiopathogenic review. *In:* Carvajal HJ, Parks DH. *Burns in children.* Chicago: Year Book Medical, 1988: 305–323.

54. Muir KF, Barclay TL, Settle JA. *Burns and their treatment.* 3rd ed. London: Butterworths, 1987: 154.

55. Rogers R. Proven methods. *Paediatr Nursing* 1990; 2 (7): 20–21.

56. Johnson CL, Underwood R. Harbourview: a view of a rehabilitation team. *J Burn Care Rehab* 1986; 7: 261–267.

57. Manger G, Speed E. A co-ordinated approach to the discharge of burned children. *J Burn Care Rehab* 1986; 7: 127–129.
58. Perkins K, Davey RB, Wallace K. Current materials and techniques used in burn scar management. *Burns* 1987; 13: 406–410.
59. Surveyor JA, Clougherty DA. Burn scars: fighting the effects. *Am J Nursing* 1983; 5: 746–751.
60. King SD, Blomberg AH, Pegg SP. Preventing morphological disturbances in burn-scarred children wearing compression face garments. *Burns* 1994; 20: 256–259.
61. Gordon M. Pruritis in burns. *J Burn Care Rehab* 1988; 9: 306–308.
62. Ross DM, Ross SA. Childhood pain: current issues, research and management. Baltimore: Urban and Schwarzenberg, 1988: 259–273.
63. Kinsella J, Booth MG. Pain relief in burns. *Burns* 1991; 17: 391–395.
64. Wallace MR. Temperament: a variable in children's pain perception. *Pediatr Nursing* 1989; 15 (2): 118–121.
65. Muir FK, Barclay TL, Settle JAD. *Burns and their treatment.* London: Butterworths, 1987: 103–104.
66. Iafrati NS. Pain on the burn unit: patient vs nurse perceptions. *J Burn Care Rehab* 1986; 7: 413–416.
67. Gaukroger PB, Chapman MJ, Davey RB. Pain control in paediatric burns — the use of patient controlled analgesia. *Burns* 1991; 17: 396–399.
68. Vanstone K. The use of entenox in a paediatric burn unit. *PATCH* 1991; 6 (1): 9–12.
69. Elliott CH, Olson RA. The management of children's distress in response to painful medical treatment for burn injuries. *Behav Res Ther* 1983; 21: 675–683.
70. Hinsch A. The psychological effects on nursing staff working in a burn unit. *A'asian Nurses J* 1982; 11 (2): 25–26.
71. Brack G, LaClave L, Campbell J. A survey of attitudes of burn nurses. *J Burn Care Rehab* 1987; 8: 299–306.
72. Perry S, Heidrich G. Management of pain during debridement: a survey of US burn units. *Pain* 1982; 13: 267.
73. Nagy S. The reactions of nurses to the pain of their patients: a personal construct analysis. Unpublished PhD Thesis, 1995.
74. Sandroff R. When you must inflict pain on a patient. *RN* 1983; 1: 35–39, 112.
75. Adler R. Burns are different: the child psychiatrist on the paediatric burns ward. *J Burn Care Rehab* 1992; 13: 32.
76. Cunningham JJ, Lydon MK, Russell WE. Calorie and protein provision for recovery from severe burns in infants and young children. *Am J Clin Nutr* 1990; 51: 553–557.
77. Hildreth MA, Herndon DN, Desai MH, Duke MA. Reassessing caloric requirements in paediatric burn patients. *J Burn Care Rehab* 1988; 9: 616–618.
78. Solomon JR. Nutrition in the severely burned child. *Progress Pediatr Surg* 1981; 14: 63–79.
79. King N, Goodwin CW Jr. Use of vitamin supplements for burned patients: a national survey. *J Am Dietetic Assoc* 1984; 84: 925.
80. Bell SJ, Molnar JA, Krasker WS, Burke JF. Dietary compliance for paediatric burned patients. *J Am Dietetic Assoc* 1984; 84: 1329–1333.
81. Souba WW, Schindler RD, Carvajal HF. Nutrition and metabolism. *In:* Carvajal HF, Parks DH. *Burns in children: pediatric burn management.* Chicago: Year Book Medical, 1988.
82. O'Neil CE, Hustler D, Hildreth MA. Basic nutritional guidelines for paediatric burn patients. *J Burn Care Rehab* 1989; 10: 278–281.
83. Bell SJ, Molnar JA, Krasker WS, Burke JF. Weight maintenance in paediatric burned patients. *J Am Dietetic Assoc* 1986; 86: 207–211.
84. Brodie B, Matern S. Emotional aspects in the care of a severely burned child. *Int Nursing Rev* 1967; 14 (6): 19–24.
85. Bernstein NR. The child with severe burns. *In:* Noshpitz JD, ed. *The basic handbook of clinical psychiatry.* Vol 1. New York: Basic Books, 1979; 465–474.
86. Woodward J. Emotional disturbances of burned children. *BMJ* 1959; 1: 1009–1013.

87. Long RT, Cope O. Emotional problems of burned children. *N Engl J Med* 1961; 264: 1121–1127.
88. Brodie LS. Stop! You're hurting me. *Nursing Aust* 1984; 2 (3): 13–15.
89. Loomis WG. Management of children's emotional reactions to severe body damage (burns). *Clin Pediatr* 1970; 9: 362–367.
90. Walls-Rosenstein DL. A school re-entry program for burned children. *J Burn Care Rehab* 1987; 8: 319.
91. Bernstein NR. *Emotional care of the facially burned and disfigured.* Boston: Little Brown, 1976.
92. Watson ACH. The disfigured child. *Update* 1983; May: 133–141.
93. Sawyer MG, Minde K, Zuker R. The burned child scarred for life? A study of the psychological impact of a burn injury at different developmental stages. *Burns* 1983; 9: 205–213.
94. Byrne C, Love B, Browne G, et al. The social competence of children following burn injury: a study in resilience. *J Burn Care Rehab* 1986; 7: 247–252.
95. Abdullah A, Blakeney P, Hunt R, et al. Visible scars and self-esteem in paediatric patients with burns. *J Burn Care Rehab* 1994; 15: 164–168.
96. Jessee PO, Strickland MP, Leeper JD, Wales P. Perception of body image in children with burns, five years after burn injury. *J Burn Care Rehab* 1992; 13: 33–37.
97. Meyer WJ, Blakeney P, Moore P, et al. Parental well-being and behavioral adjustment of paediatric survivors of burns. *J Burn Care Rehab* 1994; 15: 62–68.
98. Partridge J, Robinson E. Psychological and social aspects of burns. *Burns* 1995; 21: 453–457.
99. Mason SA. Young scarred children and their mothers — a short term investigation into the practical, psychological and social implications of thermal injury to the preschool child. *Burns* 1993; 19: 495–500.
100. McKeever P. Siblings of chronically ill children: a literature review with implications for research and practice. *Am J Orthopsychiatry* 1983; 53: 209–218.
101. Lobarto D, Faust D, Spirato A. Examining the effects of chronic disease and disability on children's sibling relationships. *J Pediatr Psychol* 1988; 13: 389–407.
102. Brownmiller N, Cantwell D. Siblings as therapists: a behavioral approach. *Am J Psychiatry* 1976; 133: 447–450.
103. Hight DW, Bakalar HR, Lloyd JR. Inflicted burns in children: recognition and treatment. *JAMA* 1979; 242: 517–520.
104. Hobbs CJ. Burns and scalds. *BMJ* 1989; 298: 1302–1305.
105. Brodie LS. *Children at risk and burn injuries.* NSW Paediatric Nurses Association Occasional Papers 1986: 17–19.
106. Hobson MI, Evans J, Stewart IP. An audit of non-accidental injury in burned children. *Burns* 1994; 20: 442–445.
107. Rosenburg NM, Marino D. Frequency of suspected abuse/neglect in burn patients. *Pediatr Emerg Care* 1989; 5: 219–221.
108. Lenoski EF, Hunter KA. Specific patterns of inflicted burns. *J Trauma* 1977; 17: 842–846.
109. Stone NH, Rinaldo L, Humphrey CH. Child abuse by burning. *Surg Clin North Am* 1970; 50: 746–751.
110. Carrigan L, Heinbach DM, Marvin JA. Risk management in children with burn injuries. *J Burn Care Rehab* 1988; 9: 75–78.
111. Weimer CL, Goldfarb W, Siater H. Multidisciplinary Approach to Working with Burn Victims of Child Abuse. *J Burn Care Rehab* 1988; 9: 81.
112. Swift W. Emotional care and support: an overview tour around burn units and centres. *Aust Nurses J* 1976; 6 (5): 31–33.
113. Lewis KF, Poppe S, Twomey J, Peltier G. Survey of perceived stressors and coping strategies among burn unit nurse. *Burns* 1990; 16: 109–112.

Chapter 14

Nursing Care of the Adolescent with Special Needs

Introduction

Gail Anderson

TREADING PATHS

Birth
childhood,
adolescence,
the future.

All those years
of guidance, love
and parenting.
Progressively confused by
conflicts and
misunderstandings.

The quest for independence
so very strong.
To be one's own person
the overwhelming,
egocentric need.
Yet, this path,
instinctually followed
so often hazy,
taken with faltering steps,
declining guidance,
befuddled with inner turmoil,
so often painful.

Painful for the individual,
family
and onlookers.
Pain to be endured
for growth.
Growth from adolescence to adult,
the margin so often blurred
in this so called sophisticated age.
An age of abbreviated childhood.

Eventually we crawl
out of the communal trough,
into the light.
Children grown into adult friends and
we watch them tread
their singular path.

Professor Neil Buchanan

Adolescent nursing requires an understanding of the biological, psychological and developmental aspects of adolescence. To be effective, one also needs to have a genuine interest in and desire to work with this dynamic population.

Providing optimal nursing care for all adolescents, and particularly for the adolescent with special needs, can be challenging and rewarding as there are many issues to be addressed in addition to the medical diagnosis and treatment.

Adolescence is a period of change, transition and first experiences. There is rapid biological, social and personal growth. Most people survive this transition process without experiencing any long-lasting adverse effects. They then enter adulthood with the skills, behaviours and attitudes necessary to survive and cope independently as healthy, functioning adults.

This chapter focuses on some of the issues and difficulties that can be faced by adolescents, which may threaten or delay mastery of adolescent developmental tasks. The information presented here represents an effort to examine *some* of these special needs and to explore how nurses can best provide holistic, age-appropriate care. Medical conditions, including anorexia nervosa, obesity and chronic illness, will be examined. As well, issues relating to psychosocial, psychological and intra-familial problems will be discussed. Remember, effective intervention for the adolescent of today will lead to decreased morbidity and mortality in the adult of tomorrow.

Anorexia Nervosa

Gail Anderson

Anorexia nervosa is a serious and complex eating disorder. It is characterised by a persistent and focused drive for thinness which leads to severe weight loss. Invariably sufferers see themselves as being fat. This is regardless of how much weight they lose and how extremely emaciated they become. Anorexia nervosa is seen most commonly in females in advanced industrialised societies.

Onset of the illness characteristically occurs in postpubertal female adolescents between the ages of 12 and 18 years of age. However, this can vary. Prepubertal girls as young as 9 years have been diagnosed and treated in Australia. These children are particularly difficult to treat due to the associated severity of mental disturbance. Young adults in their twenties have also presented for initial management. Females comprise 95% of individuals in whom anorexia nervosa is diagnosed.[1]

Most persons diagnosed with anorexia nervosa are described by their parents as having been thoughtful, obedient and perfect children. Sufferers come from all socioeconomic backgrounds, but the majority are seen in middle-class families. They are generally high academic achievers, not because they are more intelligent, but because they strive harder for achievement and perfection.

Anorexia nervosa should not be confused with the term 'anorexia', which involves a compromised or absent desire for food. Individuals with anorexia nervosa primarily control their weight by rigorously restricting food intake despite experiencing sensations of hunger. Therefore, they may feel hungry but conscious fear of weight gain overrides their hunger and prevents them from eating normally.

Other weight controlling behaviours employed can include extensive exercising, self-induced vomiting and the ingestion of emetics, diuretics, laxatives or more rarely, appetite suppressing agents.

It is common for persons suffering with anorexia nervosa to have premorbid obsessional personality traits, depression and low self-esteem. The illness has major social effects — invalidism, regression and isolation, as well as serious physical consequences including malnutrition, disordered body chemistry and endocrine dysfunction.[2]

Two specific subtypes of anorexia nervosa have been identified: individuals who remain emaciated through stringent dieting and food restriction; and individuals who cannot lose the weight they desire through dieting alone and thus resort to self-induced vomiting and abuse of laxatives and diuretics.[3] Patients who restrict food have been described as more obsessive–compulsive, stoical, perfectionistic, introverted and emotionally inhibited. Those who binge eat and purge are more likely to be compulsive, depressive, socially dysfunctional, sexually adventurous and substance misusers.[4]

Anorexia nervosa may come to be seen as a 'dieting' disorder, rather than an eating disorder. Dieting behaviour invariably precedes the development of anorexia nervosa. Factors which initiate or predispose an individual to develop anorexia nervosa are not thoroughly understood, but include an interplay of individual, family, social and cultural issues (see **aetiology**).

Caring for individuals with anorexia nervosa presents a special challenge for nurses. Management encompasses the complex and multi-determined nature of the illness. Difficulties can be experienced in managing the behaviours of these patients. Typical behaviours include initial denial of the illness, ambivalence about seeking professional help and non-compliance with management programs. Manipulative attempts to split and deceive staff and family are common, especially during the initial stages of management when patients experience difficulty in trusting others. These behaviours stem from an awareness that intervention includes encouraging weight gain. Weight gain is the one thing affected individuals fear the most and is often perceived by the patient as 'losing self-control'. As therapy progresses, and patients begin to acknowledge and deal appropriately with their thoughts and feelings, these behaviours subside.

Feeling in control is a central issue for sufferers. To be most effective, nurses need to be aware that the apparent manipulative behaviours described above are part of the illness. They are a defence against the perceived threat to a fragile sense of control. Food intake and weight may be the only things that the individual feels any control over in life. Therefore, nursing care should not be directed at 'taking charge' of the patient. It should rather encourage the patient to exert personal control over areas of their life other than those focused on losing weight. Patients should be encouraged to give full informed consent and agree to participate actively in all proposed programs of management. The rationale for intervention may need to be reiterated numerous times to the patient, particularly if their cognitive state is compromised by extreme low bodyweight.

DIAGNOSIS

Most adolescent girls are weight conscious and sensitive to their body shape, but relatively few develop the behaviours characteristic of anorexia nervosa. There is a marked distinction between healthy nutritional practices and the stringent, obsessional patterns of dietary restraint as practised by the anorexia nervosa sufferer. A principal feature of the illness is the 'morbid fear of becoming fat',[6] which refers to the complex set of attitudes to shape and weight that are not encountered in any other psychiatric disorder.

Medical assessment is necessary to exclude other causes of weight loss and to ensure an accurate diagnosis. Other causes of weight loss include psychiatric illness (e.g., major depressive disorder, obsessive compulsive disorder), and systemic illnesses (e.g., malignancy, inflammatory bowel disease).

A comprehensive psychiatric assessment is needed to clarify psychopathology. Comorbidity is a common finding. For example, a young person may be suffering from

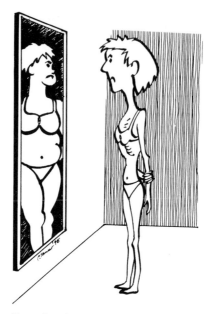

Figure 14.1 Body image distortion is a core feature of anorexia nervosa.

(Celia Tanner 1995. Reproduced with permission from the Audio-visual Department, Westmead Hospital, NSW)

both anorexia nervosa and an affective psychiatric disorder, anxiety disorder or personality disorder.

The American Psychiatric Association[5] lists the criteria (**Table 14.1**) which are widely used to determine the diagnosis of anorexia nervosa. This definition is unusual for a psychiatric condition in that the 1st criterion relates to a physical phenomenon, the 2nd is psychological, the 3rd is a distortion of perception and the 4th is one of the hormonal effects of the illness.

ANOREXIA NERVOSA IN MALES

Many features of anorexia nervosa in males are similar to those in females, with the specific exception of amenorrhoea. However, males with an onset of anorexia nervosa after adolescence have been reported to demonstrate a more severe form of the disorder.[7] Males are also thought to express different attitudes to body shape and have a worse long-term prognosis. They present different premorbid personality features, including a higher incidence of gender identity problems.[8] Anorexia nervosa has been particular noted among male homosexuals and sportspeople (e.g., jockeys).

AETIOLOGY

There is no single causal factor for anorexia nervosa. An interplay of predisposing biological, psychological, familial and experiential factors are thought to be involved in the development of the disorder. Perceived significant separation and loss, disruption of family homeostasis or new developmental demands coupled with low self-esteem are just

Table 14.1 DSM 1V criteria for diagnosis of anorexia nervosa

A. Refusal to maintain bodyweight at or above a minimally normal weight for age and height (e.g., weight loss leading to maintenance of body weight less than 85% of that expected; or failure to make expected weight gain during period of growth leading to bodyweight less than 85% of that expected).

B. Intense fear of gaining weight or becoming fat, even though underweight.

C. Disturbance in the way in which one's bodyweight or shape is experienced; undue influence of body weight or shape on self-evaluation, or denial of the seriousness of the current low bodyweight.

D. In post-menarchal females, amenorrhoea, i.e., the absence of at least 3 consecutive menstrual cycles. (A woman is considered to have amenorrhoea if her periods occur only following hormone, e.g., oestrogen) administration.

Specify type:

Restricting type: During the current episode of anorexia the person has not regularly engaged in binge eating or purging behaviour (i.e., self-induced vomiting or the misuse of laxatives or diuretics).

Binge eating/purging type: During the current episode of anorexia nervosa, the person has regularly engaged in binge eating or purging behaviour (i.e., self-induced vomiting or the misuse of laxatives, diuretics or enemas).

some of the common histories seen in clinical practice. A history of child sexual abuse is another common finding. Numerous theories have been proposed to explain the illness.

Psychoanalytic theories

Early psychoanalytic theories based on the work of Sigmund Freud focused on the oral nature of eating, which was interpreted in sexual terms. These theories postulated that the central conflict for these young women was a fear of femininity.[9,10] They presented the idea that self-starvation, or self-induced vomiting and progressive weight loss, is a defence against sexual fantasies of oral impregnation. Refusal to eat was therefore seen as a symbolic expression relating to fear of adult sexuality.

More recently, psychoanalytic theorists have attempted to explain anorexia nervosa in terms of disturbance of self-concept and the development of independence. As they grow, older children learn to function and elicit satisfaction of their needs without their parents. Difficulties in functioning on their own impede the development of self apart from the family. Adolescents suffering from anorexia nervosa maintain a dependent state and may delay separation from the family.

The illness has been described as a distorted biological solution to an existential problem with the sufferer having little in the way of more sophisticated coping devices.[11] Anorexia nervosa is therefore seen to be associated with a delay or reversal of normal maturation. Hilda Bruch, a psychotherapist, argues that anorexia nervosa has to be understood in terms of the total personality in the context of the family rather than in the narrow terms of psychosexual development.[12] She proposed that before manifesting the illness, individuals experience feelings of helplessness and ineffectiveness. These patients feel inadequate to meet the high expectations placed upon them by their families. Therefore, the rigid discipline over dietary intake, with subsequent weight loss, provides the experience of being effective and in control of at least one area of life.

Table 14.2 Common themes seen in families

1. Family rigidity.
2. Parental over-protectiveness.
3. Enmeshment (over-involvement of family members).
4. Inability to resolve conflict or avoidance of confrontation.
5. Involvement of the adolescent in unresolved parental conflict.

Adapted from Minuchin et al.[15]

Goodsitt[13] refers to a disorganisation of the self in the development of anorexia nervosa and described the sufferer as reacting and responding passively, but rarely initiating. There is then an accompanying sense of emptiness, helplessness and ineffectiveness.

Feminist theories

Feminist and sociocultural theories facilitate an understanding of the context in which society and culture interact with the individual in the development of eating disorders. For example, eating disorders have been described as the quintessential symbol of female oppression in a male-dominated culture.[14] Women are conditioned to care for others rather than themselves and, as a consequence, they feel that their own needs are less important. Women are therefore steeped in the necessity for self-deprivation, but are constantly in need of approval. Culturally, approval is generally given to the slender body shape.

Family theories

Another set of theories discusses the influence of family functioning on the development of eating disorders. Families are often intensely involved in their child's anorexia nervosa. Debate arises here as to whether aspects of family functioning may have contributed to the development of the illness, or whether these aspects are reactive to the need to focus attention on the affected child because of the eating disorder.

It is therefore important to obtain a clear history of the family functioning and an understanding of the way in which the family has attempted to resolve problems. Whilst it is important **not** to imply or assume family causality, specific dysfunctional characteristics have been identified in the families of adolescents suffering from anorexia nervosa. **Table 14.2** describes some common themes which have been noted in these families.[15]

Irrespective of the ascribed theory of causality, various degrees of depression, poor self-concept, disturbed body image (see **Figure 14.1**), and a confused sense of identity underlie much of the psychopathology of anorexia nervosa. Fortunately, these complex issues can often be addressed by therapeutic intervention.

INCIDENCE

There is considerable uncertainty and wide variation surrounding the incidence of anorexia nervosa. Reported incidence figures vary considerably from 1:100 to 1:1000 girls. It should be remembered that, as with all illnesses, anorexia nervosa presents in varying degrees of severity, which will influence incidence figures.

The overall impression from international studies is that those study designs which have used the most adequate sampling methods and rigorous diagnostic criteria have found prevalence rates of 1:1000. This is the case with a major Australian study where

5705 pupils in girls' high schools were surveyed.[16] This study concluded that it seems likely that no more than 1:1000 of the total South Australian female population 12+ years of age are suffering from anorexia nervosa of sufficient severity to qualify as cases of anorexia nervosa using the DSM-111 diagnostic criteria.[5] These results imply that while anorexia nervosa is a relatively rare disorder, there is a significant number of affected young people needing professional intervention.

PATHOPHYSIOLOGICAL MANIFESTATIONS

With increasing community awareness in recent years, most adolescents present to the health care system before they become severely physically compromised. The clinical manifestations of anorexia nervosa are a direct result of starvation. The combination of a low-energy but relatively high-protein intake and strenuous exercise ensures that weight lost is preferentially adipose tissue until the bodyweight has reached 80% of standard weight for height. At this point, physiological changes are minor, but may include amenorrhoea. As the illness progresses and protein catabolism increases, fat and muscle depletion lead to extreme emaciation and a skeletal-like appearance. Lanugo, a fine downy hair, is often seen on the patient's trunk.

Cerebral disturbance

Cognitive changes due to extremely low bodyweight can include impaired concentration and a general loss of interest in issues outside food and weight-related areas. When this occurs, patients are unable to effectively engage in psychotherapy. Therefore, in very emaciated patients, weight gain is needed before psychotherapy can begin. Non-specific abnormalities in the EEG have been noted in patients with anorexia nervosa.[17] The most frequent finding is of a generalised slow wave activity which may be related to depression. Diffuse abnormalities reflecting a metabolic encephalopathy may result from significant fluid and electrolyte disturbances.[5]

Gastrointestinal disturbance

Gastrointestinal symptoms may include delayed gastric emptying, constipation, abdominal pain and decreased intestinal motility. This leads to a sensation of fullness and early satiety after eating small amounts of food. Patients complain of feeling bloated after only small meals or snacks are eaten. Hypertrophy of the salivary glands and dental enamel erosion are sometimes noted, especially if the patient has a history of self-induced vomiting.

Electrolyte disturbance

Electrolyte disturbances rarely occur in adolescents who control their weight by dietary restriction alone. However, when protein is catabolised, water is lost largely from the intracellular compartment, taking potassium with it. The hypokalemia that results is much more severe if diuretics are abused or if vomiting is induced. Hyponatraemia, hypochloraemia, hypomagnesaemia and metabolic alkalosis may also develop in these patients. An elevated blood urea and nitrogen level may reflect a state of dehydration.

Dehydration, salt loss and consequent hypovolaemia can activate the renin-angiotensin-aldosterone system. This secondary aldosteronism, while aiding sodium conservation, will promote further loss of potassium from the kidneys.[17] Peripheral oedema is occasionally seen and has been related to eating binges[18] and hypoalbuminaemia.[19] Following weight gain, the suggested cause of oedema is enhanced sodium retention secondary to increased renal sensitivity to aldosterone and the effect of increased insulin secretion on the renal tubules.[19]

Cardiac disturbance

Sinus bradycardia and hypotension are commonly noted in patients with anorexia nervosa. Cardiac arrhythmia and conduction defects can result from electrolyte disturbances, particularly hypokalaemia, and are a rare cause of sudden death. ECG changes are usually not widely noted, however a prolonged P–R interval, prominent U waves and flattened T waves have been demonstrated on ECG in patients with very low body weights. Cardiac atrophy may occur with prolonged emaciation. Syncopal episodes may occur as a result of hypotension and an impairment of orthostatic response.

Haematological disturbance

Most haematological tests are normal in patients with anorexia nervosa, depending on the degree of emaciation. However, hypercholesterolaemia is common. Some patients have shown moderate normochromic anaemia with reversible bone marrow hypoplasia. Liver function test results may be elevated (including SGOT, LDH and alkaline phosphatase levels) due to fatty degeneration of the liver, and raised low-density lipoprotein levels. Leukopenia may occur increasing susceptibility to bacterial infections. Nutritional anaemia due to dietary iron deficiency may also occur, but is usually mild. Thrombocytopenia occurs rarely.

Metabolic and endocrine disturbance

Starvation has a profound effect on endocrine function. Amenorrhoea, in post-menarchal females, occurs early and may persist long after weight is regained. This is associated with a regression of gonadotrophin secretion to the prepubertal pattern. However, patients who are taking the oral contraceptive pill can still experience light withdrawal bleeding. Anovulation is usual in patients with anorexia nervosa, due to the altered sensitivity of the hypothalamic feedback mechanism. The hypothalamus releases inadequate lutenising hormone releasing hormone (LHRH), causing low levels of plasma lutenising hormone (LH) and follicle stimulating hormone (FSH). This is accompanied by a profound oestrogen deficiency.[20] Similarly, males have low serum testosterone levels.

The decrease in oestrogen may be responsible for the development, later in life, of osteoporosis in these patients.[20] Oestrogens are needed for maintaining bone density, which is normally increasing rapidly during puberty. Stress fractures have been noted in anorexia nervosa patients who indulge in excessive exercise. In an effort to prevent the consequences relating to decreased oestrogen levels, some health care agencies have trialled the use of the oral contraceptive pill for selected anorexia nervosa patients. However, more research needs to be undertaken on the efficacy of this practice before it is widely accepted.

Mild hypothyroidism, which serves to minimise energy expenditure, is sometimes noted. Cold intolerance, hypothermia and dry skin are common. Anorexia nervosa sufferers often wear several layers of clothing. (This bulky apparel can serve to disguise weight loss for quite some time.) Serum levels of thyroxine (T_4) are usually normal or slightly reduced. However, levels of triiodothyronine (T_3), the more active metabolite, are often depressed.[19]

If the illness is severe, and has occurred during the pubertal growth spurt, permanent stunting of premorbid potential height may occur. It is not known why the extent of growth retardation varies so much between patients.

MANAGEMENT OF ANOREXIA NERVOSA

Anorexia nervosa is best managed when an early diagnosis is made and an experienced multidisciplinary team implements and supervises a structured intervention program. Every patient has special needs. The management program for each patient should be individually designed following a comprehensive biopsychosocial assessment. The choice and course of therapy will vary depending on the circumstances of each individual.

Individual psychotherapy

Individual psychotherapy is necessary to address the multitude of psychological issues involved in initiating and perpetuating the eating disorder. Self-esteem, feelings of control expressed in healthy ways, and mastery of the normal tasks of the adolescent developmental period are some of the issues usually addressed. A variety of approaches has been used including psychoanalytic, cognitive and behavioural psychotherapy. It should be remembered that patients who have cognitive states impaired by very low bodyweight are unable to engage in meaningful psychotherapy. When this occurs, psychotherapy may need to be delayed until weight gain restores sufficient cognitive capacity.

Family therapy

Family therapy is usually considered an essential component of a management program for adolescents suffering from anorexia nervosa. It is used to improve the overall functioning of the family. Families form the major context in which individual children grow and develop. Anorexia nervosa in one family member impacts on all other family members. The focus of attention becomes the eating-disordered adolescent. The family finds coping with the effects of the anorexia nervosa overwhelming. Parents generally need help in understanding their child's behaviour and with designing new strategies to deal with this behaviour.

Any family dysfunction should be addressed in family therapy. Families also benefit from the support given during therapy as dealing with the exhibited behaviours of the child produces an enormous amount of stress and emotional upheaval. Family therapy sessions are an ideal vehicle for building rapport between the family and the treatment team. This ensures that parents understand and support the management program. Parents must give their full support and commitment to the management program. If this is not the case, the management program will be ineffective as the adolescent will attempt to undermine the program and split parents from the treatment team.

Nutritional counselling

The dietitian is a valuable adjunct to therapy. Nutritional counselling should include providing information about the re-feeding process and the physiology of dieting and weight gain. The dietitian is usually seen as having a major role in effecting a positive outcome. All issues relating to food, including prescribed amounts of food for adequate weight gain, are generally referred to the dietitian.

Postpubertal adolescents are generally expected to gain between 1 and 1.5 kg each week until they reach a healthy goal weight. Prepubertal patients are encouraged to gain between 750 g and 1 kg each week.

Medical assessment

Initial medical assessment and ongoing monitoring of the patient's condition is necessary. Patients with a compromised physical condition (see pathophysiological manifestations) may need admission to hospital. A physician specialising in the care of adolescents is the ideal person to undertake medical management. Depending on the age of the adolescent, a paediatrician or adult physician may also be consulted.

Group therapy

Structured psychoeducational group work provides opportunities for individuals to share common fears, problems and anxieties. Relevant issues that may be the focus of specific groups include: self-esteem, body image, assertiveness, relationships (social, peer and family), self-expression and effective communication.

Management programs

There are currently 3 main modes of management for anorexia nervosa patients. These are: outpatient programs; day patient programs; and inpatient programs.

Outpatient programs

Adolescents with lesser degrees of weight loss can respond positively to outpatient management, especially when they and their families are motivated to change. The best candidates for outpatient treatment have been described as those patients whose illness is of less than 4 months' duration, who have no bingeing or vomiting and who have cooperative parents who will engage in family therapy.[22] The current trend in management of anorexia nervosa is to treat all patients on an outpatient or day patient basis whenever possible. **Table 14.3** describes some common reasons why admission to hospital may become necessary.

A typical outpatient program involves a great deal of commitment from the family in terms of travelling to numerous appointments for assessments and follow-up management visits. These may include:

Initial outpatient assessment:

- Medical assessment (including full physical examination, full blood count, thyroid function tests and electrolyte levels. Electrocardiograph if severe weight loss).
- Psychiatric assessment.
- Family assessment.
- Interview with dietitian.
- Education to explain the illness and the physiological effects of starvation.
- Explanation of the proposed management program.
- Ensuring commitment to the program by patient and family.

Ongoing outpatient management:

- Regular medical assessments.
- Weight monitoring.

Table 14.3 Common reasons for hospital admission

1. Continuous weight loss despite outpatient treatment.
2. Critical physical condition — e.g., grossly abnormal biochemical or pathophysiological manifestations of starvation.
3. Severe emotional and/or cognitive compromise.
4. Risk of suicide due to depression.
5. Intolerable family situation leading to increasing conflict.
6. Co-morbidity and complexity of clinical picture.

- Individual psychotherapy (up to 3 times per week).
- Family therapy (usually every 2 to 3 weeks).
- Nutritional rehabilitation and dietetic advice as needed.
- Introduction to and ongoing group therapy (weekly).
- Continuous evaluation of care and patient's progress.

Day programs

Day programs are a relatively new concept in the management of patients suffering from anorexia nervosa. The major thrust for this style of management comes from the current economic climate and the high costs associated with hospitalisation. Some of the advantages of day programs include a decreased risk of institutionalisation, and normal social contact with family and peers can be maintained.

Day programs differ from outpatient management in that patients remain in care for approximately 8 hours each weekday. Schooling is usually maintained throughout the program in a school attached to the unit providing care. These programs are usually coordinated by a psychiatrist, along with a multidisciplinary team of caregivers. Program content varies from unit to unit, but usually includes all the features of an outpatient program as well as continuing schooling.

Inpatient management

Hospitalisation may be necessary if the patient fails, or is too ill, to respond to outpatient or day patient treatment (see **Table 14.3**). When a patient is admitted to hospital, it is usually for a protracted length of time — from 2 to 6 months, or until a specified target weight is reached. There are several negative aspects associated with admission to hospital. These include the risk of contagion or deterioration (e.g., copying the behaviours of other eating disordered patients), initial regression due to resentment at being hospitalised, especially if the adolescent is unwilling to be admitted, and cost.

Inpatient programs are usually based on a behavioural regimen using positive reinforcements consisting of rewards. Increased physical activity including structured exercise programs, and social activity such as 'gate passes' in the form of day, overnight or weekend leave from hospital are earned by gaining weight and normalising eating behaviours. Types of programs vary according to the environment in which the patient is nursed. A management program on a general adolescent unit may differ from that on a psychiatric unit or in a specialised eating disorders unit in terms of general milieu and patient mix. However, when nursing adolescents suffering from anorexia nervosa, the philosophy should be consistent with nursing care aimed at encouraging achievement of adolescent developmental tasks as well as consistent management of the illness itself.

Table 14.4 Essential aspects of nursing assessment

1. Physical assessment including weight, height, temperature, pulse, blood pressure, urinalyses.
2. Previous health history, including illnesses, allergies and previous growth and developmental history.
3. Dietary history including oral intake and patterns of eating.
4. History of types of behaviours employed to lose weight.
5. Exercise activity patterns.
7. History detailing menarchal onset and pattern.
8. Elimination pattern.
9. History of sleeping patterns.
10. Educational activities.
11. Social and peer interaction.
12. Observations of family interactions.

NURSING ASSESSMENT

A thorough nursing assessment on admission is essential to enable the construction of a therapeutic nursing care plan. The care plan should be continually updated and evaluated as new information is gleaned and should be consistently adhered to by all staff. Ideally, the nursing assessment should be performed by the primary nurse who will work closely with the adolescent during the admission. Essential aspects of the nursing assessment should include those presented in **Table 14.4**.

NURSING MANAGEMENT

Overall short-term goal

Reversal of severely compromised physical state by weight restoration (nutrition and rehydration); education about the effects of malnutrition on physical and cognitive functioning; development of a therapeutic relationship based on trust.

Overall long-term goals

Acceptance and maintenance of appropriate weight for age and height; restoration of normal growth and development; normalisation of eating behaviours; self-examination and expression of inner feelings; correction of distorted body image perception; development of positive self-esteem; prevention of relapse.

Nurses have a pivotal role in promoting positive outcomes as they are the main caregivers who supervise the patient 24 hours a day. Nursing management should emphasise a holistic approach to care, including the physiological, emotional and psychosocial issues identified during the nursing assessment. Of primary importance in the treatment of anorexia nervosa is securing the confidence and cooperation of both the patient and the family in the overall management program. This can prove particularly difficult as patients typically deny that they have a problem and may resent intervention.

Adolescents often use manipulative statements to their parents such as 'I'll know you don't love me if you make me stay here' or 'Let me go home and I'll eat'. When family resistance occurs and the adolescent is not in imminent danger physiologically, it is often wise to discharge the adolescent into the care of the family until they accept the need for intervention and cooperate with the management program. Otherwise the program will be undermined by conflicting responses to the adolescent's manipulative attempts to avoid weight gain.

The adolescents themselves take pride in their skeleton-like appearance. Particularly in the early stages of treatment, they mistakenly interpret their weight as an indicator of their self-control. If they have lost or not gained weight, they experience a sense of gratification, accomplishment and success. If weight is gained, it is perceived as a loss of control. This distorted perception leads to non-compliance with proposed management and inability to acknowledge or accept that they are ill or emaciated.

Developing and maintaining a trusting and therapeutic nurse–patient relationship is essential. The nurse is then in a position to be an agent for positive change by encouraging an increased tolerance of change in the adolescent. The nurse can act as a teacher and role model and encourage the sufferer to develop more appropriate and healthy ways of exerting control over life, including the healthy expression of personal feelings, needs and emotions.

The program of care should be clearly stated to both parents and patient in the presence of the nursing staff. It is preferable that the primary nurse be present at initial and subsequent meetings between patient, family and other professionals involved in the patient's management. This helps avoid any misunderstandings and minimises the chance of manipulation of management. Using primary nursing helps facilitate communication and consistency of care as well as providing the opportunity for the patient to develop a trusting relationship with one significant caregiver. To minimise undermining of management plans, the value of a well documented program of care cannot be overemphasised. Nursing interventions should reinforce appropriate behavioural limits and provide a sense of consistency of care and expectations.

As the issues involved in every case of anorexia nervosa are unique, and as programs are run according to the philosophy of the specific unit on which the patient is managed, the following suggested nursing interventions act as a general guide.

Eating behaviours

Food and weight are central focus issues for affected individuals. Eating is an activity performed with obsessive slowness. The patient may feel guilty if the food is eaten, and resent family and staff members who comment on their eating behaviours. Due to the difficulties experienced with eating, meal times can be particularly frustrating for the patient. It is not unusual to find the majority of the patient's uneaten food hidden under the lettuce leaf on the dinner plate, wrapped in tissues or simply left uneaten.

Patients with anorexia nervosa often attempt to manipulate nursing staff and others into compromising on issues related to their oral intake. It is important that the adolescent receive education regarding nutritional requirements and take responsibility for ordering an adequate amount of food. Three meals appropriately spaced throughout the day plus snacks should be encouraged.

The nurse needs to be observant and firm regarding acceptable behaviours at meal time. A time limit of 30 minutes to eat meals helps address disordered eating behaviours. Consistency is needed in setting and ensuring adherence to set limits. **Table 14.5** lists some suggested nursing interventions to assist in the normalisation of eating behaviours.

Table 14.5 Suggested nursing interventions with respect to eating behaviours

1. Encourage toileting before meals.
2. Restrict meal times to 30 minutes maximum.
3. Discourage disordered eating behaviours such as cutting food into minute pieces and avoiding foods previously eaten.
4. Encourage the selection of adequate amounts of food.
5. Encourage 3 properly spaced meals plus snacks each day.
6. Provide structured support at meal times.
7. Avoid extensive discussion about food at meal times by encouraging conversation about other topics of interest.
8. Act as a role model for normal eating behaviour.
9. Discourage visitors at meal times, especially in the initial stages of treatment.
10. Provide encouragement and positive feedback about progress in normalisation of eating patterns and behaviours.
11. Encourage bed rest for 1 hour after meals. Relaxation therapy or discussing feelings is beneficial at this time.

Excessive exercising behaviours

Anorexia nervosa sufferers often feel driven to over-exercise as a symptom of their illness. The purpose of the exercise is not to get fit, but rather to lose weight. Because of its driven nature, the patient does not necessarily enjoy exercising, but feels a compulsion to burn off calories. Patients can exercise, covertly in the bathroom or even while lying in bed. These behaviours are often seen in patients who use exercise as a means of achieving weight loss. Monitoring and restriction of physical activity, to conserve energy and assist weight gain, may be necessary for patients suffering from a compromised physical state.

As the patient's weight gain progresses, an exercise program consisting of toning and stretching exercises and anaerobic activity is introduced. This helps ensure that weight gained is distributed in the form of muscle rather than fat. An exercise program can also act as an incentive or reward for weight gain and compliance.

Self-esteem and body image

Anorexia nervosa sufferers often experience strong feelings of inadequacy and unworthiness. Self-doubt leaves them ill-equipped to meet the challenges of independent decision making. Activities and interactions should be directed towards increasing the adolescent's self-esteem and feeling of adequacy.

The nurse can facilitate the development of positive self-esteem and confidence by identifying strengths and reinforcing positive aspects of the patient's behaviour. Self-worth promotes a positive self-concept and enhances self-esteem. Feelings of helplessness are masked by the patient's obsession with food and weight.

A very important aspect of treatment involves encouraging the adolescent's awareness of personal *feelings* that have been displaced onto food, shape and weight-related behaviour. Having assisted patients to identify their feelings, nurses can then help to explore the reasons for, and encourage expression of, these feelings in more healthy ways.

Weight monitoring

A minimum target or goal weight for the adolescent suffering from anorexia nervosa is usually specified to both the patient and family at the onset of the treatment program. Healthy expected weight range for older adolescents is often determined by calculating the body mass index (BMI): weight (kg) divided by height (in metres^2). While these measures are often used to indicate the extent of emaciation, they should always be used in conjunction with the results of a thorough physical assessment. A BMI of 20 is considered healthy for adolescents over 16 years of age. Generally speaking, the older adolescent is considered to be emaciated if the BMI falls below 17.5 and may require hospitalisation if the BMI falls below 15. Standardised growth charts are more accurate for determining healthy weight ranges, and are particularly advocated for younger adolescents (**Appendix A**).

While underweight, patients are usually weighed from 1 to 3 times each week. Weighing should take place after toileting and at the same time of day, preferably before breakfast. Drinking fluids or eating before weighing should be discouraged. The patient should be weighed on the same scales each time, dressed only in a hospital gown. Once the target weight has been reached the frequency of weighing should be reduced to normalise behaviour. Range weighing (weighing with the scale set at the lowest acceptable weight and then at a weight 2 or 3 kg higher) should then be instituted to avoid reinforcement of the patient's preoccupation with a specific weight. Maintenance of weight within this range is generally required for 1 week before discharge from hospital.

Follow-up

Restoration of weight will correct most of the pathophysiological dysfunctions. However, refeeding is only one aspect of management. Depending on the amount of weight lost and the duration of the illness when treatment is initially sought, recovery from anorexia nervosa can take from several months to several years of intense psychotherapy. Follow-up, aimed at preventing relapse, then needs to continue for several years. Weight loss can recur following discharge from hospital and up to 80% of patients will require at least one re-admission. Furthermore, some anorexia nervosa patients go on to develop another form of eating disorder, bulimia nervosa.[23]

Management of the adolescent after discharge typically includes continuous supportive psychotherapy, family therapy, nutritional counselling, weight and physical health monitoring as well as supportive group therapy.

LONG-TERM OUTCOME OF ANOREXIA NERVOSA

Anorexia nervosa is associated with a high morbidity and mortality. Methodological shortcomings and the various measures of successful outcomes used in studies make it difficult to compare reported outcomes. However, one review of long-term follow-up studies,[24] noted that only approximately 40% of all patients recovered, 30% considerably improved, at least 20% remained unchanged or seriously impaired. There were also reported mortality rates of 5% to 10% with death most frequently resulting from gross electrolyte disturbances (especially secondary to vomiting and purgatives), cardiac arrhythmia or suicide.

More recent reviews of 4 decades of outcome research[25,26] into the course of anorexia nervosa concluded that the chronicity of the disorder had changed little over the years. The degree of reported normalisation of weight, menstruation and rate of remission and chronicity have remained constant. These findings reflect the need for more research into specific therapies or interventions that best enhance successful outcomes.

Poor prognosis has been related to late age of onset, poor childhood adjustment, impaired parental (marital and personal) psychosocial adjustments, lower social class background, probably also premorbid borderline personality structure, and being male.[11] Adolescents with a history of child sexual assault are particularly difficult to treat. The likelihood of a poor prognosis also increases with a long duration of the illness, a very low bodyweight, and persistent vomiting and laxative abuse. Early detection and intervention can therefore be a most crucial factor influencing the long-term outcome.

PREVENTION

Nurses can play a role in prevention of eating disorders by encouraging all adolescents to develop and maintain healthy eating patterns and behaviours. There should be an emphasis on the importance of good nutrition during this growth phase. There also exists a need to improve self-esteem and the overall perception many girls have of themselves. Unnecessary and inappropriate dieting should be discouraged and the psychological and emotional aspects of the cause for this behaviour should be explored and addressed.

There needs to be less social emphasis on the importance of slender body shapes and more education regarding the normality of differences. The issue of prevention of child sexual assault also needs to be continually targeted as this is a common finding in the histories of girls suffering from anorexia nervosa.

SUPPORT FOR NURSING STAFF

Providing support, supervision or debriefing sessions for nursing staff and other caregivers should be a high priority. Nursing adolescents with anorexia nervosa can be very stressful due to the high emotional demands of both patients and their families. Even the most experienced nurse can have feelings of frustration and anger when dealing with the complexities of the illness and the exhibited behaviours of sufferers. As reflected in outcome figures, there are some patients who do not respond well to management despite the best treatment currently available.

There exists a need for an appropriate outlet for discussion of the feelings that nurses experience when caring for anorexia nervosa sufferers to prevent staff burn-out. Regular case discussions and ongoing evaluation of care may help focus attention on the rationale behind nursing interventions. Staff cohesion and consistency must be maintained in order to present a united and firm front. Treatment may be jeopardised if one member of the staff bends the rules by being less firm to win the patient's favour.[26] A clear understanding of the complex issues involved in the illness and open communication between all team members is essential to enhance positive outcomes.

REFERENCES

1. Carina C, Chmelko P. Disorders of eating in adolescence: anorexia nervosa and bulimia. *Nursing Clin North Am* 1983; 18: 343–352.

2. Touyz SW, Beumont PJ. *Eating disorders: prevalence and treatment.* Sydney: Williams & Williams, 1985.
3. Suskind RM, ed. *Textbook of pediatric nutrition.* New York: Raven Press, 1981.
4. Garner D, Garner M, Rosen L. Anorexia nervosa restricters who purge; implications for sub-typing anorexia nervosa. *Int J Eating Disorders* 1993; 13: 171–185.
5. American Psychiatric Association. *Diagnostic and Statistical Manual of Mental Disorders.* 4th edition. Washington: APA, 1994.
6. Russell G. Anorexia nervosa: its identity as an illness and its treatment. *In:* Price JH, ed. *Modern trends in psychological medicine.* Vol. 2. London: Butterworths, 1970: 131–164.
7. Kiecolt-Glaser J, Dixon K. Postadolescent onset male anorexia. *J Psychosocial Nursing Mental Health Services* 1984; 22: 11–20.
8. Crisp AH, Kalucy RS, Lacey B, Harding B. The long-term prognosis in anorexia nervosa: some factors predictive of outcome. *In:* Vigersky RA, ed. *Anorexia nervosa.* New York: Raven Press, 1977: 55–65.
9. Waller JV, Kaufman MR, Deutsch F. Anorexia nervosa: psychosomatic entity. *Psychosomatic Med* 1940; 2: 3–16.
10. Moulton R. A psychosomatic study of anorexia nervosa including the use of vaginal smears. *Psychosomatic Med* 1942; 4: 62–74.
11. Crisp AH. Therapeutic outcome in anorexia nervosa. *Can J Psychiatry* 1981; 26: 232–235.
12. Bruch H. Four decades of eating disorders. *In:* Garner D, Garfinkel P, eds. *Handbook of psychotherapy for anorexia nervosa and bulimia.* New York: Guilford Press, 1985.
13. Goodsitt A. Self psychology and the treatment of anorexia nervosa. *In:* Garner DM, Garfinkel PE, eds. *Handbook of psychotherapy for anorexia nervosa and bulimia.* New York: Guilford Press, 1985: 55–82.
14. Eichenbaum L, Orbach S. *Outside in, inside out, a feminist psychoanalytic approach to women's psychology.* Harmondsworth: Penguin, 1982.
15. Minuchin S, Rosman BL, Baker L. *Psychosomatic families: anorexia nervosa in context.* Cambridge, MA: Harvard University Press, 1978.
16. Ben-Tovim D, Morton J. The epidemiology of anorexia nervosa in South Australia. *Aust NZ J Psychiatry* 1990; 24: 182–186.
17. Bhanji S, Mattingly D. *Medical aspects of anorexia nervosa.* London: Butterworth, 1988.
18. Mira M, Stewart P, Abraham S. Medical complications of disordered eating. *In:* Abraham S, Llewellyn-Jones D, eds. *Eating disorders and disordered eating.* Sydney: Ashwood House. 1987: 106–110.
19. Russell JD. Eating disorders. *Mod Med Aust* 1991; 34 (6): 108–129.
20. Warren M. Anorexia nervosa and related eating disorders. *Clin Obstet Gynecol* 1985; 28: 588–597.
21. Rigotti NA, Nussbaum SR, Herzog DB, Neer RM. Osteoporosis in women with anorexia nervosa. *N Engl J Med* 1984; 311: 1601–1606.
22. Halmi KA. Treatment of anorexia nervosa. *J Adolescent Health Care* 1983; 4: 47–50.
23. Touyz SW, Beumont PJ. The management of anorexia nervosa in adolescents. *Mod Med Aust* 1991; 34 (11): 86–97.
24. Garfinkel PE, Garner DM. Anorexia nervosa. A multidimensional perspective. New York: Brunner/Mazel, 1982.
25. Steinhausen H, Rauss-Mason C, Seidel R. Follow-up studies of anorexia nervosa: a review of four decades of outcome research. *Psychological Med* 1991; 21: 447–454.
26. Garfinkel PE, Garner DM, Kennedy S. Special problems of inpatient management. *In:* Garner DM, Garfinkel PE, eds. *Handbook of psychotherapy for anorexia nervosa and bulimia.* New York: Guildford Press, 1985: 344–350.

Table 14.6 A simplified list of the causes of obesity[2]

---

1. Increased Energy Ingestion

   a) true hyperphagia — hypothalamic damage
                          — altered feedback of metabolic fuels on feeding centre
                          — acquired
                          — inherited ⎱
                                    ⎰ e.g., Prader-Willi syndrome
                          — congenital ⎰
   b) 'relative' hyperphagia — social
                          — behavioural
                          — psychological

2. Decreased Energy Expenditure

   a) altered mobility (decreased activity) — immobilization
   b) metabolic changes — diet-induced thermogenesis
                          — 'futile cycles'
                          — decreased basal metabolic rate (e.g., low activity of Na/K ATP'ase)

3. Endocrine Causes

   a) Diabetes Mellitus (Type II)
   b) Cushing's Disease — glucocorticoids
   c) Acromegaly
   d) Hypothyroidism
   e) Hypogonadism
   f) Hyperprolactinaemia

Obesity

Gail Anderson

Obesity is an *excessive* accumulation of fat throughout the body, usually as a result of caloric intake exceeding energy expenditure. While many adolescents are overweight, relatively few (approximately 5% to 15%) suffer from true obesity. Adipose tissue is the body's store for energy and it increases if food intake exceeds the energy demands of the body.

Individuals may not overeat by family standards, but may eat too much for personal requirements.[1] Other common factors thought to dispose adolescents to obesity include decreased activity levels (reduced energy output) or an altered metabolic rate. Some obese adolescents do maintain an excessive dietary intake which can be either relative hyperphagia, due to factors such as stress or depression, or true hyperphagia, due to hypothalmic damage.[2]

There are 3 main types of obesity in adolescence: increased total body fat with normal lean muscle mass; increase in both total body fat and lean body mass; and normal or increased body fat with large fat deposits in inappropriate places.

THEORIES OF OBESITY

While theories of obesity abound, no single theory has adequately accounted for all presentations of obesity in adolescents. Biologically based theories argue that genetic inheritance plays a major role, and that people are biologically programmed to fat.[3] The

Table 14.7 Classification of obesity[10]

BMI	Grade of obesity	Grade of obesity
<20	Underweight	
20–24.9	Healthy weight	0
25–29.9	Overweight	1
30–39.9	Obese	2
>40	Morbidly obese	3

fat cell theory[4] proposed that a critical period of development, with major consequences for one's adult weight, occurs somewhere between birth and 5 years of age. It has also been suggested that there are 2 peaks for the onset of adolescent obesity, one between birth and 4 years of age and another at 7 to 11 years of age.[5]

Environmentally based theories suggest obesity is a normal response of persons in certain subgroups of society to the perceived expectations of their social milieu[6] and that decreasing activity levels lead to increasing prevalence of obesity in young people.

RISK FACTORS

Reported risk factors for obesity in adolescence include a genetic predisposition, an obese childhood, membership of a lower social class, with sedentary television viewing.[7] Prolonged grief, deprivation of affection, low self-esteem and lack of success or interests may all lead to excessive eating as a source of satisfaction or consolation.

Compliance with nutritional recommendations is often poor in adolescents. A study of adolescents in Australia, Europe and North America[8] reports that eating habits of adolescents are characterised by missed meals, 'snacking', a fondness for fast and take away foods, the questioning of parental nutritional values and the consumption of alcohol and soft drinks. Foods most preferred by adolescents contain high energy from both fat and simple carbohydrate. Since nutritional needs vary, excessive intake of these foods can result in a considerable positive energy balance with consequent weight gain. Given their sensitivity to personal physical appearance, once adolescents gain weight they often avoid sporting and physical activities, which would assist in reducing body fat. Obesity is more prevalent in females, possibly due to the increased oestrogen output of puberty which fosters an increase in the size rather than the number of cells.[9]

ASSESSMENT OF OBESITY

Ideal bodyweight ranges for adolescents under 16 years of age are usually derived from standardised growth charts giving average weight for age, height and sex. However, great individual variability exists in the height and weight of normal, healthy adolescents. Growth spurts during adolescence cause rapid weight gain and linear growth.

General observation or 'eyeball method' is a fairly reliable way to recognise obesity. Another simple estimate of body fatness for adolescents over 16 years of age can be obtained by calculating the body mass index (BMI), also known as Quetelet's index. This is calculated by dividing the individual's weight (in kilograms) by their height (in metres)^2. To help classify different weight ranges (using BMI), the criteria given in **Table 14.7** have been defined for both males and females.[10]

The waist-to-hip ratio may also prove a useful measurement in some older adolescents. Those with high waist/hip ratios (or upper body segment obesity) are thought to be more at risk for metabolic complications of obesity, ischaemic heart disease and hypertension.[1]

PSYCHOLOGICAL EFFECTS

Society currently dictates that slimness is desirable. Obese adolescents, particularly those in the early or middle stage of adolescent development, can be extremely aware of a sense of difference and isolation from peers. This is especially so because adolescence is a time when acceptance within the peer group and the socialising power of peers become paramount. Rejection by the group can leave the adolescent with lingering doubts about their self-worth. The consequence of any associated low self-esteem and poor body image can lead to difficulties in social relationships, school performance, emotional adjustment and personality development.

PATHOPHYSIOLOGICAL EFFECTS

A variety of physiological and metabolic processes are influenced by obesity. Obesity during childhood can lead to accelerated bone growth and skeletal maturation, which may cause a failure to reach potential adult height, especially in girls. Growth hormone levels are decreased, despite accelerated growth.[11] Early menarche in females, and decreased levels of testosterone in males, may also occur and can complicate the psychological and psychosocial aspects of personal development.

Obesity can contribute to obstructive sleep apnoea and excessive snoring. This can then cause a general lack of energy which diminishes cognitive ability. In extreme cases, the adolescent can have difficulty concentrating on school work and other important tasks. This lack of energy can also discourage the adolescent from exercising adequately.

A major problem of obesity during childhood and adolescence is that the precursors of nutritionally related adult diseases can be established. This can compromise future health in areas relating to cardiovascular disease (hyperlipidemia with increased cholesterol and triglyceride levels), hypertension, orthopaedic problems (osteoarthritis, slipped femoral epiphyses and exaggerated lumbar lordosis), gynaecological problems (ovarian malignancy and menstrual problems), diabetes mellitus (Type 2) and gall bladder disease. There is a positive correlation between levels of obesity and the potential risk for these disorders. Subsequently, these can become risk factors of their own and can potentially cause shorter life expectancy.

Prevention, early detection and appropriate intervention programs will assist in arresting and reversing the medical and psychological sequelae of obesity in adolescents.

NURSING ASSESSMENT

The nursing assessment of an obese adolescent should reveal the adolescent's perception of issues and problems of concern to them. It may be wise initially to defer questions about appetite and food intake. Precedence should be given to questions about general health, relationships with peers, parents and significant others, school, interests, activities, perceptions of body image and sense of identity. This gives the adolescent the feeling that the nurse is interested in them as a worthwhile individual. It also enables the nurse to determine the approximate stage of the adolescent's development, where they

Table 14.8 Essential aspects of nursing assessment

1. Previous health history.
2. Physical assessment including:
   a) the adolescent's overall appearance
   b) weight and height, (patient and family)
   c) Urinalyses (particularly screening for diabetes mellitus)
   d) blood pressure
   e) presence of skin irritation
   f) presence of scoliosis or orthopaedic abnormality
   g) presence of dysmorphic features.
3. History of previous growth and development.
4. History of activities of daily living with particular reference to physical activity and interests.
5. History detailing menarchial onset and pattern.
6. Exploration of body image and self-concept.
7. Perception of peer and family relationships.
8. History and observation of family interaction.
9. History of sleeping pattern.
10. Elimination pattern.
11. Academic achievements.
12. Dietary history including typical oral intake and patterns of eating (should include alcohol and soft drink consumption).

are at in terms of achievement of adolescent developmental tasks, and any risk factors in psychosocial development. One can then formulate a comprehensive nursing care plan to provide for the holistic needs of the adolescent. **Table 14.8** lists some essential aspects of a nursing assessment.

NURSING INTERVENTION

Short-term nursing goals should address any immediate physiological concerns such as hypertension, shortness of breath, elevated blood sugar levels; encourage activity, provide individual and family education relating to optimal health and nutrition; encourage small, achievable increments of change.

Long-term nursing goals should consist of encouraging strategies to normalise any inappropriate food intake and eating patterns; instigate a good exercise program; promotion of effective coping strategies to improve psychosocial adjustment; working with the family to encourage maintenance of change in the diet of the whole family.

Adolescent developmental stage and obesity

Of ultimate importance in the nursing management of any adolescent with obesity is the establishment of a good nurse–patient relationship based on trust and understanding of the aetiological factors involved. Having established this relationship, the nurse is then in a position to encourage, educate and support adolescents in *their* decision and efforts to lose weight. To be successful, the adolescent must have the desire and commitment to losing weight, and the family need to be committed to change. Specialised eating disorder units are often the best source of comprehensive management for adolescents with obesity.

For some adolescents, excessive eating fulfils a serious need. Therefore, the relative importance of psychological factors should be determined before instituting any dietary restrictions. While long-term holistic outcomes, rather than short-term weight loss, should remain the focus of nursing intervention, adolescents need immediate successes to continue change. This can be provided by setting accomplishable tasks with appropriate rewards.

Self-concept, body image and self-esteem

Given the opportunity of a trusting nurse–patient relationship, the adolescent will be able to express his or her personal feelings and concerns. Education and supportive counselling may assist the adolescent with motivation to improve current life-style, eating and activity patterns.

Other concerns of the adolescent should be openly discussed. Addressing these concerns and providing encouragement may convey a sense of optimism and assist motivation to change. New interests or activities may yield friends, support and recognition. However, developing these new interests may prove difficult if self-esteem is low.

Relationships

If needed, individual counselling for the adolescent may prove more helpful than a group approach. However, some adolescents may respond well to small group sessions which provide a support network and help reduce feelings of difference from peers. New ideas, encouragement and competition may result. Opportunities to form relationships and have partners for activities and sports may be a positive outcome of group activities.

Family therapy

Family therapy may also prove beneficial in certain circumstances. Parents may gain assistance in setting limits appropriately without being intrusive. Focusing on positive rather than negative traits and behaviours of their child, trusting their child as new eating and exercise behaviours are learnt, and allowing the adolescent to gain control of weight are positive outcomes.[12] Family communication and relationships may also need addressing in family therapy.

Exercise programs

Exercise may be the best prescription for obesity. Exercise programs should be encouraged as a priority intervention. Graded programs can be individually designed and supervised by a physiotherapist in the first instance, to help motivate the young person.

Modification of diet

Often, the adolescent will have tried many types of weight reduction programs and diets such as those advertised in magazines. If previous attempts to lose weight have proved unsuccessful, the adolescent may have developed feelings of hopelessness associated with their inability to succeed. Reassurance and education are a major part of the nursing role.

The modification of diet is a sensitive issue and this should involve the whole family. The adolescent need not be singled out as requiring a special and very different diet to the rest of the family. Dietary modification usually requires implementation and monitoring by a specialist dietitian who is cognisant of the developmental needs and tasks of adolescence as well as the nutritional needs of adolescents during periods of accelerated growth.

The focus of dietary intervention should be on normalising, rather than restricting, food intake and patterns of eating. Good weight loss is slow and steady, targeting fat rather than muscle. Regular meals, a reduction in fat intake and an increase in complex carbohydrate intake are important elements.

A combination of dietary modification with provision of adequate calories for growth and development, increasing exercise and activity levels, improving the adolescent's self-esteem and an emphasis on changing abnormal eating patterns (behaviour modification) are the main components of treatment. Long-term success in weight control depends on acquiring and maintaining new and healthier eating and exercise habits.

Prevention

Prevention of obesity is always better than cure. Observation of growth charts in childhood and puberty with sudden changes of extreme weight gain should alert the nurse to the need for investigation into food intake and patterns of eating, activity levels, psychosocial and emotional status.

REFERENCES

1. Caterson I. Obesity — current thoughts and management. *Mod Med Aust* 1990; September: 60–68.
2. Caterson I. Obesity — the metabolic basis. *In:* Touyz SW, Beumont PJV, eds. *Eating disorders: prevalence and treatment.* Sydney: Williams & Wilkins, 1985.
3. Nisbett RE. Hunger, obesity and the ventromedial hypothalamus. *Psychological Rev* 1972; 79: 433–452.
4. Knittle JL. Obesity in childhood: a problem in adipose tissue cellular development. *J Paediatr* 1972; 81: 1048–1059.
5. Mossburg HO. Obesity in children; a clinical prognostical investigation. *Acta Paediatr* 1948; 35: Supplement 2.
6. Goldblatt PB, Moore ME, Stunkard AJ. Social factors in obesity. *JAMA* 1965; 192: 97–100.
7. Gortmaker SL, Dietz WH Jr, Cheung LW. Inactivity, diet and the fattening of America. *J Am Diet Assoc* 1990; 9: 1247–1252, 1255.
8. Trunswell AS, Darnton-Hill I. Food habits of adolescents. *Nutrition Rev* 1981; 39 (2): 73–88.
9. Dusek JB. *Adolescent development and behaviour.* New Jersey: Prentice-Hall, 1987.
10. Garrow JS. *Obesity and related diseases.* Edinburgh: Churchill Livingstone, 1988.
11. Hammer L. Obesity. *In:* Schwartz M, ed. *Clinical paediatrics.* Chicago: Year Book Medical Publishers, 1987.
12. Rees JM. Management of obesity in adolescence. *Med Clin North Am* 1990; 74: 1275–1292.

General Risk-taking Behaviour

Gail Anderson

One of the most important issues that nurses working with adolescents need to understand is that all adolescent behaviour is purposeful. It is generally meeting a need. If we look beyond the behaviours presented by adolescents, we are usually able to discover the reasons why adolescents behave the way they do. It is only then that effective intervention, if warranted, can be instituted.

For example, when caring for adolescents with perceived problem behaviours, we need to ask ourselves several questions:

- Is this behaviour abnormal?
- What need is this behaviour meeting?
- What has initiated the behaviour?
- What maintains and perpetuates the behaviour?
- Why is this behaviour occurring now?
- What effect does this behaviour have on the adolescent?
- What effect does this behaviour have on those persons close to the adolescent?

As abstract thinking develops, adolescents question parental and societal values. They often rebel against previously accepted limits and rules of childhood and this is a sign of beginning emancipation of the adolescent from their family. This constructive phenomenon of asserting the self assists the adolescent in developing personal identity and autonomy. As maturing individuals, adolescents need to develop their own value systems and be able to answer confidently the question 'Who am I?'. To function and cope independently in an adult society, they need to find their own individual identity outside of their family of origin.

This is achieved in highly individual ways. Many factors influence an adolescent's individuation from their family, including: genetic factors; family constitution and support; peer interaction; personal attitudes; health; intellect; educational opportunities and achievements; goals and career aspirations; social and cultural environment; and life experiences.

Adolescence is a time of many first autonomous experiences. As the search for personal identity and independence continues, the adolescent's behaviour and moods may fluctuate and change dramatically. Adolescents may become involved in risk-taking behaviours in an attempt to prove to themselves the validity, or otherwise, of certain values. They experiment with their abilities and limitations.

Conflict often revolves around the questioning and testing of limits of freedom set for adolescents by parents and authority figures. Some theories of development view conflict[1,2] or social opposition to parents[3,4] as necessary for normal development. A degree of conflict can therefore be viewed as positive and potentially productive.

Effective and insightful parenting can assist the adolescent to develop age-appropriate independence and personal autonomy within the safe and caring environment of their home. However, some parents have difficulty accepting that their child is now at a stage where she or he is endeavouring to individuate and preparing to face the world outside of parental control. If parents are not sensitive to the changing developmental needs of their adolescent, risk-taking behaviours outside of the safe environment of the home may be more pronounced.

Some risk-taking behaviours during adolescence are not necessarily negative or maladaptive. Quantum leaps in personal growth and learning can occur by making mistakes. Self-esteem can be increased by achieving that which took a personal risk. However, adolescent risk-taking behaviours should always be evaluated in the context of adolescent norms as set: by the family; by the peer group; by the school; and by society or the particular culture from which the adolescent originates.

Engaging in risk-taking behaviours during adolescence therefore serves many functions. These have been summarised as follows:[5]

- Taking personal control of one's own life.
- Expressing opposition to adult authority and conventional society.
- Dealing with frustration, anxiety, inadequacy or failure.
- Gaining admission to a peer group and demonstrating identification with the peer subculture.
- Confirming personal identity; affirming maturity.
- Marking a developmental transition into young adulthood.

Belief in a shield of invulnerability from untoward consequences is common during the adolescent developmental period. David Elkind[6] defined the belief held by young adolescents that they are unique, somehow omnipotent and invulnerable as 'personal fable'. He proposed that this is a normal cognitive function and has the positive effect of allowing adolescents to believe that any goal is attainable. However, Elkind also acknowledged the negative consequences of this belief, as when young adolescents engage in potentially serious risk-taking behaviours. This sense of invulnerability can lead adolescents to believe that they are protected from the consequences of their behaviour (e.g., 'That won't happen to me.'). Examples include the sexually active adolescent who does not use contraception or safe-sex practices thinking 'I won't get pregnant or catch a STD'. Or the unlicensed adolescent who speeds down the highway in father's car believing that he will not be caught by the police. Adolescents often think that getting caught only happens to others. Therefore, adolescent perceptions of the risks involved in certain behaviours are often unrealistic.

Nursing intervention

Nursing intervention strategies, when needed, are aimed at assisting adolescents to answer the question 'Who am I?'. After establishing good rapport, the nurse can assist adolescents to find their uniqueness by encouraging the adolescent to question and understand themselves.

The following are suggested interventions for nurses assisting the adolescent who is experiencing an identity crisis:[7]

- Explore with the adolescent the question 'Who am I?'.
- Help the adolescent think in future terms:
  a. Where will you be in five years?
  b. What do you want to be like then?
  c. Who is the ideal you?
  d. Who is the real you?
- Explore intimacy needs and how best to appropriately meet them.
- Help them to recognise their emotional states and their actions stemming from them.
- Discuss sexuality issues comfortably.
- Build self-esteem by recognising the positive contribution of the adolescent to the therapy process.
- Confront and eliminate inappropriate acts and self-degrading remarks.
- Encourage positive 'I' statements, e.g., 'I am good at. . . .'.

Nurses can also educate and support the parents regarding normal adolescent development and behaviours. Some families are very enmeshed. Having invested years of emotional and financial support in their child, parents may have difficulty in allowing the maturing person to separate from them.

UNUSUAL RISK-TAKING BEHAVIOURS

Violent or antisocial rebellious behaviours are not typical of acceptable risk-taking behaviours during the adolescent period and they can be pathological. The consequences, for the minority of adolescents who constantly engage in illegal, dangerous or self-destructive risk-taking behaviours, are often associated with negative outcomes. These include undesirable effects on the adolescent's health, impedance of positive psychosocial development and delay in mastering adolescent developmental tasks.

Negative risk-taking behaviours can be motivated by factors such as depression with underlying suicidal ideation. Seeking peer approval, or submitting to peer pressure, can indicate a powerful psychological need to feel accepted and to 'belong'. Research has demonstrated a positive correlation between susceptibility to peer pressure and injurious risk taking.[8] It has also been shown that ability to resist negative peer pressure appears to be directly related to positive family attachment.[9]

Authoritative, but flexible parenting, characterised by open communication, has been associated with increased competency in the adolescent and less susceptibility to antisocial influences. Parenting of adolescents involves a combination of constant support and encouragement along with a firm enforcement of fair and unambiguous rules. This is also a good standard for nurses in caring for adolescents. One should never condone negative risk-taking behaviours.

SEXUAL RISK TAKING

Human sexuality is an integral and natural part of adolescent development. When working with adolescents, one is confronted with sexuality and sexual risk-taking behaviours. Nurses are frequently in a position to give accurate information and advice. Thus, up-to-date knowledge and a general understanding of issues relating to adolescent sexuality are essential in order to deal effectively and appropriately with these issues.

In New South Wales, girls can consent to sexual intercourse at 16 years of age. With the mean age of onset of menarche at 12.9 years, it is on average, 4 years between the age of sexual maturity and the beginning of sexual activity.[10] Early sexual activity is often associated with increased risk of sexually transmitted diseases, gynaecological cancer and unplanned or unwanted pregnancy. Girls who become sexually active at an early age may be suffering from severe depression and may seek comfort and consolation in this way as it can provide them with a feeling of closeness.[11] Incest or child sexual abuse can also lead to sexual acting-out behaviours in the young adolescent.

Sexually active adolescents constitute only 18% of all women capable of conception, but account for 40% of all illegitimate births and 31% of abortions.[12] This lack of safe sex practices constitutes a major health risk. AIDS prevention is an area of grave concern for the adolescent population.

Sexuality and assertiveness do not necessarily go hand in hand. Many adolescents are not yet mature enough to be assertive in relationships and insist on the use of a condom.

Nursing intervention

Open discussion of sexual activity and contraception in a non-judgmental and informative way is imperative. The purpose of sex education continues to be:[13]

- To promote healthy sexual relationships.
- To encourage responsible decision making.

- To reduce unintentional pregnancies.
- Sexual protection.

Information should be offered that enables the adolescent to recognise the wide range of normality, the options available and the ramifications of each. Nurses need to be aware of the various contraceptive devices and empower the adolescent with assertive skills to encourage condom use, not only as a method of contraception, but also as a potential life-saving measure. Sexually active females should also be made aware of the need for regular gynaecological check-ups and Pap smears.

As well as providing essential information and practical advice, nurses should assess the adolescent for risk factors of early sexual behaviours such as depression, low self-esteem, childhood sexual abuse, or dysfunctional family systems. Appropriate referral for counselling and follow-up should be offered.

ALCOHOL AND SUBSTANCE ABUSE

Many adolescents experiment with drugs and alcohol. For some, this is simply out of curiosity, and this does not necessarily signify an emotional health problem. For others, however, drug use may stem from a seeking of peer approval and acceptance. Or, it may be a way of self-medicating to obliterate feelings of depression, helplessness or alienation. Drug and/or alcohol use associated with the following behaviours raise is a cause of concern about the welfare of the adolescent:

- Deterioration in school/work performance.
- Criminal activity.
- Communication problems within the family.
- Runaway behaviour.
- Sexual promiscuity.
- Marked aggression.

A major cause of drug abuse in adolescents is thought to be the lack of a satisfactory emotional environment.[14] From this perspective, drug abuse can be viewed as the adolescents' attempts to meet their own emotional needs. Significantly higher percentages of non-drug-using adolescents report close or good relationships with parents.[15] This is particularly true when non-users are compared with adolescents who have significant experience with drugs and alcohol. Drug and alcohol abuse is associated with physical illness, accidents and even suicide.

Nursing assessment

Nurses need to be knowledgeable, and feel comfortable, talking about issues relating to drug and alcohol use. If the nurse feels uncomfortable talking to adolescents about drug and alcohol use, then the adolescent will feel uncomfortable. This can lead the adolescent to evade the truth. Personal beliefs, value systems and attitudes towards drug and alcohol use should not interfere with an objective assessment. Non-judgmental, open and empathetic responses will give the adolescent 'permission' to discuss issues of concern.

During both inpatient or outpatient assessment, adolescents should be asked about drug and alcohol use. The nurse should identify the type of drugs/alcohol used, how much, how often and under what circumstances. It is important to explore: the adolescent's perception of their drug/alcohol use; the effect it has on the adolescent's life; and the adolescent's knowledge of the risks involved.

The adolescent's general functioning at home, school, socially, and within the peer group should also be ascertained. What interests does the adolescent have? How does the adolescent deal with stress? What strategies are used for problem solving? How do they perceive their self-worth and competency? Family interaction and functioning may also shed light on the true nature of the issues involved.

Nursing interventions

Nursing goals should include assisting the adolescent to make responsible choices about drug and alcohol use. After helping the adolescent to identify and discuss any stressors and issues of concern, the nurse is in a position to teach healthy problem-solving strategies. The adolescent may need to learn to react to stress without resorting to drugs and/or alcohol. Education and health promotion are important nursing roles and can be used as a lever in motivating the adolescent to seek and accept treatment. Referral to a specialised drug and alcohol unit catering for the developmental needs of adolescents may be required.

A team approach often provides the most effective intervention. The level of motivation for treatment is extremely important in order to achieve a favourable outcome. Unless the adolescent recognises and accepts change is needed, efforts by others to assist will be frustrating and ineffective. It should be remembered that it is ultimately the adolescent who must assume responsibility for compliance with on-going management.

REFERENCES

1. Erikson E. *Identity, youth and crisis.* New York: Norton, 1968.
2. Piaget J. Piaget's theory. *In:* Mussen P, ed. *Carmichael's manual of child psychology.* New York: Wiley, 1970: 703–732.
3. Freud A. Adolescence. *Psychoanalytic Study Child* 1958; 13: 255–278.
4. Minuchin P. Families and individual development: provocations from the field of family therapy. *Child Dev* 1985; 56: 289–302.
5. Jessor R. Adolescent development and behavioural health. *In:* Matarazzo J, Weiss S, Alanherd J, Weiss SM, eds. *Behavioural health: a handbook of health enhancement and disease prevention.* New York: Wiley, 1983.
6. Elkind D. Egocentrism in adolescence. *Child Dev* 1967; 30: 1025–1034.
7. Beck K, Rawlins R, Williams S. *Mental health — psychiatric nursing: a holistic life-cycle approach.* Missouri: Mosby, 1988.
8. Kandel D. On processes of peer influences in adolescent drug use: a developmental perspective. *In:* Brook J, Lettieri D, Brook D, eds. *Advances in alcohol and substance abuse.* New York: Hayworth, 1985: 139–163.
9. Baumrind D. A developmental perspective on adolescent risk taking in contemporary America. *In:* Irwin C, ed. *Adolescent social behaviour and health: new directions for child development.* San Francisco: Jossey-Bass, 1987: 93–125.
10. Clarke S. Adolescent health and the general practitioner. *Mod Med Aust* 1991; March: 62–73.
11. Raphael B. Adolescent sexuality: psychological and psychiatric aspects. *In:* Bennet D, ed. *Problems associated with adolescents at work and at play.* Sydney: Australian Association for Adolescent Health, 1985.
12. Snider SL, Slapp G. Adolescent contraception. *In:* Schwartz M, ed. *Clinical pediatrics.* Chicago: Year Book Medical Publishers, 1987: 95–99.
13. Mausner J, Gerzon H. Report on a phantom epidemic of gonorrhoea. *Am J Epidemiol* 1967; 85: 320–331.
14. Saltman J. *The new alcoholics: teenagers.* New York: Public Affairs Committee, 1975.

15. Harford TC. A national study of adolescent drinking behaviour, attitudes and correlates. *J Stud Alcohol* 1976; 37: 1747–1750.

Runaway Behaviour

Gail Anderson

A brief, *impulsive* episode of running away from home, particularly in early adolescence, may not necessarily indicate significant behavioural problems or emotional turmoil. It may result from a search for 'adventure', or peer pressure. Following an argument with parents, the act of running away may be a manipulative behaviour used in an attempt to negotiate more flexibility concerning family rules, or greater freedom.

However, planned, repeated or prolonged episodes of running away from home can be indicative of major behavioural or emotional health problems. Some young people who run away have a background of social alienation and parental estrangement and may share common motivations in their flight from situational stresses with which they can not cope.[1] Serious consequences in the achievement of normal adolescent developmental tasks, optimal health and future adult functioning may result.

One needs to explore the reason behind runaway behaviour. Running away can be an expression of despair, anger and the wish to be loved.[2] Many young people run from actual, or perceived, abusive home situations. Physical, emotional and sexual abuse are not uncommon precipitants. Adolescents may act out their hostile feelings by running away from what they perceive to be an unbearable home situation. Such adolescents often withdraw from their peer group or become involved with groups of adolescents with similar backgrounds and philosophies. They then may become misunderstood, socially alienated, discontinue schooling and lack any career aspiration or means to achieve financial independence. Finally, they become homeless and exist doing whatever they find is necessary for survival.

LIFESTYLES ASSOCIATED WITH HOMELESSNESS

Homeless children have been defined as those people under 18 years of age who have a lifestyle dominated by insecurity and transience of shelter.[3] This includes not only those surviving openly on the streets, but also those squatting in abandoned buildings, accommodated in short-term refuges and those moving about with no fixed address.

Frequently associated with a homeless lifestyle is involvement in petty or greater crime. Homeless adolescents are largely vulnerable to exploitation, drug use, prostitution, sexual promiscuity and violence.[3,4] Contributing to this lifestyle is the current issue of rising youth unemployment and difficulties associated with getting a job. Gaining meaningful employment is particularly difficult for homeless adolescents, who have few appropriate resources, and often poor literacy and numeracy skills.

MAJOR HEALTH PROBLEMS

In their struggle for survival, homeless adolescents may suffer from a large variety of physical, emotional and psychological problems. Some commonly reported health problems include:

- asthma and respiratory infections
- skin infections
- poor nutrition and hygiene
- dental caries
- sexually transmitted diseases
- unwanted or unplanned pregnancies
- behavioural disorders
- drug dependence
- depression and attempted suicide.[3-6]

Sexually transmitted diseases

Studies of homeless and 'at risk' youth in America[7-9] report prevalence rates of chlamydia at between 8% and 35%, and for gonorrhoea between 5% and 8%. One youth health service in Sydney has reported that 85% of pap smears of homeless girls show evidence of human papilloma virus.[3] More worrying perhaps is the result of a recent survey of 92 homeless Australian children,[4] which revealed only 46.2% of females and 50% of sexually active males regularly used condoms. The potential for infection with HIV in this group is therefore of great concern.

Present educational programs may not reach this group, whose activities place them at particular risk for infection. They may miss out on information given through schools and the media, and their sense of invulnerability may isolate them from the general community's fear of disease.[10]

Drug use

Most street kids smoke cigarettes, drink alcohol and use a variety of illegal and legal drugs depending on the amount of money they have.[4] Amphetamines, which rate second after cannabis as the most frequently used illicit drug, present a significant health risk. These are generally used intravenously and, because of the excitability effect, may contribute to a propensity to violence and sexual activity.[4]

Poor nutrition

Hunger is a common problem for this population. Furthermore, when they do eat, homeless children often eat from fast food outlets. Few homeless children eat adequate, balanced diets and most foods consumed contain inadequate amounts of vegetables and meats and excessive amounts of grains or starch.[5] A common background of childhood deprivation, coupled with poor nutrition in adolescence, may explain anecdotal reports of shorter than average stature for this group.[6]

Mental health

The most common mental health problems experienced by homeless adolescents are depression and self-destructive behaviour, including suicide.[6] One Australian study[4] reported that 83% of the sampled homeless adolescents felt life was not worth living. Suicide attempts had been made by 76.9% of the females and 59% of the males surveyed. Psychosomatic complaints, resulting from a combination of social, psychological and biological variables, often cause symptoms of illness. Stomach aches, headaches and general aches and pains are commonly reported by homeless children.

NURSING INTERVENTIONS

While they may be psychologically compromised, homeless youth still struggle with the maturational crises of development and the search for identity, meaning and security.[11] The major emphasis of nursing interventions needs to focus on providing the adolescent with contacts and skills that will facilitate this search.

Appropriate intervention for health, emotional and existential problems deserve a high priority. A sensitive and non-judgmental approach is needed as the adolescent is often the victim of circumstance. The key intervention can be a therapeutic long-term relationship with one significant, stable and consistent adult. However, establishing rapport with this population can prove difficult. Because of life events, the homeless adolescent may not have developed the intrinsic ability to trust others. The itinerant lifestyle may also impede any long-term relationship.

The nurse can assist the adolescent by taking an active and directive approach. Practical help may be necessary in the first instance in terms of accommodation, food and financial assistance. Free and confidential individual counselling, health assessments, and supervised peer group activities in a relaxed, informal setting may encourage adolescents to set some personal, achievable goals.

Nurses need to have a general knowledge of the wide variety of available community services to which these adolescents may be referred for specialised help and assistance. Youth refuges provide sanctuary in the form of short or long-term accommodation, support and referral services. Youth health or 'drop in' centres provide health care assistance, counselling, group activities, information and referral services.

The Family Planning Association provides clinical, educational and informational programs on sexually related issues. Youth Access (Commonwealth Employment Service) offers vocational counselling and assistance with social security benefits, education and training advice, employment placement and acts as a referral agent for legal matters and crisis accommodation. The Department of Community Services offers a wide variety of services, including fostering or placement of adolescents under the age of 18 years, adolescent support services and family mediation services.

Other community family medication or counselling services are available to assist reconciliation of these disaffiliated youth with their families. Some larger community health centres are now catering for the needs of adolescents by setting up special multidisciplinary 'adolescent teams'.

Family reunification

Family reunification is one option worth exploring with the adolescent. However, parents and adolescents generally require professional counselling to help with unresolved conflicts and issues which may have pre-empted the runaway behaviour. Some homes are realistically unsuited to adolescent needs and therefore family reunification is not always an optimal solution. Placement in foster care, group homes or supported independent living arrangements are options that may prove preferable to returning to an unsuitable home environment.

Ideally, all these services should be located and offered at one agency. Youth health services in Australia are currently striving to provide comprehensive health care which is easily accessed by homeless young people in an adolescent-friendly and supportive environment.

REFERENCES

1. Brennan T, Huizinga D, Elliott DS. *The psychology of runaways.* Lexington: DC Heath and Company, 1978.
2. Lewis M, Lewis DO. *Paediatric management of psychological crisis.* Chicago: Year Book Medical, 1973: 43.
3. Burdekin B. *Our homeless children.* Report on the National Inquiry into Homeless Children by the Human Rights and Equal Opportunity Commission. Canberra: AGPS, 1989.
4. Howard J. Dulling the pain: two surveys of Sydney street youth. Paper presented at the Ninth National Behavioural Medicine Conference, Sydney, 1991.
5. Wood D, Valdez R, Hayashi T, Shen A. Health of homeless children and housed poor children. *Paediatrics* 1990; 86: 858–866.
6. Council on Scientific Affairs. Health care needs of homeless and runaway youths. *JAMA* 1989; 262: 1358–1361.
7. Jaffe L, Siqueira L, Diamond S, Diaz A, Spielsinger N. Chlamydia trachomatis detection in adolescents. *J Adolescent Health Care* 1986; 7: 401–404.
8. Braverman P, Viro F, Brunner R, Gilchrist M, Rauh J. Screening asymptomatic adolescent males for chlamydia. *J Adolescent Health Care* 1990; 11: 141–144.
9. Smith, P., Phillips, L., Faro, S., McGill, L. & Wait, R. (1988) Predominant sexually transmitted diseases among different age and ethnic groups of indigent sexually active adolescents attending a family planning clinic. *Journal of Adolescent Health Care* 9: 291–295.
10. Remfedi, G. (1988) Preventing the sexual transmission of AIDS during Adolescence. *Journal of Adolescent Health Care* 139–143.
11. MacKenzie, R. (1988) The Health Consequences of Homelessness. *In:* Bennett, D. and Williams, M. (Eds) New Universals: Adolescent Health in a Time of Change. (For the Australian Association for Adolescent Health) Queanbeyan: Brolga Press.

Adolescent Suicide

Gail Anderson

Suicide rates among Australian adolescents have steadily risen in recent years. After accidents, suicide is the second highest cause of death of Australians aged 15 to 24 years.[1] These figures reflect only official 'successful' suicide rates. It has been estimated that the true rate of suicide is at least twice the official rate.[2] There are a number of recorded 'accidental' deaths that may in fact be disguised suicides. For example, an adolescent may be fatally injured during a motor vehicle accident, fall, or drowning which was actually an undetected, premeditated suicide attempt.

There are no accurate figures on the number of attempted suicides in adolescents. However, it is believed that for every successful suicide there are between 20 to 100 attempts.[3] Many suicide attempts go undetected. It has been estimated that as few as 12% ever come to medical attention.[4]

Suicide is rare before 12 years of age. Incidence figures increase with the age of the adolescent or young person, particularly between the ages of 15 and 24 years. One of the proffered reasons for this is that younger children have less cognitive maturity. In particular, they have less complex planning ability, foresight, awareness of self as seen by others, and a less mature concept of death as universal and irreversible.[5] Unless socially exposed, younger children also have less knowledge of methods or materials necessary to achieve suicide.

Females attempt suicide more frequently than males with a ratio of 3:1. However, the successful suicide rate among males is much higher. This is due to the male's propensity to resort to more lethal means of death such as firearms and hanging. Males are also more likely to act upon problems impulsively and aggressively. They are less inclined than females to seek help, especially for 'emotional' problems. Females generally, but not always, use less violent means such as the intentional ingestion of drugs.

PREDISPOSING FACTORS

Why do young people contemplate suicide? The answer to this question is multifaceted and complex. Predisposing factors include inherited and acquired personality traits, life experiences, psychosocial circumstances and an inability to cope with the increasing pressures on the youth of today. They also involve the interaction of individual predispositions with demographic and sociocultural factors.[5]

Brent[6] provides a good summary of the psychiatric features noted in depressed and suicidal children and adolescents. Many depressed children and adolescents 'act out' their emotional disturbance and exhibit behavioural disturbances at home, at school or socially. They may be labelled as conduct disordered or as having antisocial behavioural problems. Masked depression in adolescents can manifest itself in many ways. Feelings of hopelessness, despair concerning the future and personal worthlessness can help distinguish suicidal or potentially suicidal adolescents.

RISK FACTORS

Increasing pressures on youth today such as rising unemployment, drug and alcohol availability and abuse, exposure to violence and abuse, homelessness and family breakdowns, can lead to feelings of helplessness, depression and low self-esteem. As a consequence of this, some youth may see suicide as a solution to their existential distress.

Exposure of a vulnerable adolescent to suicide at home, in the community, at school or in the media can increase the risk of 'copy cat' or cluster suicides. The recent trend following the suicide of a school peer is to debrief whole classes of youth attending the school. Individuals who are thought to be at risk of 'copy cat' behaviour are then provided with individual ongoing counselling in an effort to prevent similar outcomes.

Studies of self-poisoning in adolescence[7,8] show that stressful situations such as family arguments, rejection by peers, the breakdown of a love affair or some significant failure can precipitate a suicide attempt. Persistent feelings of being unwanted, unloved, worthless, rejected and socially alienated can also precipitate a suicide attempt in a vulnerable adolescent.

A suicide attempt by an adolescent can imply a breakdown in the system of mutual supports in the family that guides and protects while also promoting autonomy.[9] Family pathology including abuse, chronic marital and family conflict, or parental psychiatric disorder can lead to the adolescent feeling that life is intolerable. This is particularly so if there is an accompanying lack of availability of other significant support for the adolescent. Family therapy is often helpful in addressing these situations.

Suicidal thoughts and behaviours can be associated with specific psychiatric disorders such as bipolar disorders (e.g., manic depression) and schizophrenia. Attention

Table 14.9 Some key issues in assessing the risk of adolescent suicide

1. Suicidal ideation (particularly if the adolescent has a plan).
2. Previous suicide attempt.
3. Exposure to suicide (family, school, recent media).
4. Depressed, hopeless mood.
5. Poor self-concept.
6. Impulsivity, aggression, low frustration tolerance.
7. Breakdown in a perceived significant relationship.
8. Difficulty with making friends or peer acceptance.
9. Extreme unrealistic parental pressure to achieve.
10. Chronic unresolved family conflict.
11. Unemployment and financial difficulties.
12. Alcohol or substance abuse by the adolescent or family.
13. Prolonged grief over the death of someone significant.
14. Chronic illness, disability or disfigurement.
15. Mental illness or psychosis in the adolescent or family.
16. History of physical or sexual abuse.
17. Perceived humiliating or painful life experiences.
18. Rigid, authoritarian, overpermissive or absent parents.
19. Running away or antisocial behaviours.

should be drawn to the adolescent who seems to suddenly recover from a known or suspected depression. Calmness and tranquillity can be evident once the decision to commit suicide has been made. The nurse should be alert to sudden changes in mood and discuss these changes with the adolescent.

Most adolescents have thoughts about the meaning of life and death as their abstract thinking evolves. However, morbid preoccupation with death and dying warrants careful evaluation. Those adolescents who plan their death, show a strong wish to die, time the suicide so as not to be discovered, leave a note, or choose an irreversible method to take their life are more likely to be successful.[10] However, adolescents using less lethal means of suicide, such as an insufficient dose of drugs to cause death, may be unaware of the associated low lethality. They may have had a strong wish to die, but inadequate knowledge at the time to attempt this successfully.

Table 14.9 lists some key risk factors associated with suicidal behaviour in adolescents. These risk factors should be kept in mind when assessing vulnerable adolescents. They should alert the nurse to the possibility that the adolescent may be covertly contemplating suicide. However, these factors are generally inconclusive standing alone, and need to be taken seriously in conjunction with an adolescent's individual personality, circumstances and coping ability.

NURSING ASSESSMENT AND INTERVENTION

Short-term nursing goals should include identifying adolescents at risk; providing a secure environment to assist the adolescent through the immediate suicidal crisis without self-harm; conveying hope for improvement; and mobilising therapeutic resources such as psychiatric consultation. It is important to inform responsible members of the health care team within which framework nursing care is provided.

Long-term nursing goals should include helping to increase the adolescent's feelings of positive self-esteem, self-worth and problem solving skills; ensuring appropriate follow-up.

How does the nurse assess or recognise adolescents at risk? Nurses need to take an active role in identifying suicidal adolescents and initiating preventative and therapeutic intervention. Predicting suicidal risk is not always easy. The presence of factors that are associated with suicide potential should alert the nurse to question carefully for suicidal ideation. Given the correlation between adolescents with intent to commit suicide, and/or with a plan and those who actually do attempt suicide,[11] adolescents with suicidal ideation should be considered to be at high risk of acting upon their intent.

Suicidal ideation in adolescents should be taken seriously and evaluated thoroughly. Decisive action is essential as one cannot risk ignoring what might be a final plea for help. Successful intervention begins with prevention. Any adolescent who is considered at risk should be questioned about suicidal ideation. Talking directly and openly about suicide emphasises its seriousness and gives the adolescent 'permission' to tell you that something is wrong. Discussing suicide in this way does not 'put the idea into their heads' or pre-empt a suicide attempt. It shows them that you have been actively listening to their distress.

Obtaining information relating to the adolescent's thoughts, emotions and lifestyle provides insight into general functioning, relationships and coping abilities. The following suggestions are not exhaustive, but provide some examples of issues that can act as a guide to questioning.

- Persistent feelings of sadness?
- Feelings of hopelessness?
- Negative attitudes to the future?
- Significant peer problems?
- Social withdrawal?
- Academic problems? (e.g., difficulty concentrating)
- Appetite and sleep changes?
- Present thoughts about harming self?
- Previous attempts or threats to hurt self?
- Frequent thoughts about death?
- Wish to die?
- Problem-solving strategies?

Nursing interventions

By talking sensitively and in a caring manner the nurse can convey hope that the situation can improve. At the same time the nurse should avoid promises of confidentiality as they will need to be broken to protect and effectively manage the suicidal adolescent. A good rule when working with adolescents is to tell them initially the standards of confidentiality you adhere to. For example, you might say: 'What we talk about will remain confidential unless I think you are in danger, or unless I need some advice on how best to help you'. In this case, you would need to discuss your concerns about the adolescent with the health care team with whom you work. The adolescent should be made aware of your intention prior to your doing this, so that trust is maintained. This clearly shows the adolescent that you have their best interest at heart. Specific exceptions to confidentiality should always include child physical, emotional and sexual abuse, which are notifiable to the Department of Community Services, and suicidal or homicidal behaviours or ideation.

Table 14.10 Brief summary of suggested nursing interventions

1. Organise a psychiatric consultation. Medication and/or psychotherapy may be necessary. Individual psychotherapy with adolescents is complex and demands specialised experience.
2. Assure the adolescent that the seriousness of their distress is recognised.
3. Don't allow the suicidal adolescent to be left or sent home alone without constant surveillance.
4. Facilitate the belief that helpful solutions can be reached and that suicide is not the best solution.
5. Foster a therapeutic relationship based on trust by being honest, dependable and consistent.
6. Assist the adolescent to develop a positive self-concept and increased feelings of self-worth. Acknowledge and positively reinforce strengths, achievements and talents.
7. Facilitate the appropriate expression of feelings and thought and release of tension in healthy ways.
8. Talk about and model effective coping skills.
9. Encourage the creation of a supportive network.
10. Asses the strengths and assets of the family and encourage involvement in family therapy if appropriate.
12. Social skills training may be instituted, especially for enhancing confidence.
13. Ensure appropriate follow-up is arranged.

Gibbs[12] discusses potential difficulties in communication with suicidal patients and suggests some techniques to enhance communication and assessment. Close observation and documentation of behaviour, and communication of relevant information to other significant health care workers, is essential to ensure effective management. A summary of potential nursing interventions when dealing with the suicidal adolescent is listed in **Table 14.10**.

SUMMARY

Nurses have a responsibility to ensure that the adolescent's distress is taken seriously and that follow-up care is offered. A psychiatric assessment is advisable, particularly for clarification and diagnosis. If the adolescent is suffering severe depression, antidepressant medication may be warranted. Family therapy can be beneficial, especially when family dysfunction contributes to and perpetuates feelings of hopelessness.

Many suicidal adolescents give warning of their intent, either verbally or non-verbally. Adolescents who are thinking of committing suicide may want to live, but find this too painful without the resources of professional help and guidance. By building a good therapeutic relationship with the adolescent, the nurse can assist gradual changes with remediation of personal, social and problem-solving skill deficits. The existence of one meaningful and consistent relationship with the suicidal adolescent may be a key to preventing the contemplated suicide.

REFERENCES

1. Australian Bureau of Statistics. *Causes of death. Australia.* Canberra: ABS, 1988. [Catalogue No. 3302.1.]
2. Ellard J. Depression and suicide. *Bull Postgraduate Committee Med University of Sydney* 1983; 39 (4): 29–39.

3. Hart B. Youth suicide: Prevention Taskforce Position Paper. *Bull National Clearing House for Youth Suicide* 1989; 8 (1): 48–53.
4. Smith K, Crawford S. Suicidal behaviour among 'normal' high school students. *Suicide Life Threatening Behaviour* 1986; 16: 313–325.
5. Dudley M, Waters B. Adolescent suicide and suicidal behaviour. *Mod Med Aust* 1991; September: 90–95.
6. Brent D. Depression and suicide in children and adolescents. *Pediatric Rev* 1993; 14: 380–388.
7. Hawton K, O'Grady J, Osborn M, Cole D. Adolescents who take overdoses: their characteristics, problems and contacts with helping agencies. *Br J Psychiatry* 1982; 140: 118–123.
8. Hawton K, Osborn M, O'Grady J, Cole D. Classification of adolescents who take overdoses. *Br J Psychiatry* 1982; 140: 124–131.
9. Hodas GR. Suicide attempt. *In:* Schwartz M. *Clinical paediatrics.* Chicago: Year Book Publishers, 1987.
10. Brent DA. Suicide and suicidal behaviour in children and adolescents. *Pediatr Rev* 1989; 10: 269–275.
11. Pfeffer CR. *The suicidal child.* New York: The Guildford Press, 1986.
12. Gibbs A. Aspects of communication with people who have attempted suicide. *J Advanced Nursing* 1990; 15: 1245–1249.

The Adolescent with a Chronic Illness

Sandra Wales

Adolescence is the period between puberty and adulthood and is usually a healthy and active time of life (see Chapter 4). However, approximately 12% of adolescents are faced with the burden of coping with a chronic illness,[1] in addition to the need to master the usual adolescent developmental tasks.

CHRONIC ILLNESS AND ADOLESCENCE

A chronic illness is a permanent or long-term condition with residual disability.[1] The condition may be diagnosed at birth or later in childhood or adolescence, and may be caused by genetic factors, medical illness or injury. Common chronic illness affecting adolescents include epilepsy, cerebral palsy, asthma, cystic fibrosis, diabetes and juvenile rheumatoid arthritis.[1] Adolescents may also suffer from cardiovascular disorders, inflammatory bowel disease, malignancies or from accidental trauma.

Regardless of the cause, a chronic illness usually involves a long period of supervision, observation and rehabilitation.[1] At a time when adolescents are attempting to become independent of their families and establish themselves as adults, the enforced dependence of a chronic illness can be devastating.

The presence of a chronic illness has the potential to cause many physical and psychosocial problems for adolescents and their families. While many chronically ill adolescents develop normally, chronic illness places the adolescent at risk of being unable to achieve their developmental goals.[2]

The importance of each of these goals varies according to the stage of adolescence. Body image, for example, is particularly important during early adolescence because of the physical changes occurring during this period. The development of social skills and the need for independence become increasingly significant during mid adolescence. This is a time when peer groups are more influential and adolescents are sometimes rebelling against parents and authority figures in their efforts to gain independence and a sense of identity. Career decisions are often made in late adolescence when choices about education and training need to be faced.

Adolescents with a chronic illness often have frequent, and sometimes long, periods in hospital, which make it difficult for them to attain emotional and economic independence. The degree of impairment can lead the adolescent to being more dependent on adults and having less control over their lives than their friends. Conflicts during this time may often arise because of differences in the expectations of adolescents and of those close to them.

Many adolescents have a strong desire to look and behave the same as their peers and chronic illness tends to give them a sense of being different. Their intense need to be like their peers may result in a failure to adhere to their treatment regimen. For example, the diabetic adolescent who does not adhere to the diet or the adolescent with cystic fibrosis who suppresses a cough for fear of embarrassment.

POTENTIAL DEVELOPMENTAL DEFICITS DUE TO CHRONIC ILLNESS

The problems faced by the chronically ill adolescent may lead to a number of developmental deficits such as a poor body image, a low self-esteem, poor social skill development, greater emotional dependence, prolonged economic dependence and increased difficulties in developing a strong sexual identity.[3]

Development of a comfortable body image

Body image is very important to an adolescent, especially during early adolescence.[1] Young adolescents are aware of the process of their physical maturation. They are also aware of the importance of attaining their own identity, of which body image is an important part. Physical changes that occur as a result of an illness, such as a delay in the onset of puberty or the development of physical deformities, can intensify normal adolescent concerns about body image. Being 'different' from their peers has the potential to disturb the development of a comfortable body image.

Development of self-esteem

There is the potential for the development of a low self-esteem in chronically ill adolescents. Low self-esteem may result from the limitations imposed on the adolescent by chronic illness, and by adolescents' tendency not to take these limitations into account thus setting unrealistic goals for themselves.

Development of social skills

Social interaction, particularly with peer groups, becomes extremely important in mid-adolescence. The adolescent who feels 'different', may not participate in social activities, and consequently becomes socially isolated and rejected by peers. The situation may be exacerbated by the need for frequent hospitalisation, leading to absences from school and peer group activities. Fewer opportunities for social interaction may affect the development of their social skills. The adolescent is the more likely to become lonely and maybe depressed. Alternatively, there is a potential for chronically ill or disabled adolescents to take dangerous risks by attempting to deny their 'differences' or disabilities.[4]

Development of emotional and economic independence

One of the major developmental tasks that adolescents face is the achievement of independence from the family. Adolescents tend to 'experiment' with independence. They may observe the reactions of others as they try to exert control over their environment. Sometimes this creates conflict between the adolescent and authority figures such as parents, teachers and medical staff.

When illness occurs, such conflicts may increase as the adolescent also tries to deal with additional restrictions imposed by the illness. An adolescent's need for control and independence may lead to non-compliance with recommended treatment. For example, adolescents who refuse medications or do not attend to therapy regimens often do so in an attempt to take control of their situation.

Dependence, however, may also bring certain advantages for adolescents with a chronic illness. For example, when parents are in control, adolescents are relieved of the responsibility of making decisions about their treatment.

School absences associated with the disease may lead to educational deficits, which reduce career opportunities. Progression of the disease or disability may not permit the adolescent to enter the workforce or to maintain a job. Economic independence may then become much more difficult, or even impossible, to achieve.

Formation of a sexual identity

Many adolescents feel a great need to develop and explore their sexual desires and feelings. A chronically ill adolescent has the same needs, but because of social isolation and parental overprotection or the nature of the disability, may have greater difficulty in developing a sexual identity. Such adolescents may present as sexually aggressive or promiscuous. They are often vulnerable and may become targets for sexual exploitation.[1]

STRESSORS ASSOCIATED WITH CHRONIC ILLNESS

Having an organic illness can be a great stressor and may predispose the adolescent to display signs of stress. Stress occurs when people perceive the environment as taxing their resources to deal with it and consequently as threatening their well-being.[5] Although stress can be a stimulus for personal growth, it is not beneficial when it is associated with unresolved conflicts.[1] Stress which occurs over a long period may result in disease, disability or death.

At varying stages of life, we all experience stress, due to changes and events that put us under pressure. Adolescence is a period of great change. These changes include physical and hormonal alterations, changes in values, roles, standards, goals and expectations of peers and parents. Adolescents' ability to cope with and adapt to change depends on their experiences, coping abilities, level of health and social support. Periods of stress and conflict can commonly occur with the changes because of poor self-esteem, poor coping and social skills and/or lack of support and guidance from adults.

Stress can influence many of the body's systems, causing an actual physical problem. Presentations such as dizzy spells, headaches, stomach ache, chest pain, joint pains or diarrhoea may reflect acute or chronic stress. An adolescent may also present with conditions such as irritable bowel syndrome, migraine or eating disorders. Stress may also be associated with conversion symptoms and psychosomatic disorders. Adolescents with such symptoms may be expressing their unconscious inability to cope with events.

Sources of stress should be investigated when the symptoms are not consistent with an organic illness and investigations do not produce a diagnosis. The adolescent's physical and emotional problems need to be assessed. Emotional difficulties may trigger and exacerbate these disorders. The adolescent may be unaware of the underlying emotional basis of their disease and their stress needs to be addressed in a non-confrontational manner. Family involvement is often an important part of treatment.

Specific psychological disorders have been associated with stress. These include anxiety disorder and depressive disorder.

Anxiety disorder

Anxiety is usually caused by being fearful or tense. Anxiety disorder may be triggered by the adolescent not wanting to confront a new situation. The fear may make them over-dependent on parents. Fear may also trigger feelings of anger and loss of control. The adolescent may present as feeling restless and fearful and having poor sleeping and eating patterns.

Anxiety can cause tachypnoea and palpitations. In extreme cases hyperventilation may cause respiratory alkalosis which, in turn, may cause the adolescent to 'fit' or become unconscious.[6]

Learning to relax and cope with anxiety-producing situations is important for adolescents. Inducing hyperventilation can give them a better understanding of what is happening to them. Allowing the adolescent to discuss feelings and encouraging independence also helps build self-confidence and may therefore lessen anxiety.

Depressive disorder

Depression is a state of general dissatisfaction or unhappiness. It is associated with a loss of interest in usual activity, poor self-esteem, and pessimism.[7] Depression may be acute or chronic. A depressed adolescent may present with loss of appetite, poor sleeping patterns, behavioural problems, substance abuse and/or suicidal thinking.

Depression can also be masked by psychosomatic illness. The adolescent suffering from major depression usually needs to be managed in family therapy or individual psychotherapy. Pharmacotherapy is sometimes needed, depending on the severity of the illness.

ADOLESCENTS' RESPONSES TO CHRONIC ILLNESS

The adolescent's ability to adjust to both adolescence and the disease is influenced by factors such as the degree of the impairment, the age of onset of the illness, the visibility of the condition, the course of the illness and the extent and nature of treatment side effects.[1]

Adolescents whose chronic illness dates back to early childhood may adjust and cope better than those who are diagnosed during adolescence. Adjusting to the onset of a chronic illness during adolescence may affect the experience of adolescence and therefore the reaction to the disease.

A visible disorder, such as a burn or spina bifida, may emphasise adolescents' differences from their peers. When the disorder is invisible, such as diabetes, the adolescent might chose to ignore the disease or may perceive the disease severity differently to those making clinical assessments. The result may be a failure to comply with treatment regimens and an increase in stress from efforts to appear 'normal'.[4]

The prognosis of the illness and individuals' views of the stability of their health can provoke anxiety. Adolescents may be fearful about any change in their health status, even if it is an improvement, and have difficulty making the necessary adjustments.

Coping mechanisms

There are many responses or defences adolescents make in their efforts to cope with a chronic disease. There is no set pattern or single response which enables the adolescent to cope. Coping mechanisms include denial, compensation, intellectualisation, projection, aggressive behaviour, withdrawal and depression.[8]

Denial is a common reaction to a chronic illness.[9] This can be useful as it allows adolescents to cope with the illness at their own rate. However, adolescents may also deny their limitations or the need for treatment. This may lead to risk-taking behaviour or non-compliance.

Compensation is the process of making up for a deficit. It may be one of the more adaptive ways of coping with a disability. For example, the adolescent who has a learning disability may compensate by being the class clown. Such coping becomes maladaptive when the adolescent overcompensates and fails to achieve his/her academic potential.

Many adolescents intellectualise or rationalise the effects of the disease. This may be exemplified in the adolescent who appears to be nonplussed with the facts of the disease process and does not show any emotion. It is as if the impact of the diagnosis has not been fully realised. An apparent lack of emotion, however, does not necessarily equate with a lack of coping.

Adolescents may get frustrated and angry about their illness and the limitations imposed by it. They may be ashamed of their helplessness. Their anger may be projected onto caregivers and health workers.

Withdrawal may also be a response. Adolescents may not comply with treatment so they can return to the relatively safe and non-judgmental environment of the hospital. This may lead to regression when adolescents feel the need to be dependent and protected. They may thus vacillate between dependence and independence. They may become depressed and, in some cases, may display suicidal tendencies.

Adolescents may also show their rebellion by becoming aggressive. This may be a way of coping with other underlying problems, such as loneliness and hopelessness. Aggression may also be displayed as attention-seeking behaviour. Such behaviour should lead nurses to evaluate the adolescent's unmet emotional needs.

RESPONSES OF FAMILIES TO CHRONIC ILLNESS IN AN ADOLESCENT

Chronic illness during adolescence may impact on families in many ways. Some families find the chronic illness an emotional and financial drain. This may lead to anger, resentment and guilt or overprotection,[10] and family dysfunction. Relationships within the family may be changed.

It may be difficult for some parents to 'let go' of their chronically ill child, making it difficult for the adolescent to achieve their developmental goals and leading to over-dependence. Alternatively, parents may try to place demands on their child which cannot be achieved because of the disability/illness. This may hinder the development of a healthy self-esteem.

The family may need assistance coping with the chronic disease. This is particularly true if the diagnosis is recent, as parents may be mourning the loss of their healthy child.

A chronically ill brother or sister may have a great impact on the lives of siblings. Some may feel they have to take second place and can resent the amount of time parents spend with the ill child. They may be quite unprepared for the mental or physical changes that occur to their brother or sister.

The family should be involved with the health care team as part of the management of the ill adolescent. The family may need time to adjust to increased contact with and dependence upon the medical team.

CARE OF ADOLESCENTS WITH CHRONIC ILLNESS

When assessing and establishing a plan of care, the nurse should take into consideration the individual's response to the chronic illness and the adolescent's developmental stage. The nurse should encourage the adolescent to take an active part in the management of the illness. For example, adolescents may manage their medications, learn to use equipment to assist with mobility and agility and attain necessary skills for day-to-day life. Participation in decision making can increase their independence and self-esteem.

Hospitalisation can be particularly stressful for adolescents.[11] Grouping adolescents together, ideally in an adolescent ward, can help reduce this stress for a number of reasons.[10] At no other time in a person's life is it so necessary to depend on peers for support.[11] An adolescent ward increases the opportunity for peer group interaction. Peer interaction provides support, has a therapeutic role for the adolescent[10] and may reduce the adolescent's perception of being 'different'.

The expertise of a multidisciplinary team can address many issues an adolescent faces. The health team should be aware of the social contacts and family situation.

Adolescents need privacy.[12] The invasive nature of some treatments and the need for assistance can lead to a lack of privacy. The adolescent's rights to privacy should be acknowledged and responded to if possible, by ensuring curtains are drawn during procedures, bathing facilities are adequate and there is provision for private conversations.

School personnel should be involved in the overall management of the adolescent in an attempt to minimise disruption to education. Employment agencies often have special job training schemes available to people with a chronic disabling illness.

Health education is important as it can assist to enhance the adolescent's knowledge of the illness and its management. The nurse, however, cannot assume that a knowledgeable adolescent will necessarily comply with treatment plans. Compliance can be encouraged by involving the adolescent and making the treatment plan as uncomplicated as possible. The nurse could explain the anticipated outcome, allow choices if possible, use contracts and avoid fear as a long-term motivator.

Nor should it be assumed that compliance with one aspect of the regimen determines compliance with the rest of the treatment. The adolescent can often do selected parts of treatment on a particular day because that is all they feel like doing. If non-compliance is present, it is necessary to renegotiate the plan of care with the adolescents and also to reassure their parents.[12]

Adolescents oscillate between dependence on family and peers and independence. It is necessary for both family and peers to be available to the chronically ill adolescent, but it is also important that they are not too intrusive or controlling.

The nursing of adolescents with chronic illnesses requires the nurse to be able to advocate, counsel, advise and provide a high standard of nursing care to a wonderful, challenging and rewarding group of patients. It must be remembered that adolescence is difficult for many adolescents. Chronic illness can be an added burden.

REFERENCES

1. Bennett D. The adolescent with a chronic disability. *Mod Med Aust* 1986; November: 34.
2. Gerben S. Psychological and social care for the chronically ill adolescent; the role of the hospital. *In:* Bennett D, Williams M, eds. *New universals: adolescent health in a time of change.* ACT: Brolga Press, 1988.
3. Zelter I. Chronic illness in the adolescent. *In:* Shenker I. *Topics in adolescent medicine.* Vol. 1. New York: International Medical Book Corp, 1978: 226.
4. Blum R. The chronically ill adolescent. *In:* Bennett D, Williams M, eds. *New universals: adolescent health in a time of change.* ACT: Brolga Press, 1988: 64.
5. Lazarus R, Folkman M. *Stress appraisal and coping.* New York: Springer Verlag, 1984.
6. Gabriel H, Hofmann A. Emotional problems with physical manifestations. *In:* Hofmann A, Greydanus D, eds. *Adolescent medicine.* 2nd ed. Norwalk: Appleton-Lange, 1989: 579.
7. Hodgman C. Depression, suicide, out-of-control reactions, and psychoses. *In:* Hofmann A, Greydanus D, eds. *Adolescent medicine.* 2nd ed. Norwalk: Appleton-Lange, 1989: 581.
8. Hoffman A. The impact of chronic illness in adolescent coping behaviour. *Acta Paediat Scand* 1975; 256 (Suppl): 29.
9. Bennett D. Adolescent health in Australia: an overview of needs and approaches to care. Sydney: Australian Medical Association, 1984: 18.
10. Wolfish M. General management of chronically ill and handicapped adolescents. *In:* Shen J. *The clinical practice of adolescent medicine.* New York: Appleton-Century-Crofts, 1980: 29.
11. Deynes M, Altshuler A. Illness: the adolescent. *In:* Scipien GM. *Comprehensive paediatric nursing.* 2nd ed. New York: McGraw-Hill, 1979: 481.
12. Blum R. The disabled adolescent: an orientation. *In:* Hofman A. *Adolescent medicine.* 2nd ed. Norwalk: Appleton-Lange, 1989: 29.

Appendix A   Percentile Growth Charts

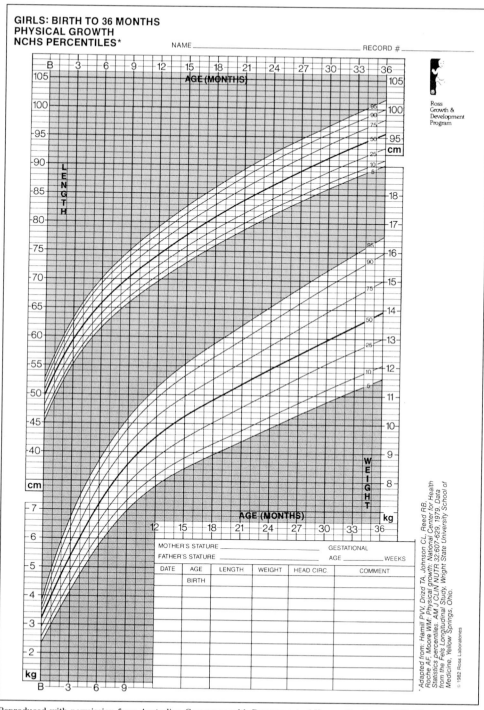

GIRLS: BIRTH TO 36 MONTHS
PHYSICAL GROWTH
NCHS PERCENTILES*

NAME _____ RECORD # _____

Ross
Growth &
Development
Program

MOTHER'S STATURE _____ GESTATIONAL
FATHER'S STATURE _____ AGE _____ WEEKS

DATE	AGE	LENGTH	WEIGHT	HEAD CIRC	COMMENT
	BIRTH				

* Adapted from: Hamill PVV, Drizd TA, Johnson CL, Reed RB, Roche AF, Moore WM: Physical growth: National Center for Health Statistics percentiles. AM J CLIN NUTR 32:607-629, 1979. Data from the Fels Longitudinal Study, Wright State University School of Medicine, Yellow Springs, Ohio.

© 1982 Ross Laboratories

1

Percentile Growth Charts — *continued*

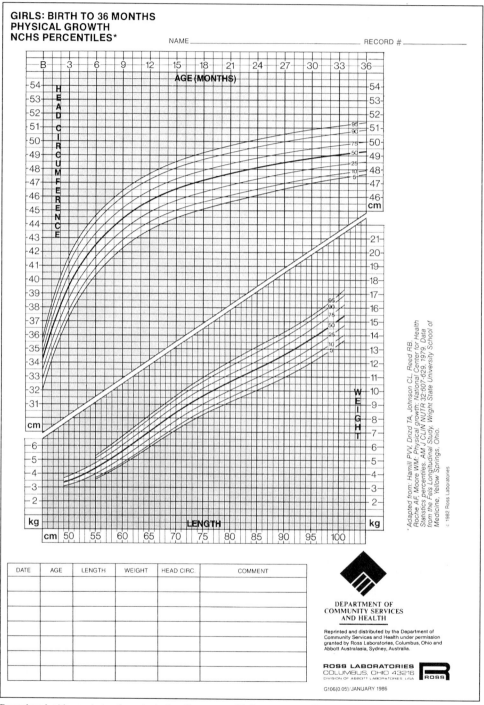

GIRLS: BIRTH TO 36 MONTHS
PHYSICAL GROWTH
NCHS PERCENTILES*

NAME _____ RECORD # _____

DATE	AGE	LENGTH	WEIGHT	HEAD CIRC.	COMMENT

*Adapted from: Hamill PVV, Drizd TA, Johnson CL, Reed RB, Roche AF, Moore WM: Physical growth: National Center for Health Statistics percentiles. AM J CLIN NUTR 32:607-629, 1979. Data from the Fels Longitudinal Study, Wright State University School of Medicine, Yellow Springs, Ohio.

© 1982 Ross Laboratories

DEPARTMENT OF
COMMUNITY SERVICES
AND HEALTH

Reprinted and distributed by the Department of Community Services and Health under permission granted by Ross Laboratories, Columbus, Ohio and Abbott Australasia, Sydney, Australia.

ROSS LABORATORIES
COLUMBUS, OHIO 43216
DIVISION OF ABBOTT LABORATORIES, USA

G106(0.05)/JANUARY 1986

Reproduced with permission from Australian Commonwealth Department of Human Services and Health.

Percentile Growth Charts — *continued*

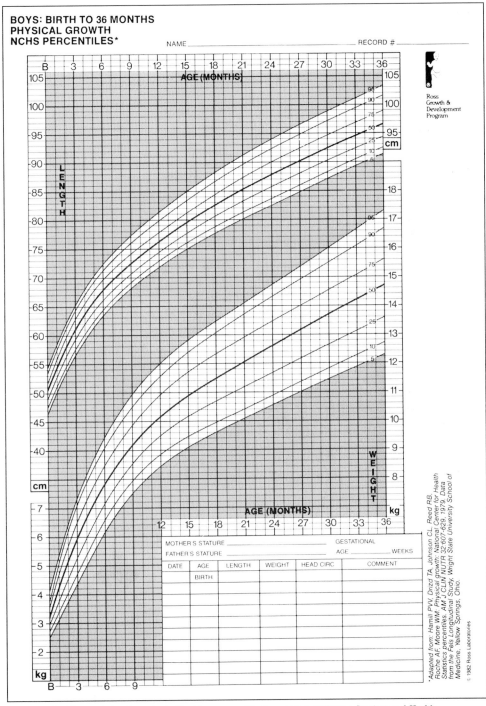

BOYS: BIRTH TO 36 MONTHS
PHYSICAL GROWTH
NCHS PERCENTILES*

NAME _____ RECORD # _____

Reproduced with permission from Australian Commonwealth Department of Human Services and Health.

Percentile Growth Charts — *continued*

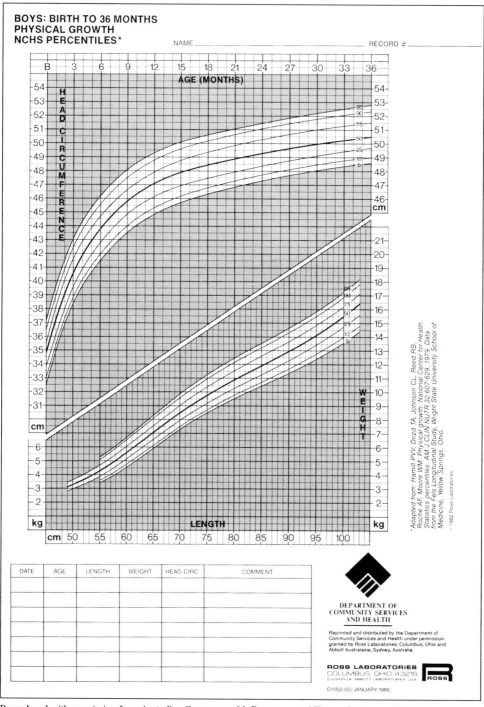

Reproduced with permission from Australian Commonwealth Department of Human Services and Health.

Percentile Growth Charts — *continued*

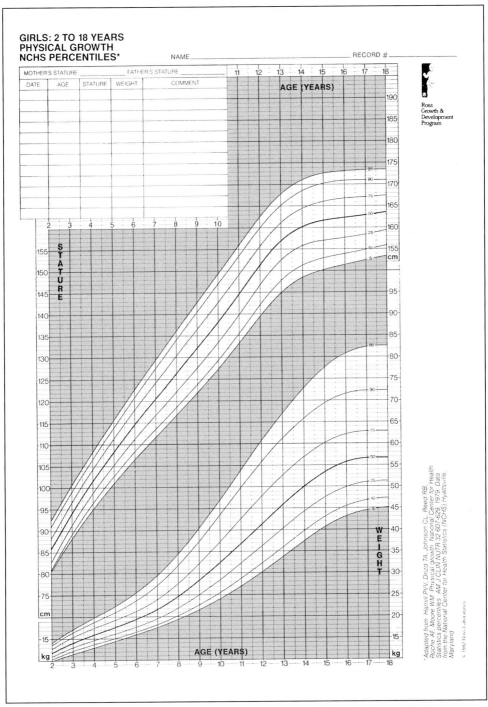

Reproduced with permission from Australian Commonwealth Department of Human Services and Health.

Percentile Growth Charts — *continued*

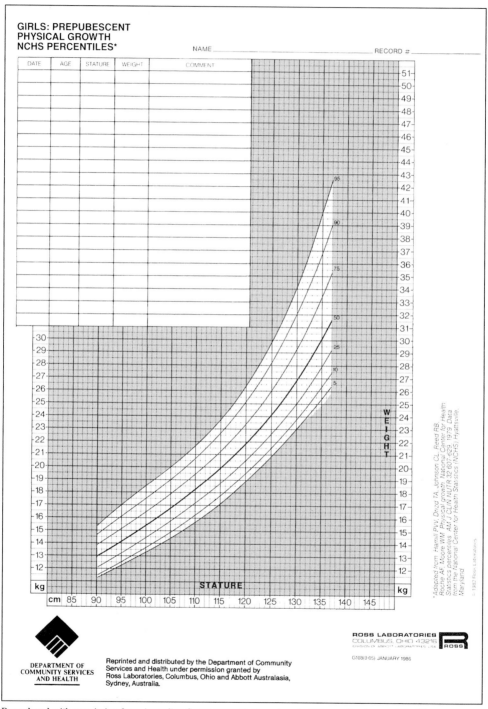

Reproduced with permission from Australian Commonwealth Department of Human Services and Health.

Percentile Growth Charts — *continued*

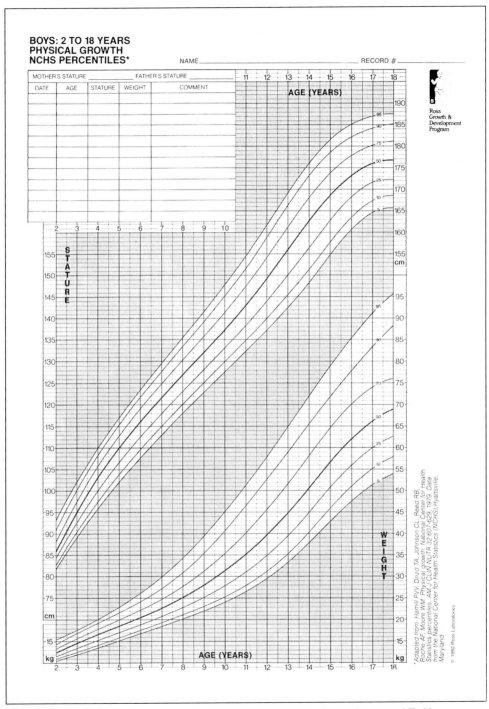

Reproduced with permission from Australian Commonwealth Department of Human Services and Health.

Percentile Growth Charts — *continued*

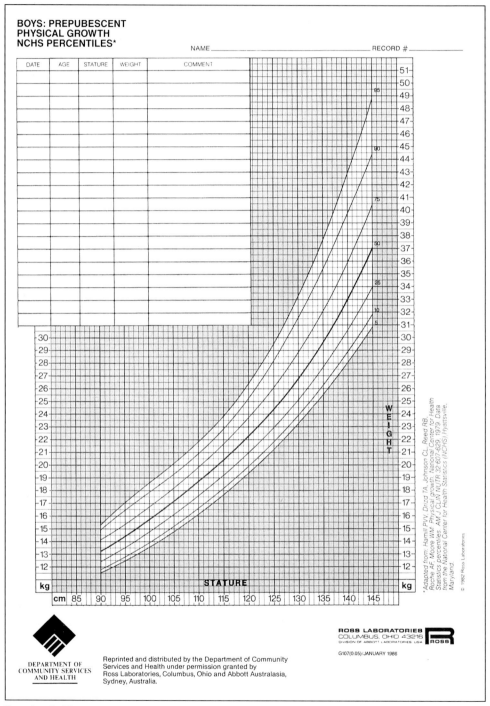

BOYS: PREPUBESCENT
PHYSICAL GROWTH
NCHS PERCENTILES*

NAME_____ RECORD #_____

DATE	AGE	STATURE	WEIGHT	COMMENT

ROSS LABORATORIES
COLUMBUS, OHIO 43216
DIVISION OF ABBOTT LABORATORIES USA

G107(0.05)/JANUARY 1986

*Adapted from: Hamill PVV, Drizd TA, Johnson CL, Reed RB, Roche AF, Moore WM. Physical growth: National Center for Health Statistics percentiles. AM J CLIN NUTR 32 607-629, 1979. Data from the National Center for Health Statistics (NCHS) Hyattsville, Maryland.

© 1982 Ross Laboratories

DEPARTMENT OF
COMMUNITY SERVICES
AND HEALTH

Reprinted and distributed by the Department of Community
Services and Health under permission granted by
Ross Laboratories, Columbus, Ohio and Abbott Australasia,
Sydney, Australia.

Reproduced with permission from Australian Commonwealth Department of Human Services and Health.

Appendix B   Neurological Observation Charts
Glasgow Coma Chart (Modified)

Westmead and Parramatta Hospitals and Community Health Services

BEST COMA SCORE
0 - 6 months	:10
>6 - 12 months	:12
>1 - 2 years	:13
>2 - 5 years	:14
>5 years	:15

Title   Family Name   M.R.N.

Given Names   C.M.O.

Address   Street   Age   Sex   H.I.S

Suburb   Postcode   Adm. date.

Binding Margin - No Writing

PAEDIATRIC NEUROLOGICAL OBSERVATION CHART

Date

LEGEND	Record best responses as ●		Time

Eye Opening:			Eye Opening	Spontaneously	4
Eyes closed by swelling = C	G L A S G O W	B E S T		To speech	3
				To pain	2
				None	1
Verbal:			Verbal	Oriented	5
Endotracheal tube or tracheostomy = T	C O M A	R E S P O N S E		Words	4
				Vocal Sounds	3
				Cries	2
				None	1
Motor:			Motor	Obeys Commands	6
Record the best arm response	S C A L E			Localises	5
				Withdrawal from pain	4
				Abnormal flexion to pain	3
				Extension to pain	2
				None	1

COMA	Best Eye Opening
	Best Verbal
SCORE	Best Motor
	TOTAL

Record Right (R) and Left (L) separately if there is a difference between the two sides	L I M B	A	Normal power
		R	Mild weakness
		M	Severe weakness
		S	No power
	P O W E R	L	Normal power
		E	Mild weakness
		G	Severe weakness
		S	No power

+ Brisk	PUPIL	Right	Size (mm)
s Sluggish			Reaction
- None	REACTION	Left	Size (mm)
o Untestable			Reaction

Pupil Scale
●1 mm
● 3 mm
⬤ 5 mm
⬤ 7 mm

OTHER COMMENTS

MR.115A   ANY CHANGE MUST BE REPORTED IMMEDIATELY   10/89

Reproduced with permission from Westmead Hospital and Community Services.

9

Neurological Observation Charts — *continued*

THE ADELAIDE PAEDIATRIC COMA SCALE
— EXPECTED NORMAL SCORES —

			BIRTH	>6 MONTHS	>12 MONTHS	>2 YEARS	>5 YEARS
Eyes Open	4	Spontaneous					
	3	To Speech					
	2	To Pain					
	1	None					
Best Verbal Response	5	Orientated					
	4	Words					
	3	Vocal Sounds					
	2	Cries					
	1	None					
Best Motor Response	6	Obeys Commands					
	5	Localises					
	4	Withdrawal from pain					
	3	Abnormal flexion to pain					
	2	Extension to Pain					
	1	None					
		TOTALS					

The above chart shows the expected normal scores for different age groups, as follows:

Eye Opening
No modification of the adult scale was needed in this category. The normal score, for all age groups, is 4.

Best Verbal Response
We assume that during the first 6 months of life the normally conscious infant will cry or grunt spontaneously or when disturbed; the expected normal score is therefore 2.

Between 6 and 12 months, the normal infant babbles and begins to vocalise; the expected normal score is 3.

After 12 months, recognisable and relevant words are expected, and the normal score is 4.

By 5 years, orientation, defined as awareness of being in hospital, or ability to give his/her name, is expected; the normal score is 5.

Best Motor Response
Motor responses are recorded in a 6 point scale. However, the paediatric scale recognises that before the age of 6 months, the best normal response is withdrawal from pain; this scores 4.

In the period 6 months to 2 years, it is assumed that the normal infant will localise pain but will not obey commands; the normal score is 5.

Beyond 2 years, the normal score is 6.

Thus the normal aggregate scores at different ages are as follows:

Birth – 6 months	: 10
>6 – 12 months	: 12
>1 – 2 years	: 13
>2 – 5 years	: 14
>5 years	: 15

Binding Margin—No Writing

Reproduced with permission from Women's and Children's Hospital, Adelaide.

Appendix C Vaccination Schedule

NHMRC Standard Childhood Vaccination Schedule
(August 1994)

AGE	DISEASE	VACCINE
2 months	Diphtheria, tetanus and pertussis	DTP - Triple antigen
	Poliomyelitis	OPV - Sabin vaccine
	Haemophilus influenzae type b (Hib) (Schedule 1 or 2)**	Hib vaccine (a or b or c)*
4 months	Diphtheria, tetanus and pertussis	DTP - Triple antigen
	Poliomyelitis	OPV - Sabin vaccine
	Hib (Schedule 1 or 2)**	Hib vaccine (a or b or c)*
6 months	Diphtheria, tetanus and pertussis	DTP - Triple antigen
	Poliomyelitis	OPV - Sabin vaccine
	Hib (Schedule 1 only)**	Hib vaccine (a or b)*
12 months	Measles, mumps and rubella	MMR
	Hib (Schedule 2 only)**	Hib vaccine (c)*
18 months	Diphtheria, tetanus and pertussis	DTP - Triple antigen
	Hib (Schedule 1 only)**	Hib vaccine (a or b)*
Prior to school entry (4-5 years)	Diphtheria, tetanus and pertussis	DTP - Triple antigen
	Poliomyelitis	OPV - Sabin vaccine
10-16 years	Measles, mumps and rubella	MMR
Prior to leaving school (15-19 years)	Diphtheria and tetanus	ADT - Adult diphtheria and tetanus
	Poliomyelitis	OPV - Sabin vaccine

* Abbreviations for Hib vaccines - (a) is HbOC ['HibTITER']; (b) is PRP-T ['Act-HIB']; (c) is PRP-OMP ['PedvaxHIB'].

** There are two different schedules for Hib vaccines. Schedule 1 Hib vaccination applies to the use of HbOC and PRP-T. The selected vaccine is given at 2, 4, 6, and 18 months. Schedule 2 Hib vaccination refers to the use of PRP-OMP. This vaccine is given at 2, 4, and 12 months.

Note that a 4th Hib vaccine (PRP-D; 'ProHIBit') is approved for use as single injection for children over 18 months of age.

All of the vaccines in the standard schedule, except OPV, are given by deep subcutaneous or intramuscular injection. OPV is given orally. OPV should never be injected.

NHMRC National Health and Medical Research Council

iMMUNiSATiON

NH&MRC, The Australian immunisation procedures handbook 5th ed. The Council Canbera 1995. Commonwealth of Australia copyright, reproduced with permission.

Index

*All index entries numbering from **page 695** onwards occur in **Volume 2***